NONINVASIVE IMAGING OF CARDIAC METABOLISM

DEVELOPMENTS IN CARDIOVASCULAR MEDICINE

Recent volumes

Hanrath P, Bleifeld W, Souquet, J. eds: Cardiovascular diagnosis by ultrasound. Transesophageal, computerized, contrast, Doppler echocardiography. 1982. ISBN 90-247-2692-1.
Roelandt J, ed: The practice of M-mode and two-dimensional echocardiography. 1983. ISBN 90-247-2745-6.
Meyer J, Schweizer P, Erbel R, eds: Advances in noninvasive cardiology. 1983. ISBN 0-89838-576-8.
Morganroth J, Moore EN, eds: Sudden cardiac death and congestive heart failure: Diagnosis and treatment. 1983. ISBN 0-89838-580-6.
Perry HM, ed: Lifelong management of hypertension. 1983. ISBN 0-89838-582-2.
Jaffe EA, ed: Biology of endothelial cells. 1984. ISBN 0-89838-587-3.
Surawicz B, Reddy CP, Prystowsky EN, eds: Tachycardias. 1984. ISBN 0-89838-588-1.
Spencer MP, ed: Cardiac Doppler diagnosis. 1983. ISBN 0-89838-591-1.
Villarreal H, Sambhi MP, eds: Topics in pathophysiology of hypertension. 1984. ISBN 0-89838-595-4.
Messerli FH, ed: Cardiovascular disease in the elderly. 1984. ISBN 0-89838-596-2.
Simoons ML, Reiber JHC, eds: Nuclear imaging in clinical cardiology. 1984. ISBN 0-89838-599-7.
Ter Keurs HEDJ, Schipperheyn JJ, eds: Cardiac left ventricular hypertrophy. 1983. ISBN 0-89838-612-8.
Sperelakis N, ed: Physiology and pathophysiology of the heart. 1984. ISBN 0-89838-615-2.
Messerli FH, ed: Kidney in essential hypertension. 1984. ISBN 0-89838-616-0.
Sambhi MP, ed: Fundamental fault in hypertension. 1984. ISBN 0-89838-638-1.
Marchesi C, ed: Ambulatory monitoring: Cardiovascular system and allied applications. 1984. ISBN 0-89838-642-X.
Kupper W, MacAlpin RN, Bleifeld W, eds: Coronary tone in ischemic heart disease. 1984. ISBN 0-89838-646-2.
Sperelakis N, Caulfield JB, eds: Calcium antagonists: Mechanisms of action on cardiac muscle and vascular smooth muscle. 1984. ISBN 0-89838-655-1.
Godfraind T, Herman AS, Wellens D, eds: Calcium entry blockers in cardiovascular and cerebral dysfunctions. 1984. ISBN 0-89838-658-6.
Morganroth J, Moore EN, eds: Interventions in the acute phase of myocardial infarction. 1984. ISBN 0-89838-659-4.
Abel FL, Newman WH, eds: Functional aspects of the normal, hypertrophied, and failing heart. 1984. ISBN 0-89838-665-9.
Sideman S, Beyar R, eds: Simulation and imaging of the cardiac system. 1985. ISBN 0-89838-687-X.
Van der Wall E, Lie KI, eds: Recent views on hypertrophic cardiomyopathy. 1985. ISBN 0-89838-694-2.
Beamish RE, Singal PK, Dhalla NS, eds: Stress and heart disease. 1985. ISBN 0-89838-709-4.
Beamish RE, Panagio V, Dhalla NS, eds: Pathogenesis of stress-induced heart disease. 1985. ISBN 0-89838-710-8.
Morganroth J, Moore EN, eds: Cardiac arrhythmias. 1985. ISBN 0-89838-716-7.
Mathes E, ed: Secondary prevention in coronary artery disease and myocardial infarction. 1985. ISBN 0-89838-736-1.
Lowell Stone H, Weglicki WB, eds: Pathology of cardiovascular injury. 1985. ISBN 0-89838-743-4.
Meyer J, Erbel R, Rupprecht HJ, eds: Improvement of myocardial perfusion. 1985. ISBN 0-89838-748-5.
Reiber JHC, Serruys PW, Slager CJ: Quantitative coronary and left ventricular cineangiography.
1986. ISBN 0-89838-760-4.
Fagard RH, Bekaert IE, eds: Sports cardiology. 1986. ISBN 0-89838-782-5.
Reiber JHC, Serruys PW, eds: State of the art in quantitative coronary arteriography. 1986. ISBN 0-89838-804-X.
Roelandt J, ed: Color Doppler Flow Imaging. 1986. ISBN 0-89838-806-6.
Van der Wall EE, ed: Noninvasive imaging of cardiac metabolism. 1986. ISBN 0-89838-812-0.
Liebman J, Plonsey R, Rudy Y, eds: Pediatric and fundamental electrocardiography. 1986. ISBN 0-89838-815-5.
Hilger HH, Hombach V, Rashkind WJ, eds: Invasive cardiovascular therapy. 1987. ISBN 0-89838-818-X
Serruys PW, Meester GT, eds: Coronary angioplasty: a controlled model for ischemia. 1986. ISBN 0-89838-819-8.
Tooke JE, Smaje LH: Clinical investigation of the microcirculation. 1986. ISBN 0-89838-819-8.
Van Dam RTh, Van Oosterom A, eds: Electrocardiographic body surface mapping. 1986. ISBN 0-89838-834-1.
Spencer MP, ed: Ultrasonic diagnosis of cerebrovascular disease. 1987. ISBN 0-89838-836-8.
Legato MJ, ed: The stressed heart. 1987. ISBN 0-89838-849-X.

NONINVASIVE IMAGING OF CARDIAC METABOLISM

Single Photon Scintigraphy, Positron Emission Tomography and Nuclear Magnetic Resonance

edited by

E.E. VAN DER WALL

Department of Diagnostic Radiology, Yale University
New Haven, Connecticut, U.S.A.

Department of Cardiology
Leiden University, The Netherlands

1987 **MARTINUS NIJHOFF PUBLISHERS**
a member of the KLUWER ACADEMIC PUBLISHERS GROUP
DORDRECHT / BOSTON / LANCASTER

Distributors

for the United States and Canada: Kluwer Academic Publishers, P.O. Box 358, Accord Station, Hingham, MA 02018-0358, USA
for the UK and Ireland: Kluwer Academic Publishers, MTP Press Limited, Falcon House, Queen Square, Lancaster LA1 1RN, UK
for all other countries: Kluwer Academic Publishers Group, Distribution Center, P.O. Box 322, 3300 AH Dordrecht, The Netherlands

Library of Congress Cataloging in Publication Data

Noninvasive imaging of cardiac metabolism.

(Developments in cardiovascular medicine ; 55)
Includes index.
1. Heart—Muscle. 2. Metabolism. 3. Radioisotopes in cardiology. 4. Magnetic resonance imaging.
I. Wall, E. van der. II. Series: Developments in cardiovascular medicine ; v. 55.
QP113.2.N66 1986 616.1'20757 86-9752
ISBN 0-89838-812-0 (U.S.)

ISBN 978-94-010-7976-1 ISBN 978-94-009-3287-6 (eBook)
DOI 10.1007/978-94-009-3287-6

To my father

For Barbara

Table of contents

Preface

F.J.Th. WACKERS

Metabolic imaging: The future of cardiovascular nuclear imaging?

Since cardiovascular nuclear imaging emerged as a new subspecialty in the mid-1970s, the field has gone through an explosive growth. Radionuclide techniques became readily recognized as important new diagnostic aids in the armamentarium of the clinical cardiologist. Initially, cardiovascular nuclear imaging focused on static myocardial imaging using either thallium-201 or technetium-99m-pyrophosphate for diagnosing acute myocardial infarction. Shortly thereafter, multigated equilibrium radionuclide angiocardiography became the most widely used noninvasive method for assessing cardiac function. Furthermore, attention and clinical application shifted towards the use of radionuclide techniques in conjunction with exercise testing, either with thallium-201 myocardial perfusion imaging or technetium-99m left ventricular function studies. The future of cardiovascular nuclear imaging appeared exciting and promising. However, around 1980 pessimists predicted the premature demise of cardiovascular nuclear imaging with the introduction of digital subtraction angiography and nuclear magnetic resonance imaging. These doomsayers have been proven wrong: in 1985 cardiovascular nuclear imaging is thriving and, in many centers, even expanding. Although digital substraction angiography and magnetic resonance imaging provided exquisite anatomic detail, for practical evaluation of patients with ischemic heart disease — in the Coronary Care Unit or exercise laboratory — nuclear techniques appeared to be more practical.

Presently, the clinical usefulness of equilibrium radionuclide angiocardiography in patients with acute myocardial infarction or chronic cardiac disease is well established. In addition, a number of studies have demonstrated that nuclear techniques have great value in providing functional and prognostic information in ischemic heart disease.

Rather than aiming at further improvement of image resolution for providing greater anatomic detail, radionuclide methods are to be used for which they are uniquely suited: detection of (rapid) changes in count densities. Rapid assessment of left ventricular function during exercise and acute interventions by first-pass angiocardiography, or assessment of myocardial perfusion at exercise by planar or tomographic thallium-201 imaging are typical applications of radionuclide techniques that cannot be duplicated by other noninvasive methods.

Another most appropriate use of radioactive tracers, the subject of this monograph, appears to be labeling of natural substrates of myocardial metabolism. The fascinating promise of metabolic imaging is the possibility to explore the fundamental metabolic aspects of the various diseases. The important clinical issue of differentiating between reversible and irreversible myocardial ischemia probably can only be answered unequivocally by monitoring radiolabeled substrates of metabolism. Furthermore, it is conceivable that, in particular in cardiomyopathies metabolic imaging will provide important new insights. Initially, imaging of myocardial metabolism appeared to be the exclusive domain of positron emission tomography. However, more recently, investigators have been successful in developing radioiodine labeled substrates that can be imaged using conventional gamma cameras.

In the present volume Dr. van der Wall has succeeded in bringing together the authoritative expertise of several of the pioneers and leaders in the field of myocardial metabolic imaging. The emphasis of most work is on radiolabeled free fatty acids and radiolabeled glucose, but also nuclear magnetic spectrometry of metabolic processes is being discussed. Free fatty acids are a key substrate in myocardial metabolism for production of adenosine triphosphate. Although myocardial accumulation of various iodine-labeled compounds of free fatty acids can be imaged with the conventional gamma camera, it is evident that substantial work still needs to be done in evaluating the relationship between uptake and clearance of labeled free fatty acid and whether they accurately reflect myocardial free fatty acid metabolism. The present volume provides a particularly useful and timely overview for those working in the field of nuclear cardiology, interested in myocardial metabolic imaging. Nuclear techniques are indeed uniquely suited to explore the pathophysiology of myocardial metabolism in a variety of myocardial diseases. As such, metabolic imaging is one of the most promising and exciting new directions in cardiovascular nuclear imaging.

List of contributors

Barrett, E.J.,
Department of Internal Medicine, Yale University School of Medicine, 333 Cedar Street, New Haven, CT 06510 USA
Co-authors: R. Zahler and M. Laughlin

Comet, M.,
Laboratory of Medical Biophysics, Grenoble University Hospital, Domaine de la Merci, 38799 Le Tronche, Grenoble, France

De Landsheere, C.M.,
Cyclotron Research Center, Liege University, Bât 830 Sart Tilman, B-4000 Liege, Belgium

Elmaleh, D.R.,
Department of Nuclear Medicine, Massachusetts General Hospital, Boston, MA 02114, USA
Co-authors: E.E. van der Wall, E. Livni, D. Miller and H.W. Strauss

Fox, K.A.A.,
Cardiovascular Division, Department of Internal Medicine, Washington University School of Medicine, 660 South Euclid Avenue, Box 63110, St. Louis, MO 63110, USA. Co-authors: R.M. Knabb, S.R. Bergmann and B.E. Sobel

Knapp, F.F.,
Nuclear Medicine Group, Oak Ridge National Laboratory, P.O. Box X, Oak Ridge TN 37831, USA
Co-authors: K.R. Ambrose, P. Angelberger, A.B. Brill, R. Dudczak, M.M.

Goodman, K. Kubota, R. Schmoliner, P. Som, K. Yamamoto and Y. Yonekura

Otto, C.A.,
Department of Natural Sciences, University of Michigan-Dearborn, Dearborn, MI 48128 USA

Paans, A.M.J.,
Department of Nuclear Medicine, Groningen University Hospital, Oostersingel 59, 9713 EZ Groningen, The Netherlands
Co-author: W. Vaalburg

Reske, S.N.,
Institute for Clinical and Experimental Nuclear Medicine, Bonn University, Sigmund Freud Strasse 25, D-5300 Bonn 1, FRG

Van der Wall, E.E.,
Department of Diagnostic Radiology, Yale University School of Medicine, 333 Cedar Street, New Haven, CT 06510, USA
presently at: Department of Cardiology, Leiden University Hospital, Rijnsburgerweg 10, 2333 AA Leiden, The Netherlands

Van Echteld, C.J.A.,
Laboratory of Experimental Cardiology, Interuniversity Cardiology Institute, Utrecht University Hospital, Catharijnesingel 101, 3511 GV Utrecht, The Netherlands
Co-author: T.J.C. Ruigrok

Van Eenige, M.J.,
Department of Cardiology, Free University of Amsterdam, De Boelelaan 1117, 1007 MB Amsterdam, The Netherlands
Co-authors: F.C. Visser, C.M.B. Duwel and J.P. Roos

Visser, F.C.,
Department of Cardiology, Free University of Amsterdam, De Boelelaan 1117, 1007 MB Amsterdam, The Netherlands
Co-author: G. Westera

Wackers, F.J.Th.,
Department of Diagnostic Radiology, Yale University School of Medicine, 333 Cedar Street, New Haven, CT 06510, USA

Westera, G.,
Department of Nuclear Medicine, Free University of Amsterdam, De Boelelaan 1117, 1007 MB Amsterdam, The Netherlands
presently at: Clinic and Policlinic for Nuclear Medicine and Radiotherapy, Zürich University Hospital, CH-8091 Zürich, Switzerland
Co-authors: F.C. Visser and E.E. van der Wall

Introduction

E.E. van der WALL

Human cardiac disease such as coronary disease, hypertensive heart disease and cardiomyopathy, is mostly diagnosed and treated in an advanced stage when structural or anatomical derangements are already present. However, disease starts at the biochemical level and hence metabolic disorders of the myocardium will precede the anatomical and functional abnormalities. Therefore, new diagnostic techniques have been developed to provide insight into the *in vivo* myocardial biochemistry and to assist in designing adequate therapeutic regimens in clinical practice.

Although the interest for cardiac metabolism dates from decades ago, it was only recently that scintigraphy with radiolabeled metabolic substrates became available for noninvasive metabolic studies of the normal and diseased myocardium. These metabolic substrates can be labeled with both single-photon and positron emitting radioisotopes and they both provide, in a different way, a lot of information about the biochemical processes in the myocardium.

Several centers in Europe have very successfully focused their attention on the development and application of metabolic tracers in the past decade. Also in the USA this investigative field has recently become the subject of great interest in well-known medical centers and the number of metabolism-oriented laboratories is expanding rapidly.

This book is intended to assist the experimental and clinical cardiologist, the radiochemist and the nuclear medicine physician in understanding the intricate metabolic processes of the (patho)physiological myocardium. Each chapter has been written by an expert in the field from either Europe or the USA. The first chapter gives a survey of the presently available radionuclides for the detection of human heart disease. Most chapters deal with the use of the various radioiodinated free fatty acids (single-photon emitters) and in two chapters the value of positron emission tomography with labeled metabolic substrates is discussed. Also two chapters have been exclusively dedicated to the most recently developed diagnostic imaging modality, i.e. nuclear magnetic resonance. By spectral analysis of myocardial tissue, valuable information of cardiac metabolism can be obtained with nuclear magnetic resonance. In the last chapter a very useful comparison is made between positron emission tomography and the magnetic resonance technique.

I hope this book will be a valuable contribution to the progress in noninvasive cardiac diagnosis and that it enhances our understanding of human heart disease.

1. Radiopharmaceuticals for cardiovascular nuclear medicine

D.R. ELMALEH, E.E. van der WALL, E. LIVNI, D.D. MILLER and H.W. STRAUSS

Introduction

Clinical nuclear cardiology has available currently only a small number of labeled agents. These agents do not include radiopharmaceuticals produced by research centers that have medical cyclotron facilities. The cardiovascular radiopharmaceuticals can be divided into six major groups: 1) tracers for cardiac blood pool studies; 2) agents for perfusion scintigraphy; 3) metabolic substrates and their analogs; 4) infarct avid agents; 5) specific cardiac receptor ligands; and 6) labeled cardiac antibodies, leukocytes and norepinephrine storage analogs. Two radionuclides, thallium-201 and technetium-99m, have assumed pre-eminence in cardiovascular nuclear medicine because their physical characteristics and biological behavior are best suited for imaging with readily available equipment. The spatial resolution of the 'system' for the average cardiovascular nuclear medicine study, (radiopharmaceutical, collimator, camera, and computer) at the depth of the heart is approximately 1 cm full width half maximum (FWHM). Against this background, new radiopharmaceuticals suggested for the evaluation of the heart must offer an improvement in dosimetry, resolution, or provide data on a previously unmeasurable parameter.

The direction of development of both gamma- and positron-labeled radiopharmaceuticals has changed tremendously in the last few years from that of nonspecific agents to ones with a biochemical rationale for their behavior. The new generation of radiopharmaceuticals in conjunction with more sophisticated detection devices and data analysis systems should provide a clearer interpretation for radiocardiology diagnostic procedures.

Cardiac blood pool agents

Blood pool studies can be recorded either during the initial passage of radiopharmaceutical through the heart or after the tracer has reached an initial equilibration in the blood pool [1-3] (Table 1). These two circumstances place different constraints on the radiopharmaceutical: a) first pass imaging requires the tracer to reside in the blood pool only long enough to traverse the chamber(s) of interest in a fashion that is representative of the flowing blood; b) equilibrium blood pool radiopharmaceuticals should have an unchanging volume of distribution over the time of observation.

A. First pass

a. Short biological half-life in the blood

The most common radiopharmaceuticals for evaluation of the right and left heart on first pass studies are technetium-99m (^{99m}Tc) labeled sulfur colloid (SC) and ^{99m}Tc DTPA [4]. Following administration ^{99m}Tc SC is cleared from the blood into the reticuloendothelial system, with a half-time of less than 3 min, while ^{99m}Tc DTPA is cleared with a half-time of less than 5 min by diffusion into the extracellular fluid and excretion via the kidneys. These mechanisms of biological clearance result in a radiation burden to the liver of approximately 3 rads/10 mCi of ^{99m}Tc SC, and a dose to the bladder which may be as low as 0.3 rads or as high as 5 rads depending on the interval of voiding after injection with ^{99m}Tc DTPA [4]. The radiation burden to the genito-urinary system can be minimized if the patient is urged to void several times in the first hour after the study. When administered in doses of 10 mCi, these agents can provide peak count rates (recorded with conventional anger cameras equipped with all-purpose parallel-hole collimation) in the range of 100,000 counts per

Table 1. Cardiac blood pool agents

Radiopharmaceutical	T ½ Nuclide	Ventricular Function First pass	Ventricular Function Equilibrium	KeV energy
Krypton-81m	13 s	+	+	190
Iridium-191m	4.7 s	+		129
Gold-195m	30.5 s	+		262
Rubidium-82	75 s	+		511
Xenon-133	5.3 days	+	+	81
Indium-113m	100 min	+		392
(Tc-99m)-Pertechnetate	6 h	+		140
(Tc-99m)-red blood cells	6 h	+	+	140
(C-11)-carboxyhemoglobin	20 min		+	511
(O-15)-carboxyhemoglobin	2 min		+	511

T ½ = physical half-life.

second with state of the art cameras. These data acquisition rates are sufficient to measure ejection fraction (EF) and regional wall motion of both the right and left ventricle.

The inert noble gas, xenon-133 (^{133}Xe, t½ physical = 5.7 days) dissolved in saline may be used to perform rapid, sequential determinations of right heart function [5]. When xenon encounters the pulmonary capillaries approximately 85% rapidly diffuses into the air space and is excreted. To prevent contamination of the surroundings with xenon released from the lungs, the patient's exhaled air is either passed through a charcoal filter to trap the xenon or exhausted through a vent system. Sequential high photon flux studies, with injected doses of 50-80 mCi, can be performed with a radiation burden to the patient of less than 0.5 rads/study.

b. Short physical half-life
In addition to tracers with a short biological half-life, agents with a short physical half-life such as ^{195m}Au (t½ = 30 s) [6-8], ^{81m}Kr (t½ = 13 s)[9] or ^{191m}Ir (t½ = 4.7 s) [10] may be successfully employed to record data with this technique.

Unique problems of ultrashort-lived generator-produced radionuclides: The short physical half-lives of these agents require that the radionuclides be eluted directly from the generator into the patient. This places severe constraints on the quality control procedures that can be performed prior to administration of a dose. Although this problem must be addressed with all of the generator systems, the severity of the problem increases when the half-life of the parent nuclide is of long duration compared to that of the daughter. For example, in the rubidium/krypton (^{81}Rb/^{81m}Kr) generator, the half-life of parent ^{81}Rb is only 4.7 h. Breakthrough of the ^{81}Rb parent into the eluate containing the daughter ^{81m}Kr with 13-s half-life will result in a relatively modest radiation burden to the patient. The (^{81}Rb/^{81m}Kr) system manifests this problem only when the generator is filled with liquid in order to elute the ^{81m}Kr in a form suitable for intravenous or intra-arterial injection. When the generator is used for inhalation, the ^{81m}Kr is evolved as a gas and ^{81}Rb breakthrough is not a problem. On the other hand, with the mercury/gold (^{195}Hg/^{195m}Au) and the osmium/iridium (^{191}Os/^{191m}Ir) infusion systems, where the parent half-lives are much longer (^{195}Hg t½ = 60 h and ^{191}Os t½ = 14 days) than those of the daughters, each microcurie of the parent in the eluate results in a greater radiation burden to the subject.

In the case of technetium-labeled agents the lot of material is quality controlled, and the activity of the specific dose destined for the patient is assayed prior to injection. The ultrashort-lived radiopharmaceuticals cannot be handled in this manner, since the assay time of several seconds to minutes results in a marked decrease in activity. The quality control of these short-lived agents is usually accomplished by performing two elutions: the first into an ionizaton chamber to measure the activity and half-life. Parent breakthrough is manifest as an apparent increase in the half-life of the agent. The initial activity measured represents the daughter, while activity remaining after the daughter has decayed through ten half-lives represents breakthrough of the parent. If the dose eluted is sufficient for the proposed measurement and parent breakthrough is acceptable, the next dose is administered to the patient.

(b_1) *Krypton-81m:* In 1968 Yano and Anger [9] proposed the use of the rubidium-81/krypton-81m generator system to image the blood pool. The cyclotron-produced 4.7 h half-life ^{81}Rb [alpha particle bombardment of a ^{79}Br (alpha, 2n)] is adsorbed onto a column, and the inert gas ^{81m}Kr 13 s half-life will be produced. The daughter ^{81m}Kr decays to Kr-81, a radioactive nuclide with a half-life of 10E6 years. The long half-life of the progeny does not represent a radiation hazard to the recipient of the ^{81m}Kr. If the column of the generator is filled with dextrose, the resulting solution of dextrose/^{81m}Kr can be injected intravenously to determine right ventricular function [11-13] and pulmonary perfusion, or intra-arterially to determine regional cerebral perfusion or myocardial perfusion [14-16]. If the generator is opened to the air, the resulting gas can be inhaled to define regional ventilation. The 190 keV energy of the ^{81m}Kr is well suited for imaging with low or medium energy collimators available on most scintillation cameras. Due to its short effective half-life ($T\frac{1}{2}$ effective = [$T\frac{1}{2}$ biological $\times$ $T\frac{1}{2}$ physical)/($T\frac{1}{2}$ biological + $T\frac{1}{2}$ physical)] ^{81m}Kr is particularly useful for the repetitive evaluation of right ventricular function. The short effective half-life comes from the combination of short physical half-life and short biological half-life due to the evolution of the radionuclide from the blood into the alveolus during its passage through the lung. As a result, no significant activity enters the left heart. The short effective half-life results in a low radiation burden per mCi, which permits a large dose to be administered per injection. The resulting photon flux allows high count density data to be recorded during the initial passage of radionuclide through the right heart.

Since right ventricular function varies with the respiratory cycle, it may be preferable to measure right ventricular ejection fraction (RVEF) during several respiratory cycles, rather than during a single inspiration or expiration, as is currently done during first pass studies. This can be accomplished by recording a gated collection during a continuous infusion directly into the patient's vein over a 30-60 s interval instead of using the bolus injection technique. The calculated RVEF with this approach is typically higher than that calculated from equilibrium blood pool studies.

Right heart studies with ^{81m}Kr require high doses of ^{81}Rb on the infusion generator. The costs of producing the parent radionuclide, coupled with its short physical half-life make this an expensive nuclide. To market the generator which is primarily intended for use with inhalation imaging, at a reasonable price, the manufacturer elected to make it with 5 mCi of rubidium on the column. As a result, the photon flux available is low compared tot that theoretically achievable. The detected photon flux of about 5000 counts/second available from infusions of ^{81m}Kr from this generator are less than 25% of that from ^{99m}Tc during an equilibrium study. These low photon fluxes generate 'noisy' images, which preclude the determination of regional wall motion of the right ventricle. If larger generators become available, ^{81m}Kr will be useful for the determination of right heart function.

(b_2) *Iridium-191m:* Although the ^{191}Os generator was originally described in 1968 by Yano and Anger [9] for the determination of pulmonary perfusion, it was not until the recent work of Treves [17-19] that a practical generator for human use was developed. ^{191m}Ir has a 4.7 s half-life with gamma, photons of 129 keV and X-rays of 65 keV, and decays to ^{191}Ir, a stable agent. Due to the short half-life of the nuclide, the actual quantity of ^{191}Ir produced is small, and is considered to be nontoxic. The parent, reactor-produced ^{191}Os has a half-life of 15 days. The short half-life of the iridium product makes it difficult to characterize the chemical form of this Group VIII element. The radionuclide is associated with a radiation burden of 3-5 rads/mCi while providing a high photon flux. The majority of the radiation burden stems from the 'breakthrough' of the parent ^{191}Os into the ^{191m}Ir eluate. Improvements in the column material recently suggested by Brihaye *et al.* [20] indicate that the radiation burden may be reduced by 10 to 100 fold. The combination of high photon flux and exceptionally low radiation burden are well suited to the pediatric population for evaluating shunts and ventricular function.

Although the agent can be used in adults, the intrathoracic transit time of 8-10 s is relatively long compared to the 4.7 s half-life. As a result, right heart data is recorded with a photon flux 2 to 4 fold greater than that of the left heart. To visualize the left heart well, the count rate from the right heart must be very high. This high photon flux may actually present a problem for Anger scintillation cameras, since count rates in excess of 100,000 counts/second result in larger detector dead time of the camera, and a nonlinear relationship between activity in the field of view and counts recorded. The multicrystal gamma camera or the multiwire proportional chamber described by Lacy *et al.* [21] are able to take advantage of the very high count rates offered by ^{191m}Ir, since these instruments can process maximum count rates of 500,000-800,000 counts/second.

(b_3) *Gold-195m:* The radionuclide ^{195m}Au is a 30.5 s half-life daughter of the 40.5 h cyclotron produced ^{195}Hg. Gold-195m has a 262 keV gamma photon which is 68% abundant. The chemical form of the gold eluted from the column is not well characterized, but it is likely that this Group IB nuclide is ionic. The half-life of ^{195m}Au is long with reference to the central circulation time and permits high quality studies of the left and right heart to be recorded. The combination of short half-life and high photon energy led Mena *et al.* [22] to suggest that ^{195m}Au could be co-injected with thallium-201 (^{201}Tl) at the time of bicycle exercise studies to permit an evaluation of global and regional function in conjunction with assessment of myocardial perfusion. In the procedure described by Mena, the ^{195m}Au first pass ventricular function study was recorded followed by a 5 min wait for the gold to decay, the camera was then repeated for ^{201}Tl and myocardial perfusion data were collected.

As with other short half-life generator produced radionuclides, the radiation burden to the patient is primarily due to 'breakthrough' of the parent ^{195}Hg. Since mercury compounds localize in the kidneys, the radiation burden from breakthrough increases the renal dose. Although improvements in the generator column and eluate have resulted in a marked decrease in this problem, a limit of 300 mCi total dose is usually employed to minimize the radiation burden to the kidneys.

An additional problem, unique to the ^{195m}Au generator system, is the decay of ^{195m}Au to a long-lived daughter, ^{195}Au (T½ physical 190 days). This decay process is continuously underway on the generator, resulting in a high concentration of ^{195}Au in the initial eluate from the generator. Biodistribution studies in animals suggest that ^{195}Au localizes in the kidneys, and adds to the potential radiation burden from breakthrough of the parent ^{195}Hg. To minimize the build up of ^{195}Au, the column should be pre-eluted within 10 min of use.

The economics of manufacturing these generator systems depends on the availability of the target material to make the parent, the irradiation time required for a specific yield, the complexity of the procedure to separate the parent nuclide from the irradiated target, and the anticipated number of units sold. In general the cost/hour of cyclotron bombardment is greater than that for exposure to neutron flux in a reactor. These factors lead to the conclusion that the cost of the Os/Ir generator will be far lower than that of either the Hg/Au or the Rb/Kr generator. As a result of this consideration, it is likely that this generator system will receive increased attention.

B. Equilibrium

Equilibrium blood pool radiopharmaceuticals should have an unchanging volume of distribution over the time of observation. The label can be applied either to a macromolecule e.g., albumin [23], low density lipoproteins [24], or to a cell e.g. red blood cells [25]. The macromolecular labels have the advantage of kit formulation, ready availability and adequate quality control prior to administration.

a. Macromolecular ligands

The macromolecular radiopharmaceuticals have an effective half-time in the blood of less than 4 h. This makes it increasingly difficult to define subtle changes in regional wall motion when patients are evaluated for several hours (to define the effects of drug therapy, ect.). The radiation burden from a 20 mCi dose of ^{99m}Tc labeled albumin is less than 2 rads to the liver.

b. Red blood cells (RBC)

Both *in vitro* en *in vivo* approaches are available to bind ^{99m}Tc to RBC. Both methods employ a means of reducing technetium from the +7 state to a lower valence and accomplish binding of the reduced technetium to the beta chain of hemoglobin. The details of pertechnetate transport across the red cell membrane are only beginning to come to light, and most likely involve an anion transport enzyme, the band 3 transport protein [26]. Studies of ^{99m}Tc binding to the beta chain of hemoglobin versus time indicate that an interval of 10 min is required to accomplish a tight bond between the hemoglobin and the technetium-99m [27]. During this interval, other ligands can remove the ^{99m}Tc from the red cell and decrease the labeling efficiency. To minimize this problem the *in vitro* method [28] incubates anticoagulant-treated whole blood with stannous ion. The stannous ion changes the albumin in plasma as well as the red cells. If ^{99m}Tc is added at this point, the majority of the activity would bind to the albumin. Therefore the plasma is removed by centrifugation prior to addition of the activity. Technetium-99m pertechnetate is then added. The pretinned, pertechnetate-incubated red cells are then rewashed to remove unbound ^{99m}Tc, resuspended and reinjected.

An alternative approach utilizes a systemic injection of stannous ion (usually in the form of stannous pyrophosphate, DTPA, or diphosphonate) followed by withdrawal of 1-5 ml of blood into a syringe containing an anticoagulant (either sodium citrate [29] or heparin [25]) and pertechnetate. Following intravenous injection of the stannous-containing ligand, the stannous ion is rapidly cleared from the blood. It appears that optimal labeling requires an interval of about 20 min between injection of stannous ion and the subsequent incubation of the red cells with pertechnetate. Shorter or longer incubation results in a decrease of labeling efficiency. Incubation of the pretinned blood/pertechnetate mixture *in vitro* for 10 min is required to form a strong bond between the technetium and the beta chain of hemoglobin. Since more than 95% of the ^{99m}Tc is bound to red cells when this labeling method is employed, the contrast between the cardiac blood pool and surrounding structures is about 3:1 [25,27]. The red cells labeled either *in vivo* en *in vitro* have an effective half-life in the blood of approximately 6 h and minimal concentration in the liver, but are associated with a high concentration in the spleen, probably due to the high hematocrit in this organ. The radiation burden to the spleen from a 20 mCi administered dose of ^{99m}Tc labeled red cells is approximately 2 rads. The loosely bound technetium is excreted in the urine and causes visualization of the bladder. The stomach, salivary and thyroid glands are not seen, suggesting that the loosely bound technetium is not in the form of pertechnetate.

Labeled red blood cells may be employed for both first pass and equilibrium studies. Some laboratories record a 'gated first pass study' that is a gated data collection during the initial passage of radiopharmaceutical through the central circulation [1,30]. This can be particularly useful in determining right heart function. The data recorded following equilibration of the radiopharmaceutical provide a high contrast image of blood containing structures, but details of the borders of any one chamber may be observed by overlap from other chambers or great vessels [1-3]. As a result, combining the data from a first pass study (either gated or sequential) and an equilibrium study provides the best opportunity to define cardiac structure and function.

These measurements provide information on murmurs, cyanotic heart disease, and ischemic heart disease [31-38]. In the last few years some reports have compared the use of radionuclides such as xenon-133 to technetium-99m [39-42]. The tracers showed good correlation for first pass and right ventricular ejection fraction data. The xenon-133 studies have good reproducibility. Xenon-133 could be also used to evaluate myocardial blood flow (see section on blood flow agents).

In principle the same studies could be performed with greater accuracy using the positron agent carbon monoxide (^{11}CO or $C^{15}O$). The technique also provides regional information via the three-dimensional measurements of different levels of the heart.

Agents for perfusion scintigraphy

A number of agents have been used or investigated for the evaluation of myocardial blood flow (Table 2) [43,44]. Myocardial perfusion can be determined either following intravenous administration of radiopharmaceuticals which are avidly concentrated in the myocardium (based on the Sapirstein principle [45]) or following intracoronary injection of inert gases such as xenon-133 [46-48] or particulate agents such as macro-aggregated albumin [49].

Sapirstein principle

The initial distribution of radiopharmaceuticals which have a high extraction will be proportional to relative perfusion. This principle was first described by Leon Sapirstein [45] and bears his name. The Sapirstein principle does not require a radionuclide to belong to a particular class of agents in order to serve as an indicator of regional perfusion, but instead defines a kinetic pattern — e.g., high extraction by the organ of interest and rapid clearance from the blood (e.g., high extraction elsewhere in the body). If a radiopharmaceutical meets these criteria, it will be distributed in proportion to regional perfusion. Several classes of radiopharmaceuticals fall into this category: microspheres, thallium, rubidium, ^{13}N-labeled ammonia, labeled fatty acids and the recently described

Table 2. Myocardial perfusion agents

	Half-life	keV	Intra-venous	Intra-coronary
1. *Monovalent cations*				
a. Gamma				
Thallium-201 (^{201}Tl)	74 h	69,83	+	
Potassium-43 (^{43}K)	22.4 h	373, 619	+	
Cesium-129 (^{129}Sc)	32.1 h	375	+	
Rubidium-81 (^{81}Rb)	4.7 h	511, 190	+	
^{131}I-phosphonium (^{131}I-Ph)[a]	8 days	364	+	
^{131}I-ammonium (^{131}I-A)[a]	8 days	364	+	
b. Positron				
^{13}N-ammonia ($^{13}NH_4^+$)	10 min	511	+	
Potassium-38 (^{38}K)	7.6 min	511	+	
Rubidium-82 (^{82}Rb)	75 s	511	+	
Cesium (^{128}Cs)	36.2 min	511	+	
Manganese-52 (^{52}Mn)[b]	20 min	511	+	
Butanol (^{11}C)	20 min	511	+	
$H_2{}^{15}O$ (labeled water)	2 min	511		+
2. *Inert gas*[c]				
Xenon-133 (^{133}Xe)	5.3 days	81,204		+
Xenon-127 (^{127}Xe)	36.4 days	203, 172, 375		+
Krypton-81m (^{81m}Kr)	13 s	190		+
Krypton-85m (^{85m}Kr)	4.4 h	150, 305		+
3. *Others*				
[^{99m}Tc-DMPE]	6 h	140	+	
[^{99m}Tc-isonitriles]	6 h	140	+	
[^{99m}Tc-phospines]	6 h	140	+	
[^{99m}Tc-Diars]	6 h	140	+	
Ga-68-1, 1, 1-tris (5-methoxy-cycladiaminomethyl) ethane	68 min	511	+	
Ga-67 "	3.24 days	93, 184, 296 388	+	
^{11}C-methylbumine microspheres	20 min	511		+
^{99m}Tc-albumin microspheres for ventilation perfusion scintigraphy	6 h	140		+
Xenon-133 (^{133}Xe)	5.3 days	81, 204		+
^{99m}Tc-MAA (macroaggregates)[c]	6 h	140		+
Iridium-191m (^{191m}Ir)	5.8 s	129		+

[a] In principle ^{123}I could be used (T½ 13 h, 159 keV).
[b] Divalent cation available as generator ^{52}Fe- ^{52}Mn.
[c] The flow measurements with the inert gases and ^{99m}Tc-MAA are mostly invasive since they require intracoronary injection.
DMPE = dimethyl phospheno-ethane complex
Diars = diarsenical complex

technetium-99m isonitriles. Agents that are not highly extracted, such as labeled glucose or cesium, cannot be used to determine regional perfusion.

If the regional extraction of an agent falls below 50%, or if the residence time of the agent in the blood is prolonged such that the half-time of clearance in the blood is greater than 5 min, the agent will not follow the definition of a Sapirstein tracer and cannot be employed to define regional perfusion. The determination of regional perfusion with the monovalent cations is dependent on their maintaining a high extraction in the myocardial bed. Under reasonable physiological circumstances this is true, but when myocardial perfusion is markedly increased by vasodilators the extraction of the indicator may be reduced [50].

Monovalent cations

The monovalent cations potassium, rubidium, cesium and thallium concentrate in the myocardium to a sufficient degree to permit myocardial imaging [2]. The intravenous injection of monovalent cations such as cesium-129, rubidium-81, potassium-43, or thallium-201 is followed by their rapid extraction into tissue throughout the body. Although metabolic aspects of these monovalent radionuclides can complicate the interpretation of the blood flow measurement, the early myocardial distribution of activity is proportional to regional blood flow in the organ and to the total cardiac output received. The late images obtained with ^{201}Tl, for example, are affected by the redistribution of the tracer and its metabolism, and their interpretation should give an idea about myocardial tissue viability and integrity [42-44]. These agents enter the myocardium by the energy requiring sodium-potassium-ATPase pump mechanisms [51-52]. They differ in their physical half-lives, gamma emissions, and in the their time course of myocardial concentration and release. In a single transit through the coronary bed, the extraction of thallium is 88%, potassium and rubidium between 65 and 75%, while that of cesium is only 33% [2]. Since the myocardial extraction and total body extraction are usually similar, the time course of blood clearance and myocardial concentration will differ for each agent. The most rapid concentration in the myocardium occurs with thallium, followed by that of potassium and rubidium, while that for cesium is far slower. The importance of the time needed for localization stems from the need to maintain a 'steady-state' during the interval of radionuclide concentration in the myocardium. Within three circulatory periods, the majority of monovalent cationic myocardial tracers with high extraction fraction (thallium-201, rubidium-81-82, and potassium-43-38) has concentrated in the myocardium.

Myocardial kinetics

Once in the myocardium, the ionic radionuclides slowly leak out, with half-times ranging from 1.5 h for ^{43}K [2] to 4-6 h for ^{201}Tl [52]. The factors controlling the rate of loss from the myocardium are not fully understood, but include: 1) the presence of regional ischemia (slower loss from the ischemic segment [52]);

2) the level of exercise at the time of tracer administration (increased loss from patients achieving higher levels of exercise [53]); and 3) the plasma insulin levels (increased rate of loss from both ischemic and normal segments in animals infused with a glucose-insulin-potassium solution [54]).

The biological half-life of thallium in human subjects has been measured at over 10 days and results in a radiation burden of approximately 2 rads/2 mCi to the kidneys. Thallium-201 is not an ideal radionuclide for scintillation camera imaging because the resolution of conventional Anger scintillation cameras for the 70-80 keV energy of the mercury X-ray is about half that for the 140 keV photons of ^{99m}Tc. The 70-80 keV scintillation is about half as bright as that for the 140 keV. This lower intensity light flash results in a greater uncertainty in the positioning signal generated in the detector, and hence a lower resolution image (FWHM of approximately 6 mm). On the other hand, the energies of the rubidium and potassium nuclides are too high to permit efficient detection with the Anger camera and require high energy collimators to reduce scattered photons. These collimators generally have a lower sensitivity and lower resolution than lower energy collimators.

Positron emitting radionuclides blood flow agents

Three positron emitting radionuclides have been suggested for myocardial perfusion imaging: cyclotron-produced ^{13}N labeled ammonia (physical T½ of 10 min) [55, 56], cyclotron-produced potassium-38 (physical T½ of 7.6 min) labeled $H_2{}^{15}O$ (physical T½ of 2 min [57]) and generator-produced rubidium-82 (physical T½ of 75 s) [58, 59]. Although these agents can be imaged with a conventional Anger camera or a modified multicrystal camera, the best images are recorded with positron ring devices. The positron instruments combine high sensitivity and high resolution for myocardial imaging. Recent studies by Gould *et al.* [60] suggest that reductions of luminal diameter of less than 50% can be detected when these radionuclides are administered in conjunction with dipyridamole vasodilatation. The regional distribution of both ammonia and rubidium have excellent correlations with that of microspheres.

Rubidium-82 is a daughter of cyclotron-produced ^{82}Sr [^{85}Rb (p,4n), T½, 25 days]. The production of the parent ^{82}Sr requires a high energy cyclotron, and is accompanied by the production of small quantities of ^{85}Sr as a radiocontaminant. Since strontium radionuclides localize in bone and have a long biological half-life, the generator system has been refined to minimize the 'breakthrough' of the parent in the eluate. The generator is tested for breakthrough by the prior elution method describes above. A maximum of 0.001 μCi ^{82}Sr/mCi ^{82}Rb results in a radiation burden of 0.019 rads/mCi to the kidney and 0.001 rads/mCi to the total body [61].

Rubidium-82, a member of Group IA, is eluted from the generator as a monovalent cation. Myocardial imaging with this radionuclide requires fast acquisition of data. The images recorded during the first 1-2 min after intravenous administration depict the blood pool distribution of the radionuclide (if images are recorded with gating, ejection fraction and regional wall motion can be determined), while images recorded after 2 min depict regional perfusion. Reasonable quality images can be recorded for 4 to 6 half-lives after infusion, i.e. 1 to 2 half-lives consumed with blood clearance and the remainder for myocardial perfusion.

Intracoronary measurements
At times it is desirable to define myocardial perfusion in the catheterization laboratory by direct intracoronary injection. Under these circumstances, either the inert gases such as ^{133}Xe [46-48], or particulate agents such as macroaggregated albumin, can be employed [49]. Following intra-arterial administration the inert gas tracers leave the capillaries and enter tissue in direct proportion to their relative solubility in the tissue compared to that in blood (partition coefficient). Thereafter, the clearance of the tracer from the tissue is dependent on the rate of perfusion. Since the myocardial clearance of xenon usually has a half-time of less than 1 min, a scintillation camera must be present in the catheterization laboratory to measure the myocardial clearance. The rapid clearance of xenon makes it possible to record myocardial perfusion under several different circumstances in rapid succession, with an extremely low radiation burden to the patient (radiation burden of less than 0.1 rads to the myocardium per 0.5 mCi intracoronary injection).

The direct intracoronary administration of particulate radiopharmaceuticals in small quantities (<50,000 particles) is safe, and can be particularly useful for defining the amount and the source of collateral perfusion. In this technique either a single radiolabeled microsphere is administered directly into one coronary artery and a second labeled particulate into the other, or the two radiopharmaceuticals can be administered through the same coronary bed before and after an intervention to define the change in myocardial perfusion [62].

Since the particulate radiopharmaceuticals remain *in situ* following administration, imaging can be performed several hours following injection. The radiation burden to the myocardium is low, since only 0.1-0.2 mCi of radiolabel is required to provide a very high quality image in a short interval of imaging.

New agents

The relatively poor resolution of ^{201}Tl has led to a search for a ^{99m}Tc labeled perfusion agent. Based on the observations of Deutsch *et al.* [63-65], efforts to combine ^{99m}Tc into a lipid soluble charged complex appeared to offer the best opportunity for achieving successful myocardial concentration. Several ^{99m}Tc labeled compounds, such as the diarsenical complex of technetium-99m (DiARS) and a dimethyl phospheno-ethane complex DMPE) [66], and a hexakis complex of technetium [67] were tested in animals and found to have high myocardial uptake. The rapid myocardial concentration of these compounds fulfilled the criteria of Sapirstein tracers and a high correlation with regional perfusion was found [66]. However, when DiARS and DMPE were administered to human subjects, their myocardial concentration was extremely disappointing.

When human studies with the technetium-99m labeled hexakis-isonitrile compound were performed, however, sufficient concentration was observed in the human myocardium to permit high quality planar and tomographic images to be recorded [68]. This agent combines the properties of high lipid solubility and technetium chelation. This agent achieves a localization of up to 2% of the injected dose in the human myocardium. The mode of entry of this agent to the myocardium is not fully understood, but may depend primarily on solubility, rather than specific transport, as is the case with the monovalent cations. Following intravenous administration, the isonitrile localizes in the lungs to a sufficient degree that the myocardium cannot be visualized. The clearance from the lungs is more rapid than that from the heart, which permits myocardial visualization about 1 h after injection. Serial images recorded after the first hour indicate that myocardial clearance is slow and approximates the physical half-life of ^{99m}Tc. The metabolic fate and the relationship of the distribution of this agent to regional perfusion are under investigation.

Ultrashort-lived nuclides have been suggested for the determination of regional myocardial perfusion. Both ^{81m}Kr [14,15] and ^{191m}Ir [6,7] have been used in animal studies. These agents, administered by continuous infusion directly into the coronary bed, achieve the highest concentration in areas of greatest perfusion. Static images of the distribution of radionuclide are related to the regional distribution. Following an intervention such as pacing, the radionuclide will reequilibrate in the myocardium dependent on the redistribution of regional perfusion. Approximately three half-lives are required to obtain a new equilibrium state which reflects the regional distribution of perfusion. A second static image recorded under this circumstance can be compared to the image recorded at baseline to identify the changes in regional perfusion.

The relationship of regional perfusion to radionuclide distribution with these agents is not linear. The ^{81m}Kr enters the tissue as a result of its high permeability. The combination of short physical half-life and regional perfusion both contribute to the clearance of the radionuclide from the myocardium. As a result, the changes in regional perfusion contribute relatively little to the effective half-life of this agent (e.g., the effective half-life in normal myocardium is approximately 9 s, and if flow is doubled, the half-life decreases to 7 s, while if flow is halved the half-life increases to 10 s). On the other hand, ^{191m}Ir appears to remain in the vasculature. The effective half-life of this agent is dependent on the time required for its passage through the myocardial capillary bed. Normal myocardial transit time is approximately 8 s at rest (resulting in an effective half-time of 3 s). At high flows, the myocardial transit time may decrease to 4 s (effective half-life of 2 s), while during ischemia myocardial transit time may increase to over 16 s (effective half-life of 3.6 s). When these changes are viewed as a percentage change in regional concentration as a function of change in perfusion, the ability of the resultant image to provide a reasonable index of myocardial perfusion can be appreciated. As a result of the increase in relative change for a given change in perfusion with ^{191m}Ir, the images recorded with this agent may be easier to interpret than those obtained with ^{81m}Kr. Although ^{195m}Au has not been used for this purpose, calculation of its effective half-life in the myocardium indicates that it would provide the greatest change in regional concentration for a given change in regional perfusion. Whether this approach is useful will be determined after further clinical trials with this agent.

Blood flow measurements are useful in the following clinical situations: detection of coronary artery disease [69-75], assessment of pathology after coronary arteriography [76-78], pre- and postoperative assessment of coronary artery disease [79], and detection of acute myocardial infarction. In many instances, scans made with monovalent cations or inert gases in order to diagnose myocardial infarction have been compared with clinicopathological data and have shown good correlation [80].

Metabolic agents

In recent years developments in data analysis and instrumentation have improved our understanding of the distribution of radiotracers targeted towards myocardial metabolism. These radiopharmaceuticals should enable the differentiation of the energy consumption in the various stages of ischemia and infarction. Since both perfusion and metabolic function change with injury, studies that will evaluate the coupling or uncoupling of flow and metabolism in different diseases may determine the degree of tissue viability. Measurements of cardiac metabolism can be studied by two different approaches: 1) the use of the labeled physiologic tracer; and 2) the use of an analog that is transported in the same manner as the 'natural' metabolite, but goes through only a few steps of metabolism and is then trapped in the tissue in a chemically known form, (as in the case of 2-deoxy-D-glucose as an analog of glucose in brain tissue). This permits estimates of metabolism based on mathematical models allowing for the major changes [81].

When an analog is used as a metabolic substrate, the following must be considered in the interpretation of the data: 1) the differences in the transport properties and enzyme affinities of the analog as compared to that of the metabolite; 2) the differences between the behavior of metabolites and the analogs in a diseased state as compared to normal baseline state; 3) the toxic effect of analogs when they are enzyme inhibitors or alter the metabolic pathway, and 4) the radiation dosimetry when repetitive studies are planned.

On the other hand, metabolites present certain problems. Since the metabolite enters a biochemical pathway which may lead to the degradation of the molecule and the elimination of its radioactivity from the tissue of interest, translocation and incorporation of the activity into other tissue should be clearly defined. This necessitates alterations in the model of tracer kinetics to reflect washout and change of activity in tissue, recirculation in plasma and reextraction as other metabolites. Some of these problems can be corrected when fast and meaningful data sampling is possible [82,83]. Furthermore, the extent of change in the transport properties or the enzyme kinetics of the physiologic metabolite in each disease state should be determined. Therefore, metabolites may impose limitations similar to those of their analogs. In the following section we will review the use of some metabolites and their analogs (Table 3).

Sugars and analogs

Glucose is an important physiological substrate for the myocardium. In heart tissue this substrate can be metabolized under aerobic and anaerobic conditions through the glycolytic pathway; carbon dioxide or lactate are the resulting metabolites. Alteration in the normal rate of glucose utilization can be an indication of physiological disorder. For example, changes of glucose metabolism in the heart have been associated with hypoxia and anoxia [84]. The principles for using glucose and analogs and their tracer kinetic modeling (only for ^{14}C, ^{11}C and ^{18}F) have been reviewed many times in recent years [81, 85, 86].

In some studies the coupling or uncoupling of flow and metabolism may aid in defining the extent and severity of an ischemic injury or cardiomyopathy. Marshall *et al.* [87] studied myocardial ischemia and infarction with [^{13}N]NH_3 and [^{18}F]2-FDG and found that the changes in regional ^{18}F labeled 2-fluoro-2-deoxy-D-glucose concentrations detected with PET in patients who had had a recent myocardial infarction are consistent with regional exogenous glucose utilization and perfusion in moderately ischemic and irreversibly infarcted myocardium. It was proposed that this phenomenon could be a result of anaerobic glucose metabolism manifested as lactate production [87], whereas myocardial infarction is characterized by the loss of metabolically active myocardium.

Perloff *et al.* [88] also used [^{18}F]2-FDG, and [^{13}N]NH_3 to determine whether myocardial metabolic abnormality could be studied in the cardiomyopathy of Duchenne muscular dystrophy. In addition to the positron study, thallium-201 scans, technetium-99m multiple-gated equilibrium blood pool imaging, electrocardiograms, and other parameters were monitored. Their findings showed that [^{18}F]2-FDG activity was selectively increased in specific

Table 3. Partial list of compounds labeled with gamma and positron emitters as metabolites or their analogs

Radionuclides	Preliminary application
Sugars[a] (positron)	
^{11}C-glucose (^{11}C-Glu)	Myocardial and brain glucose metabolism[a]
^{11}C-deoxy-D-glucose (^{11}C-DG)	"
[^{18}F]-2-FDG	"
Fatty Acids (positron)	
[1-^{11}C] straight chain	Myocardial fatty acid kinetics and metabolism
[1-^{11}C] betamethyl branched chain	Myocardial perfusion and fatty acid metabolism
Fatty Acids (gamma)	
*I-straight chain	Myocardial perfusion
*I-omega-phenyl straight chain	and fatty acid metabolism
Heteroatom containing fatty acids[b]	
*I-branched chain fatty acids[c]	
^{75}Br-15-parabromophenylpentadecanoic acid	
Others	
^{13}N and ^{11}C-amino acids[d]	Evaluation of myocardial metabolism
^{13}N-glutamate and	Regional myocardial
^{13}N-alanine	metabolism
^{11}C-acetate	Myocardial metabolism
^{11}C-pyruvate	Increased uptake in ischemic regions in rabbit heart
^{11}C-L-aspartic acid	Assessment of regional myocardial metabolism in the Rhesus monkey
*I-3-quinuclidinyl-4-iodobenzilate	Muscarinic acetycholine receptor in heart
*I-phosphonium	Study the effect of structural
*I-arsonium	variations of cations on myocardial
*I-ammonium	uptake

[a] Radioiodinated and radiobrominated glucose analogs were proposed for myocardial studies but were not used in clinical investigation because of their poor *in vivo* stability.

[b] This group includes radioiodinated straight-chain, omega-iodophenyl, omega-iodovinyl or radiolabeled heteroatom such as ^{75}Se and ^{123}Te positioned at different sites of the FA chain (see text).

[c] This group includes alpha and betamethyl branched chain fatty acids alpha and betamethyl-omega-phenyl radioiodinated fatty acids.

[d] In principal ^{13}N or ^{11}C labeled amino acids that are involved in heart metabolic activity could be used. However, the biochemical rationale for the use of each amino acid metabolic activity by the heart muscle should be discussed separately depending on the amino acid of choice, the site of labeling and the label.

* I = ^{125}I, ^{131}I or ^{123}I

segments in the left ventricle whereas $[^{13}N]NH_3$ activity was selectively decreased in the same areas. This could be an indication for an accelerated regional exogenous glucose utilization, a reduction in regional blood flow, or both.

Schwaiger *et al.* [89] used $[^{13}N]NH_3$ as a perfusion indicator and ^{11}C-palmitate (see rationale in fatty acid section below) and $[^{18}F]$2-FDG as metabolic indicators in dogs after occlusion and reperfusion. Their findings indicate that there was functional recovery, paralleled by sustained metabolic abnormalities reflected by segmentally delayed clearance of ^{11}C-palmitate and increased uptake of $[^{18}F]$-2-FDG. Absence of blood flow and ^{11}C-palmitate uptake at 24 h after reperfusion correlated with extensive necrosis. Conversely, uptake of ^{11}C-palmitate and delayed ^{11}C clearance and increased $[^{18}F]$2-FDG accumulation identified reversibly injured tissue.

Schelbert *et al.* [90] used $[^{13}N]NH_3$, $[^{18}F]$2-FDG and ^{11}C-palmitate to study the relationship of flow and metabolism in myocardial ischemia in man. The ischemic regions in the heart showed reduced 1-^{11}C-palmitate and $[^{13}N]NH_3$ uptake whereas that of $[^{18}F]$2-FDG was increased. This study demonstrated that the results of changes in metabolic patterns and flow reported earlier in dogs could be observed and studied in humans.

Fatty acids and analogs

The rationale behind the use of fatty acids as potential myocardial markers is based on the fact that both at rest and during exercise, nonesterified fatty acids supply approximately 65% of the energy requirement for myocardial metabolism. The remainder of the myocardial energy needs are met by glucose (15%), lactate and pyruvate (12%) and amino acids (5%) [91-94].

Evans *et al.* [95] in 1965 first introduced a radioiodinated fatty acid as an imaging marker for the heart. They used radioiodinated oleic acid (^{131}I) to study a series of 30 dogs. The myocardium was clearly visualized on the rectilinear scans and the scans appeared different from those obtained with albumin or ionic iodide. This was quickly followed by studies in humans by Gunton *et al.* [96] who reported disappointing findings in 42 human subjects with this tracer. Of 13 patients with documented myocardial infarction, decreased fatty acid uptake was observed on scans only in five patients. This led the authors to caution that fatty acid scintigraphy is "...not a practical diagnostic method for the detection, location and estimation of size of myocardial infarcts". Based on this negative report, interest in fatty acid imaging of the myocardium waned for almost a decade.

In 1975, Poe *et al.* sought an improved method for imaging the myocardium with perfusion related tracers [97]. They reasoned that attachment of ^{123}I to a fatty acid would result in a perfusion related tracer [98] with excellent physical characteristics for imaging. This led to the synthesis of the 16-carbon unsaturated fatty acid labeled with ^{123}I at the omega position (16-iodo-9-

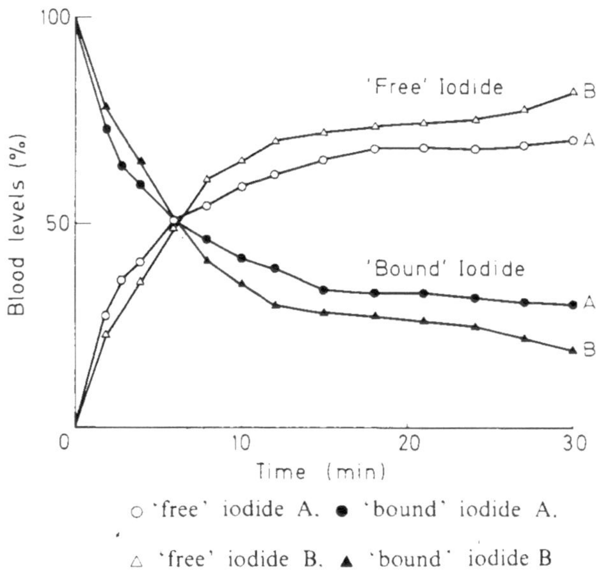

Figure 1. Relative concentrations of "bound" and "free" radioiodide separated by chromatographic analysis.

hexadecenoic acid) [97]. They compared the behavior of this agent to that of ^{11}C labeled oleic and stearic acids and potassium-43. The blood and precordial clearance of the three fatty acids were similar over the first 5 to 10 min after injection. The regional myocardial distribution of ^{123}I-hexadecenoic acid as compared to that ^{43}K in a series of dogs with coronary ligation showed a linear relationship over a wide range of flows, suggesting that the fatty acid tracer could be used as a potential flow indicator. In contrast to the work of Evans and Gunton, however, Poe observed that diagnostic quality images could be recorded during the first 10 min following injection. Poe suggested that this rate of clearance of the radiolabel from the heart, though a problem for imaging, could relate to fatty acid utilization and should be quantified [97,98].

These iodinated fatty acids are subject to enzymatic deiodination, which may occur independently of the catabolism of the fatty acid. As a result, any clearance measurement must consider elements of both fatty acid catabolism and enzymatic degradation with diffusion of the radiolabeled fragment from the myocardium (Figure 1). Although attempts have been made to correct for enzymatic degradation of iodine by measuring the distribution of ionic radioiodine [99], differences in permeability and distribution of the administered ionic radioiodine and the ionic radioiodine produced in the myocardial tissue make this correction difficult to apply.

Different groups of workers used (17-^{123}I)iodoheptadecanoic acid to measure differences in myocardial fatty acid metabolism between normal and ischemic conditions and in several types of cardiomyopathies [100]. Radioiodine has been stabilized on the phenyl of 15(p-iodophenyl) pentadecanoic acid [101-105] and the ^{123}I labeled compound has been evaluated in patients [106-109].

Van der Wall and co-workers [110-112] have shown that the radioiodinated long-chain free fatty acids, ^{123}I labeled hexadecenoic acid (16-HA) and heptadecanoic acid (17-HDA) and thallium-201 are comparable in the ability to detect areas of inadequate myocardial perfusion. The clearance rates in the ischemic areas in patients were found to be significantly lower both with ^{123}I-16-HA, and ^{123}I-17-HDA compared to normal regions (longer half-times). In contrast, clearance rates from acutely infarcted regions were consistently faster than from normal regions (shorter half-times).

Comparison of ^{131}I-16-HA and ^{125}I-17-HDA in a double label experiment in the dog heart showed that 17-HDA uptake is twice that of 16-HA and the ^{125}I to ^{131}I ratio was higher for the ischemic myocardium as compared to normal due to lower uptake of 17-HDA in ischemic myocardium. These studies conclude that 17-HDA is a better indicator of myocardial metabolism.

Feinendegen, Freundlieb and others [113-115] studied (17-^{123}I)iodoheptadecanoic acid in patients with coronary artery disease and with congestive heart failure. Infarcted zones as well as ischemic regions were indicated by reduced tracer uptake. A method for correcting iodine-123 in the blood pool and interstitial space was introduced. This improved the image quality (see chapter 2). Their studies indicate that radioiodinated fatty acids could be used to measure significant differences in myocardial fatty acid metabolism in patients with coronary artery disease.

In other patient studies ^{123}I-17-HDA was used after infusing insulin and glucose to alter the glucose level lowered fatty acid uptake. Since the uptake and washout of fatty acids seem to be influenced by other energy competing substrates like glucose, this supports the hypothesis that fatty acids are potential metabolic indicators. Additional studies [116] suggest that the metabolic turnover rates measured with ^{123}I-17-HDA could detect regional myocardial ischemia in patients.

It was thought that the problem of deiodination could be solved by using omega-p-halophenyl fatty acid analogs. Ercan *et al.* [117] investigated the biodistribution, plasma clearance and urinary excretion of omega-(p-^{123}I-phenyl)pentadecanoic acid (^{123}I-IPPA) in rats. The study included analysis of blood, urine and protein binding at various intervals after administration. The maximum uptake by myocardium occurred at 1 min and the maximal heart to blood ratios at 3 min. At any time after injection, the amount of free iodine in plasma was less than 1%, thus obviating a background problem or unnecessary radiation dose to the thyroid and whole body. The major radioactive metabolites were ^{123}I-p-hippuric acid and ^{123}I-p-iodobenzoic acid. In urine ^{123}I-p-hippuric acid was excreted almost quantitatively. The metabolism was very fast, the first metabolites being found in the blood stream 3 min post injection.

The evaluation of ^{123}I-IPPA using single tomography in dogs showed that this fatty acid concentrated in the myocardium permitting high quality tomographic sections of the heart. The rate of elimination of ^{123}I-IPPA from the canine ischemic myocardial regions was significantly prolonged when compared with unaffected control regions. Similar radiohalogenated fatty acids that could be potential heart agents were reported by Coenen *et al.* [118[.

Basamadjian *et al.*[119,120] introduced tellurium in fatty acids at the omega position. This design was improved by Knapp and Goodman *et al.* [121-126]. These investigators used tellurium, selenium and sulfur as heteroatoms in different positions on the fatty acid molecule. The initial work with ^{123}Te, which has favorable energy characteristics (159 keV) but an inadequate physical half-life ($t^1/_2$ of 120 days), indicated an acceptable biological half-life and low dosimetry. Also, tellurium has a radius comparable to that of a carbon-carbon double bond. 9-(^{123}Te)telluraheptadecanoic acid, designed as an analog for oleic acid, has high myocardial extraction and long activity retention. The unusual trapping could not be postulated from the structure of these fatty acids. A possible explanation is a fast *in vivo* oxidation of the tellurium heteroatom to produce a nonsoluble fatty acid that is very slowly removed from myocardial tissue. The toxicity of tellurium encouraged the development of other fatty acid series with selenium and sulfur, but these did not exhibit the same retention properties.

To overcome the toxicity problem, Goodman *et al.* [127,128] extended their concept to the preparation of analogs that contain cold tellurium as the heteroatom and radioiodine as the label. These investigators also stabilized the iodine on the fatty acid molecule by producing a vinyl or aryl radioiodinated derivative [125, 127, 128] with favorable properties. When prepared in high specific activity these agents should be useful for studying myocardial perfusion, since they have high myocardial extraction with good activity retention in the heart.

Branched chain iodinated fatty acids

The rationale behind the design of the betamethyl analogs of fatty acids and other branched chain fatty acids is discussed in the following section on positron labeled fatty acids. This approach was adopted for single photon tomography by introducing the radioiodine on the omega position of the fatty acid chain as a p-iodophenyl derivative. Several analogs were synthesized and tested following the production of 14-(p-iodophenyl)-3-(R,S)-methyltetradecanoic acid (IBMPTA) [129-131] and 15-(p-iodophenyl)-3-(R,S)-methylpentadecanoic acid (IBMPPA) [132].The behavior of these fatty acids was studied in rats and dogs and was compared to that of the straight chain analog 15-(p-iodophenyl)pentadecanoic acid (IPPA) [133]. The study concludes that in rats, IBMPPA has higher initial heart uptake (3.45% dose/g) than IBMPTA (1.85% dose/g) and IPPA (1.94% dose/g); however, the myocardial retention index at 60 min was similar for IBMPTA and IBMPPA as expected from their speculated metabolic behavior, and lower for IPPA which was shown to be a substrate for beta oxidation [105]. The dog and human studies with IBMPTA indicated high myocardial extraction and activity retention in the heart for a period of several hours. Methods applying IBMPTA or, in principle, IBMPPA as fatty acid markers and thallium-201 as a flow marker in the same patient should allow studies that can differentiate between flow and metabolism as in case of cardiomyopathies [133] and in the hypertensive rat model [134-136].

The betamethyl branched fatty acids showed lower extraction [130] and should not be subject to the complete beta oxidation process. Recently, Knapp *et al.* [137] synthesized the radioiodinated, beta-betadimethyl derivative, 15-(p-iodophenyl)-3,3-dimethylpentadecanoic acid (DMIPP), and studied its behavior in rats. The heart extraction of this agent and its myocardial retention index in rats was reported to be higher than those obtained with the beta-ethyl derivative.

The reason for the prolonged retention of the beta-betadimethyl derivative is not clear, since alpha and omega oxidation contribute very little to fatty acid metabolism [138] and the ^{11}C and ^{14}C betamethyl derivatives of heptadecanoic acid were found to be trapped with minimal washout at 1 h. The beta, betadimethyl, omegaaryl branched fatty acid should undergo neither the alpha nor the beta oxidation process. It should only be subject to omega oxidation. In principle, this agent should proceed only through the first thiokinase step, not be involved in other energy related steps, and be stored, whereas the betamethyl fatty acid undergoes several steps before being trapped (see below).

The ortho and para substituent effects on the physiological behavior of straight and branched chain radioiodinated fatty acids was reported recently by Machulla *et al.* [139] who proposed a careful study of the metabolism of the isomers.

Positron-labeled fatty acids

The scope of positron-labeled radiopharmaceuticals and their advantages have been reviewed many times [140-149]. In principle, labeled "physiologic"metabolic substrates, blood flow and blood volume tracers, protein synthesis and transport markers or specific receptor binding agents could be used to measure their uptake kinetics noninvasively in man. The technique goes beyond medical imaging since it allows assessment of regional biochemical changes in a quantitative manner. Rose *et al.* [150] developed approaches for the quantitative determination of the biological behavior of tracers under ideal circumstances. To calculate myocardial fatty acid utilization they took into account the behavior of the tracer in the vascular compartment, the interstitial fluid and the cellular compartment. These studies could be done under adequately controlled conditions when fast data acquisition is possible.

In vivo and *in vitro* applications of ^{11}C labeled palmitate as an indicator of fatty acid metabolism were initially reported by Weiss *et al.* [151]. With the use of radiolabeled palmitate they demonstrated that ischemia results in both decreased myocardial extraction of the fatty acid and decreased catabolism. These findings suggest that imaging with (1-^{11}C)palmitate could readily identify regions of ischemic myocardium. Animal studies by Weiss *et al.* [151, 152], Klein *et al.* [153,154], Hoffman *et al.* [155] and Ter-Pogossian *et al.* [156] using (1-^{11}C)palmitate provide the experimental basis for positron imaging as a means of studying regional myocardial fatty acid distribution. In addition these investigators have demonstrated alterations in the appearance of positron emission tomograms in patients with coronary artery disease manifested by infarction, ischemia or congestive cardiomyopathy [157-159].

To measure regional fatty acid metabolism, one needs to develop a model of the metabolism of the radiopharmaceutical so that measurements made under rigorously controlled circumstances can be quantitatively interpreted. Since palmitate is a fatty acid normally present as a metabolic substrate, the tracer enters metabolic pathways and is rapidly consumed. Recent studies by Schoen *et al.* [160,161], who employed direct intracoronary administration of (1-^{11}C)palmitate and direct myocardial monitoring, demonstrate the evolution of $^{11}CO_2$ within 30 s and a 50% clearance of the radiolabel from the heart within 2.8 min of administration. New areas of investigation are also being explored with (1-^{11}C)palmitate. Sobel *et al.* [162] evaluated myocardial fatty acid metabolism after coronary thrombolysis induced with streptokinase. The clot lysis was followed by improved regional myocardial metabolism.

The rapid metabolism of the substrate by beta-oxidation leads to the production of (^{11}C)metabolites that permit translocation of the radiolabel to any one of several sites, in either the cell or the blood. To quantify the rapid metabolism of palmitate in the myocardium requires the extremely rapid recording of sequential images, each of no more than a few seconds duration. The combination of rapid metabolic changes and the need for short imaging times makes the quantification of myocardial fatty acid metabolism with (1-^{11}C)palmitate very difficult. The evaluation by imaging of fatty acid metabolism in the heart would be significantly simplified by the use of a labeled substrate that enters the myocardium via a well delineated pathway, undergoes limited metabolism and remains *in situ* for a sufficient interval to permit the recording of high quality data. These considerations led to the development of 3-methyl-(1-^{11}C)heptadecanoate in our laboratory by Livni *et al.* [163].

The selection of branched chain fatty acids as a substrate that would be trapped is based on the analysis of the six steps required for the removal of each acetyl group from a fatty acid as acetyl-SCoA in the usual process of beta oxidation. The six steps are summarized in Figure 2. In the first step, a thioester of the fatty acid is formed by coupling HSCoA to the acyl group. This ATP dependent step takes place in the cytosol under the enzymatic catalysis of acyl-SCoA synthetase. Since the remaining steps of beta-oxidation take place in the mitochondria, where the enzymes responsible for beta-oxidation are located in the matrix, the acyl-SCoA must be transported from the cytosol through the mitochondrial membrane to the site of fatty acid oxidation. This transport is accomplished by carnitine acyl-transferase-1. In the mitochondrium carnitine acyl-transferase-2 converts the acyl-fatty acid back to the

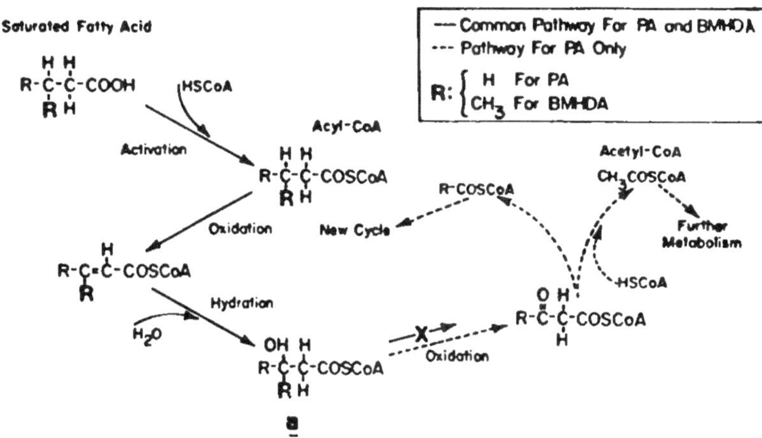

Figure 2. Metabolic pathway for ß-oxidation.

acyl-SCoA. In the third step the alpha beta unsaturated acyl-SCoA ester is produced. This reaction is catalyzed by acyl-SCoA dehydrogenase. The hydration of the acyl-SCoA by hydratase produces S-3-hydrocyacyl-SCoA. The latter is converted in the fifth step to 3-ketoacyl-SCoA, and in the last step the 3-ketoacyl-SCoA is converted to acetyl-SCoA and an acyl-SCoA that has been shortened by two carbons (catalyzed by thiolase).

The 3-methyl branched chain analog prevents the S-3-hydroxyacyl-SCoA formed in the fourth step of the process to be oxidized in the fifth step of the process to the 3-ketoacyl-SCoA. The 3-methyl fatty acid forms the betahydroxybetamethyl derivative which cannot be oxidized chemically to the ketoacyl-SCoA derivative.

To test the hypothesis a series of betamethyl fatty acids of varying chain lengths were prepared [164]. The compounds synthesized were (1-^{11}C)betamethylundecanoic acid (BMUA), betamethylpalmitic acid (BMPA), betamethylheptadecanoic acid (BMHA), betamethyloctadecanoic (BMOA) and betamethylheneicosanoic acid (BMIA). For each compound, biodistribution studies were performed in rats at various times following intravenous administration. The percentage of radioactivity released as $^{11}CO_2$ was determined by trapping $^{11}CO_2$ in KOH solution. The biodistribution studies demonstrated that the BMHA has the highest myocardial uptake and highest ratios of target (heart) to nontarget (blood, lung and liver) tissues, whereas BMUA showed lowest heart uptake at all times. The behavior of the 3-methylheptadecanoic acid was compared to that of (16-^{14}C)palmitic acid and (1-^{11}C)heptadecanoic acid.

The biodistribution studies of (1-^{14}C)BMHA showed a heart concentration for (1-^{14}C)BMHA of 2.82 and 4.18% ID/g at 5 and 60 min, respectively, while that of (16-^{14}C)palmitic acid was 2.65 and 0.89% ID/g at 5 and 60 min, respectively. As postulated (1-^{14}C)BMHA activity was retained in the heart for a period of 60 min where the normal fatty acid exhibited a fast clearance (Table 4). The observation that the modified fatty acid cleared from the myocardium at 24 h suggests that the material either back-diffuses or is metabolized by an alternate pathway.

The metabolic fate of BMHA and palmitic acid was studied in mice. The animals were sacrified 5, 15, 30 and 60 min after the injection of 5-10 mCi of either acid. The heart and blood were extracted. The organic phase of the extract was analyzed by TLC for triglycerides (TG), diglycerides (DG), free fatty acids (FFA), monoglycerides (MG) and polar lipids (PL) (Table 5). The distribution of the label between the organic (O), aqueous (A) and insoluble tissue (T) of the heart was measured (Table 6). The data in Tables 5 en 6 show

Table 4. Biodistribution of 16-(^{14}C)palmitic acid and 1-(^{14}C)betamethylheptadecanoic acid in rats expressed in % dose/g

	1-(^{14}C)BMHA			16-(^{14}C)palmitic acid	
Tissue	5 min	60 min	24 h[a]	5 min	60 min
Blood	0.44±0.18	0.22±0.08	0.88±0.07	0.09±0.03	0.09±0.01
Heart	2.45±0.63	4.18±1.05	0.40±0.08	2.65±0.75	0.89±0.22
Liver	1.85±0.39	1.96±0.21	0.50±0.08	4.84±1.13	2.01±1.02
Lung	1.40±0.34	0.92±0.22	0.47±0.09	2.78±1.56	1.89±0.12
Muscle	0.38±0.08	0.35±0.13	0.17±0.03	0.34±0.09	0.20±0.11

[a] 12 Rats: all other time points 6 rats/point.

Table 5. The distribution of (^{14}C)palmitic acid and (^{14}C)BMHA in triglycerides (TG) diglycerides (DG), free fatty acid (FFA), monoglycerides (MG) and polar lipids (PL) in heart and blood of mice

	Time (min)							
	5	60	5	60	5	60	5	60
FFA	4.8	3.6	12.1	5.3	74.8	7.0	20.3	25.1
TG	81.8	71.8	63.6	45.5	0	70.8	45.1	58.5
DG	4.8	3.8	4.7	1.7	16.6	13.8	11.1	3.7
MG&PL	8.3	18.4	15.1	39.6	6.9	6.4	17.7	12.2

Table 6. The distribution of the label between the organic, aqueous, and insoluble tissue of the heart of mice

	BMHA		palmitic acid	
	5 min	60 min	5 min	60 min
Organic	78.5	74.6	68.3	85.5
Aqueous	12.0	4.4	25.6	11.5
Tissue	9.5	20.5	6.5	3.0

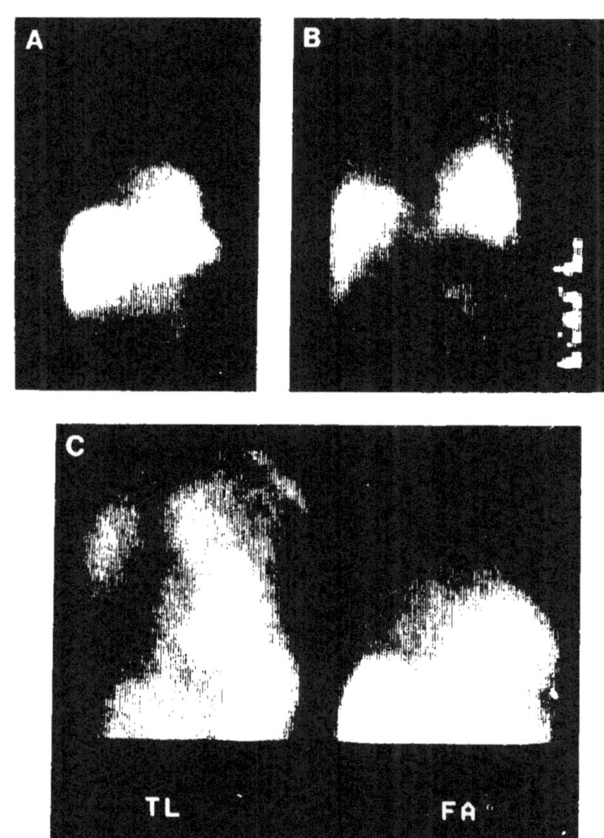

Figure 3. Heart images obtained from human normal volunteers after the intravenous administration of (A): ^{123}I-(p-iodophenyl)-3-(R,S)-tetradecanoic acid (IBMPTA) (2mCi); (B): (1-^{11}C)-betamethylheptadecanoic acid (3 mCi). The positron camera, PC-II was used to collect the 2D images; (C): Tl-201 and ^{123}I-IBMPTA in the same volunteer (immediate scans post-injection).

incorporation of both BMHA and palmitic acid into the same metabolic compartment. However, the data suggest that the fate of the modified fatty acid in blood and heart should be considered when we use these analogs.

Simultaneous single pass extraction fraction studies of (^{11}C)betamethylheptadecanoic acid and (^{14}C)palmitic acid in dogs demonstrated approximately 60% extraction for both agents.

Imaging studies in dogs with (1-^{11}C)heptadecanoic acid (HA) as compared to (1-^{11}C)betamethylheptadecanoic acid showed a fast washout of HA from the myocardium while BMHA activity was retained. Furthermore, De Landsheere *et al.* [165] compared regional myocardial uptake of (1-^{11}C)betamethylheptadecanoic acid to that of rubidium-82 and microspheres and found that the behavior of these agents is different: a mean reduction of 53% in flow was accompanied by only a 19% decrease in regional myocardial uptake of fatty acid.

Preliminary imaging studies in man with (1-^{11}C)MBHA showed high myocardial extraction with prolonged activity retention (Figure 3).

In conclusion, the similar extraction, initial biodistribution, and entry into metabolic pathways of the branched chain and unbranched fatty acids suggest that the modified fatty acid can serve as a useful analog for imaging studies.

Other metabolic agents and analogs

The availability of positron radionuclides in many centers and the development of the fast incorporation of these nuclides into metabolically active molecules initiated investigation with molecules other than fatty acids and sugars. Certain amino acids are involved in a network of energy production and/or protein synthesis in the myocardium. Their syntheses and preliminary evaluation have been reported [166-168]. Pyruvate, lactate and acetate are also being considered as agents for studying myocardial integrity [169,170] (see Table 3).

In the future studies combining metabolic activity, perfusion and heart function will strengthen the knowledge and the diagnostic accuracy of the severity of myocardial injury.

Infarct avid agents

Table 7 represents all the labeled agents that have been used for hot spot infarct imaging. The most useful among them is ^{99m}Tc-pyrophosphate (^{99m}Tc-PYP) which has proven to be diagnostically useful in patients with acute myocardial

Table 7. Infarct avid agents

	Transport	Preliminary applications
^{99m}Tc-tetracycline	Active transport	Heart lesions
^{99m}Tc-pyrophosphate	Active transport	Heart lesions
^{99m}Tc-glucoheptonate	Active transport	Heart lesions
^{99m}Tc-antimyosine antibody	Active transport	Heart lesions
^{203}Hg-mercurials	Inflammatory response to acute transmural myocardial infarction	
Radioiodinated antimyosine antibody	Active transport	Heart lesions
^{111}In-antimyosine antibody	Active transport	Heart lesions
^{111}In-autologous leukocytes	Inflammatory response to acute transmural myocardial infarction	
^{67}Ga-citrate	Inflammatory response to acute transmural myocardial infarction	

infarction. Myocytes that have been irreversibly injured undergo changes in their cell membrane which result in an increase in local permeability. These changes appear as holes in the cell membrane on electron microscopic examination. These holes cause a marked increase in cellular permeability to substances which are usually excluded from the cell entirely or only permitted to enter the cell in limited amounts. One of the electron microscopic hallmarks of acute necrosis is the presence of "dense bodies" in the mitochondria. These electron dense structures are precipitates of calcium and phosphate, and are likely related to the intense concentration of ^{99m}Tc labeled pyrophosphate in zones of severe acute myocardial injury. The formation of these dense bodies requires hours to days following coronary occlusion, and may account for the 3-day interval required for maximal myocardial concentration of the ^{99m}Tc PYP in zones of acute myocardial necrosis [171]. Zones of acute myocardial necrosis in animals can be visualized as early as 12 h after occlusion to a maximum of 10 days, a finding also observed in early patient studies. However, when patients with prior myocardial infarction were imaged over intervals of several months, between one-quarter and one-third had some degree of "persistent" PYP localization [172]. While initial studies speculated on "ongoing" myocardial necrosis, present thinking suggests that this may be due to severely damaged tissue, which has completed neither the process of necrosis nor that of healing. Regardless of its cause, the observation of "persistent positive" PYP uptake has been associated with a high risk of an intercurrent cardiac event such as sudden death or recurrent infarction. Other reports indicate that the technique has a low level of sensitivity and specificity. Several cases showed diffuse patterns of radionuclide activity and residual blood pool activity, which may be falsely interpreted as myocardial necrosis [173-181]. For differentiating myocardial uptake from persistent blood pool activity, single photon computed tomography with ^{99m}Tc-PYP showed some clinical advantages. There was improved detection and localization of myocardial infarction.

Several other ^{99m}Tc labeled agents such as ^{99m}Tc MDP and ^{99m}Tc EHDP have been tested and found to localize in zones of acute necrosis. However, comparisons suggest that ^{99m}Tc PYP achieves the highest concentration in myocardial infarction. Other ^{99m}Tc agents, such as glucoheptonate, also localize in zones of acute necrosis [182]. Glucoheptonate is particularly interesting because it has a much earlier interval of localization than ^{99m}Tc PYP - with maximal uptake within 6 h of the onset of necrosis, and virtually no concentration if injected beyond 24 h after coronary occlusion. This difference in time course suggests that this agent localizes by a different mechanism than that of PYP. Despite its earlier localization, the relative concentration of glucoheptonate in the infarct is far less than that of PYP, and the images are more difficult to interpret. For positron tomography the only hot spot agent that has been reported in the literature is $^{18}F^{-}$ [183]. The small number of positron tomography centers limits the use of this agent.

Specific cardiac receptor ligands

The labeling of beta adrenergic ligands for cardiac receptors has been developed. However, due to a high lung uptake for the labeled ligands, the imaging studies did not show their specific accumulation in heart tissue. In the last few years Gibson *et al.* have discussed the use of ligand-receptor interactions as the basis for myocardial imaging and have described the criteria for successful *in vivo* receptor binding studies [184,185]. Some degree of success has been achieved with the labeled muscarinic receptor antagonist quinuclidinyl benzilate; both this compound and quinuclidinyl benzilate methiodide (QMB) showed an accumulation of up to 2% injected dose per gram in the heart of rats, guinea pigs and rabbits, a heart to blood ratio of approximately 30, and a heart to lung ratio of approximately 4. Their accumulation in the heart was blocked 90% by preinjection of atropine.

In the last year a patient injected with ^{123}I-QMB showed myocardial extraction and clear visualization of the left ventricle after intravenous administration. The activity was retained in the myocardium. However, a thorough study of the receptor population, the effect of nonspecific binding and the use of a washout technique should be undertaken in order to make this study worthwhile. An additional study using positron tomography to study the myocardial muscarinic receptors was reported by Maziere *et al.* [186]. The use of specific activity-labeled cardiac receptor ligand may provide information on specific receptor behavior in normal and diseased states of the myocardium.

Another interesting approach is the use of insulin receptors. Insulin-labeled with ^{131}I was tested in rabbits and rats [187,188]. The kinetics of ^{131}I labeled insulin distribution in heart, liver and kidneys and in ordinary bladder did not change by administration of a 10,000 fold excess of unlabeled insulin and 5mM glucose (20%). However, the washout of activity was accelerated in the liver and kidney when preadministration of a nonlabeled hormone took place. This may indicate the involvement of binding in these organs.

Other approaches

Antimyosin

In the early phases of myocardial necrosis, when cell membrane permeability is increased, the soluble substances such as the enzymes SGOT and CPK, or the light chains of cardiac myosin, leak into the blood. Measurement of these substances in the blood are frequently used as markers of the extent of myocardial necrosis. The heavy chain of cardiac myosin, on the other hand, is insoluble and remains *in situ* until digested by leukocytes at the time of liquefaction. Antibodies directed against the heavy chain of cardiac myosin have been suggested as a means of identifying zones of acute myocardial necrosis in

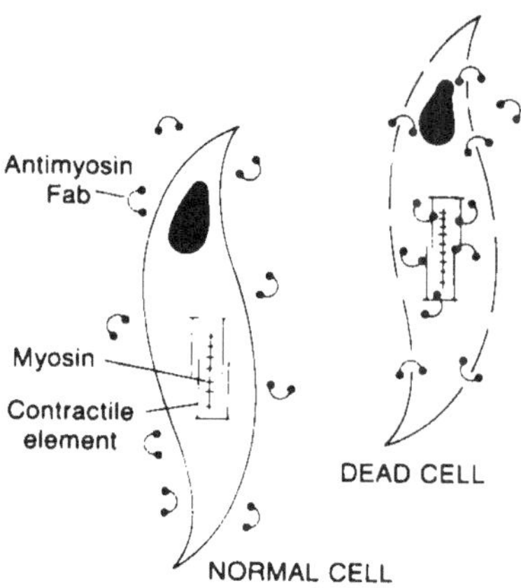

Figure 4. Labeled antimyosin antibodies concentrate exclusively in necrotic cells. They permit therefore precise localization of irreversibly damaged myocardial tissue. (From: Centocor, Malvern, PA., USA)

man. To facilitate diffusion of the antibody into the area of acute injury, the papain digested fragment, antimyosin-Fab (molecular weight approximately 50,000) was employed for studies in both animals and man (Figure 4). The antibodies were coupled to a bifunctional chelate which serves as a bridge to hold the protein on one side, and the radionuclide on the other. The bifunctional chelate approach permits labeling with either ^{99m}Tc or ^{111}Ind [189]. Studies of experimental myocardial infarction determined that the zone of necrosis could be visualized as early as 6 h following acute coronary occlusion with radiolabeled antimyosin Fab. Injection of antimyosin as late as 5 days following experimental coronary occlusion results in a positive scan. Human studies with antimyosin demonstrate a similar time course of uptake [190]. In contrast to ^{99m}Tc PYP which has a rapid blood clearance, antimyosin Fab has a blood clearance half-time of about 3 h. As a result, the earliest practical time to image a zone of necrosis following intravenous injection is 6 h. Small zones of necrosis may not become apparent for 18-24 h after injection, when blood pool concentration has reached a nadir. As a result, it may be desirable to wait until 12-18 h to image patients with the antibody. The requirement for severely damaged cell membrane, with its resultant marked increase in permeability to immunoglobulin, suggests that a "persistent positive" antibody study is unlikely to occur.

Another interesting area of research is the approach using infiltration of ^{111}Ind labeled autologous leukocytes [191]. In this study the kinetic infiltration of indium-111 labeled polymorphonuclear leukocytes occurring in the course of the inflammatory response associated with myocardial infarction was studied by external imaging in dogs subjected to closed chest anterior wall infarction.

In these dogs within 24 to 96 hours after infarction the images showed distinct areas of myocardial infarction, while these images were negative by 120 h.

Wieland *et al.* [192] proposed a radioiodinated norepinephrine storage analog, meta-iodobenzylguanidine (IMB) (a hypertensive drug). This tracer showed high localization in the heart of rats and dogs, rhesus monkey and in normal volunteers. The average myocardial uptake in normal patients was 0.63% of the injected dose at 5 min and raised to 0.76% at 2 h. The data obtained with this agent suggests the possibility of quantitating information on myocardial catecholamine uptake capacity. This agent is mostly used today in studies of the adrenals and some cancer diagnosis procedures.

Technetium-99m low density lipoproteins

Atheromatous lesions are metabolically active and undergo repetitive cycles of endothelial injury and repair. During the phase of repair, the endothelium that recovers the damaged area shows an increased permeability to low density lipoproteins which may result in incorporation of the lipoproteins into the atheromatous lesion. To determine if this could be detected by radionuclide imaging, Roberts et al (193) performed autoradiographic studies in rabbits with catheter-induced injury of the aorta. The autoradiographs demonstrated considerable increase in uptake of radioiodinated lipoproteins at the site of endothelial repair. Subsequent studies by Lees et al (24, 194, 195) showed that these atheromatous lesions can be detected in both he intact animal and man. Studies in eight patients using ^{99m}Tc-labeled low density lipoproteins showed preferred uptake in carotid, femoral, and/or coronary artery lesions. The radiopharmaceutical is prepared by dithionite reduction of TcO4 in the presence of autologous low density lipoprotein. This labeling approach has two disadvantages, 1) the six-hour half-life precludes imaging beyond 24 hours, at times when blood clearance would permit detection of zones with minimal concentration, and 2) the dithionite reduction results in the unavoidable preoduction of colloid-like material with increased concentration of the radiopharmaceutical in the liver. Despite these shortcomings, ^{99m}Tc-labeled low density lipoprotein is a promising agent for the detection of atheromatous lesions in the early phase after the onset of endothelial damage.

Future areas of research

Without doubt positron emission tomography and single photon tomography will play an important role in the improved detection of myocardial abnormalities, especially myocardial ischemia and infarction. New areas of research (for instance the study of cardiomyopathies) that were only peripheral subjects for nuclear cardiology investigations will be explored with metabolic and flow agents. The design of radiopharmaceuticals that will diagnose these functional abnormalities and that will be able to measure changes in physiology and metabolism will be the best candidates for studies. These will contribute most to the detection of myocardial tissue viability and integrity. Although positron emission tomography will be used in a small number of centers, single photon tomography and analogs of metabolites that can mimic the behavior of normal substrates of the heart muscle will be equally important. Fatty acids in combination with a flow agent should provide information about the metabolic status of the heart. These tracers could have an important impact on studies of heart disease in the same manner as amino acids could provide new information on cardiac protein synthesis. Techniques such as a ratio image of metabolism to perfusion should give an indication of the regional and total myocardial behavior. The association or dissociation of metabolism and flow should be indicative of tissue abnormalities or degree of viability. Therefore the availability of radionuclides such as ^{123}I uncontaminated with ^{124}I is very important to the future of nuclear cardiology and nuclear medicine.

Of additional interest is the use of very short half-life radionuclides for first pass studies. The use of eluates from Os-Ir and Hg-Au generators should permit repetitive studies of myocardial function. However the lack of availaability of these generators and of ^{123}I impairs the capability of nuclear medicine. The availability of technetium-99m and its imaging characteristics make this radionuclide the nuclide of choice for nuclear medicine. The development of a Tc-perfusion agent or a Tc-fatty acid agent will take several years. The technetium-labeled agents that distribute in proportion to flow will be an improvement on the diagnostic imaging capabilities of thallium-201. The development of a Tc-fatty acid that will mimic fatty acid metabolism is a remote possibility for the near future. Accordingly the contribution of Jones and Davidson to technetium chemistry is already permitting the design of molecules that are closer to the target compounds.

A widespread use of a metabolic agent could be achieved only with ^{123}I as the closest analog to the metabolic substrate or ligand. Other methods involving ligand receptor interaction or other specific biochemical approaches will require extensive investigations prior to their implementation in the routine clinical situation. Fast and simple labeling techniques as well as good quality control of the tracers injected, are additionally important factors in the application of new tracers as routine clinical procedures. Many of the tracers mentioned are useful but not applicable due to the lack of these requirements.

Acknowledgements

We would like to acknowledge Rebekah S. Taube for the editing of this manuscript and we thank the personnel (Joke van Soest) of the Leiden University Library for helping with the references.

References

1. Berger H J, Zaret B L (1981) N Engl J Med 305: 855 - 865
2. Strauss H W, Pitt B (1978) Circulation 57: 645 - 654
3. Boucher C A, Morganroth J, Pariso A F, Pohost G M, eds (1983) Noninvasive Cardiac Imaging. Chicago: Yearbook Medical Publishers Inc
4. Harbert J, da Rocha C (1984) Nuclear Medicine, 2nd edition. Philadelphia: Lea and Febiger
5. Tweddel A C, Martin W, Simpson I A, McGhie I, McKillop J H, Hutton I (1984) J Am Coll Cardiol 3: 476
6. Dymond D S, Elliott A T, Flatman W, Stone D, Bett R, Cunningham G, Sims H (1983) J Am Coll Cardiol 2: 85 - 92
7. O'Keefe J C, Dymond D S, Caplin J L, Flatman W, Banim S (1984) J Am Coll Cardiol 3: 552
8. Findlay I N, Gillen G, Wilson J, Elliot A T, Dargie H J (1984) J Am Coll Cardiol 3: 524
9. Yano Y, Anger H O (1968) J Nucl Med 9: 2 - 6
10. Cheng C, Treves S, Samuel A, Davis M A (1980) J Nucl Med 21: 1169 - 1176
11. Yano Y (1975) In: Subramanian G, Rhodes B A, Cooper J F, Sodd V J (eds) Radiopharmaceuticals. New York: The Society of Nuclear Medicine Inc, pp 236 - 245
12. Sugrue D D, Kamal S, Deanfield J E, McKenna W J, Myers M J, Watson I A, Oakley C M, Lavender J P (1983) Br J Radiol 56: 657 - 663
13. Nienaber C A, Spielmann R P, Wasmus G, Mathey D G, Montz R, Bleifeld W H (1985) J Am Coll Cardiol 5: 687 - 698
14. Selwyn A P, Steiner R, Kivisaari A, Fox K A A Forse G (1979) Am J Cardiol 43: 547 - 553
15. Selwyn A P, Forse G, Fox K A A Jonathan A, Steiner R (1981) Circulation 64: 83 - 90
16. Kleynhans P H T, Loetter M G, van Aswegen A, Herbst C P, Marx J D, Minnaar P C (1982) Eur J Nucl Med 7: 405 - 409
17. Treves S, Cheng C, Samuel A, Lambrecht R, Babchyck B, Zimmerman R, Norwood W (1980) J Nucl Med 21: 1151 - 1157
18. Treves S, Fogle R, Lang P (1980) Am J Cardiol 46: 1247 - 1255
19. Treves S, Fyler D, Fujii A, Kuruc A (1982) J Pediatr 101: 210 - 213
20. Brihaye C, Knapp FF, Butler T A, Guillaume M (1985) J Nucl Med 26: P27
21. Lacy J L, Verani M S, Packard A, Bolli R, O'Brien G M, Ball M E, Novoa M, Chodosh A, Treves S, Roberts R (1985) J Am Coll Cardiol 5: 388
22. Mena I, Narahara K A, de Jong R, Maublant J (1983) J Nucl Med 24: 139 - 144
23. Callahan R J, McKusick K A, Lamson M, Castronovo F P, Potsaid M S (1975) J Nucl Med 17: 47 - 49
24. Lees R S, Lees A M, Strauss H W, Isaacsohn J, Barlai-Kovach M, Fischman A J, McKusick K A, Garabedian H (1985) J Nucl Med 26: P35
25. Callahan R J, Froelich J W, McKusick K A, Leppo J, Strauss H W (1982) J Nucl Med 23: 315 - 318
26. Callahan R J, Rabito C A, McKusick K A, Strauss H W (1985) Proceedings of the 132 annual meeting of the American Pharmacy Association, San Antonio
27. Dewanjee M K (1974) J Nucl Med 15: 703 - 708
28. Eckelman W C, Smith T D, Richards P (1975) In: Subramanian G, Rhodes B A, Cooper J F, Sodd V J, Radiopharmaceuticals. New York: The Society of Nuclear Medicine Inc, pp 49 - 55
29. Porter W C, Dees S M, Freitas J E, Dworkin H J, (1983) J Nucl Med 24: 383-387
30. Winzelberg G G, Boucher C A, Pohost G M, McKusick K A, Bingham J B, Okada R D, Strauss H W (1981) Chest 79: 520 - 528
31. Maddox D E, Wynne J, Uren R, Parker J A, Idoine J, Siegel L C, Neill J M, Cohn P F, Holman B L (1979) Circulation 59: 1001 - 1009
32. Pitcher D, Wainwright R, Brennand-Roper D, Deverall P, Sowton E, Maisey M (1980) Br Heart J 44: 143 - 149

33. Strauss H W (1974) In: Strauss H W. Pitt B, James A E (eds) Cardiovascular Nuclear Medicine. Saint Louis: CV Mosby Company, pp 128 - 137
34. Friedmann M L, Cantor R E (1979) J Nucl Med 20: 720 - 723
35. Borer J S, Kent K M, Bacharach S L, Green M V, Rosing D R, Seides S F, Epstein S E, Johnston G S (1979) Circulation 60: 572 - 580
36. Bodenheimer M M, Banka V S, Fooshee C M, Hermann G A, Helfant R H (1979) J Nucl Med 20: 724 - 732
37. Jengo J A, Oren V, Conant R, Brizendine M, Nelson T, Uszler M, Mena I (1979) Circulation 59: 60 - 65
38. Brennand-Roper D, Wainwright R J, Maisey N M, Sowton E (1980) Br Heart J 43: 110 - 111
39. Dahlstroem J A (1982) Clin Physiol 2: 205 - 214
40. Goldberg M J, Mantel J, Friedin M, Ruskin R, Rubenfire M (1981) Am J Cardiol 47: 626 - 630
41. DeLand F H (1981) Clin Nucl Med 6(suppl): P131 - P135
42. Pitt B, Strauss H W (1976) Am J Cardiol 37: 797 - 806
43. Ritchie J L (1982) Am J Cardiol 49: 1341 - 1346
44. Berger H J, Zaret B L (1981) N Engl J Med 305: 799 - 807
45. Sapirstein L A, Moses L E (1964) In: Knisely R W (ed) USAEC Division of Technical Information. Washington DC, pp 135 - 152
46. Cannon P J, Dell R B, Dwyer E M (1972) J Clin Invest 57: 964 - 977
47. L'Abbate A, Maseri A (1980) Semin Nucl Med 10: 2 - 15
48. Holman B L, Adams D F, Jewitt D, Eldh P, Idoine J, Cohn P F, Gorlin R, Adelstein S J, (1974) Radiology 112: 99 - 107
49. Jansen C, Grames G, Judkins M P (1974) In: Strauss H W, Pitt B, James A E (eds) Cardiovascular Nuclear Medicine. Saint Louis: CV Mosby Company, pp 211 - 225
50. Weich H F, Strauss H W, Pitt B (1977) Circulation 56: 188 - 191
51. Strauss H W, Harrison K, Langan J K, Lebowitz E, Pitt B (1975) Circulation 51: 641 - 645
52. Pohost G M, Alpert N M, Ingwall J S, Strauss H W (1980) Semin Nucl Med 10: 70 - 93
53. Massie B M, Wisneski J, Kramer B, Hollenberg M, Gertz E, Stern D (1982) J Nucl Med 23: 381 - 385
54. Wilson R A, Okada R D, Strauss H W, Pohost G M (1983) Circulation 68: 203 - 209
55. Bergmann S R, Hack S, Tewson T, Welch M J, Sobel B E (1980) Circulation 61: 34 - 43
56. Phelps M E (1983) Ann Int Med 98: 339 - 359
57. Bergmann S R, Fox K A A, Rand A L, McElvany K D, Ter-Pogossian M M, Sobel B E (1982) Circulation 66: II - 148
58. Mullani N A, Gould K L, Goldstein R A, Gaeta J M, Smalling R W, Ekas R D, Hartz R K (1984) Circulation 70: II - 249
59. Grover M, Schwaiger M, Ramirez B, Schelbert H R (1984) Circulation 70: II - 124
60. Gould K L, Schelbert H R, Phelps M E, Hoffman E J (1979) Am J Cardiol 43: 200 - 208
61. Kearfott K J (1982) J Nucl Med 23: 1128 - 1132
62. Gould K L, Lipscomb K, Hamilton G W (1974) Am J Cardiol 33: 87 - 94
63. Deutsch E, Glavan K A, Sodd V J, Nishiyama H, Ferguson D L, Lukes S J (1981) J Nucl Med 22: 897 - 907
64. Deutsch E, Bushong W, Glavan K A, Elder R C, Sodd V J, Scholz K L, Fortman D L, Lukes S J (1981) Science 214: 85 - 86
65. Nishiyama H, Deutsch E, Adolph R J, Sodd V J, Libson K, Saenger E L, Gerson M C, Gabel M, Lukes S J, Vanderheyden J-L, Fortman D L, Scholz K L, Grossman L W, Williams C C (1982) J Nucl Med 23: 1093 - 1101
66. Sullivan P J, Werre J, Elmaleh D R, Okada R D, Kopiwoda S Y, Castronovo F P, McKusick K A, Strauss H W (1984) Int J Nucl Med Biol 11: 3 - 10
67. Pendleton D B, Delano M L, Sands H (1984) J Nucl Med 25: P15

68. Holman B L, Jones A G, Lister-James J, Davison A, Abrams M J, Kirshenbaum J M, Tumeh S S, English R J (1984) J Nucl Med 25: 1350 - 1355
69. Trobaugh G B, Ritchie J L, Hamilton G W (1978) In: Ritchie J L, Hamilton G W, Wackers F J Th (eds) Thallium-201 Myocardial Imaging. New York: Raven Press, pp 81 - 99
70. Wainwright R J, Maisey N M (1978) Hosp Update 4: 673 - 686
71. Hamilton G W (1979) J Nucl Med 20: 1201 - 1205
72. Diamond G A, Forrester J S (1979) N Engl J Med 300: 1350 - 1358
73. Vogel R A, Kirch D L, LeFree M T, Rainwater J O, Jensen D P, Steele P P (1979) Am J Cardiol 43: 787 - 793
74. McKillop J H, Murray R G, Turner J G, Bessent R H, Lorimer A R, Greig W R (1979) J Nucl Med 20: 715 - 719
75. Dash H, Massie B M, Botvinick E H, Brundage B H (1979) Circulation 60: 276 - 284
76. Detre K M, Wright E, Murphy M L, Takaro T (1975) Circulation 52: 979 - 986
77. DeRouen T A, Murray J A, Owen W (1977) Circulation 55: 324 - 328
78. Ritchie J L, Trobaugh G B, Hamilton G W, Gould K L, Narahara K A, Murray J A, Williams D L (1971) Circulation 56: 66 - 71
79. Wainwright R J, Brennand-Roper D A, Maisey M N, Sowton E (1980) Br Heart J 43: 56 - 66
80. Wackers F J Th, Becker A E, Samson G, Sokole E B, van der Schoot J B, Vet A J T M, Lie K I, Durrer D, Wellens H (1977) Circulation 56: 72 - 78
81. Sokoloff L (1985) In: Reivich M, Alavi A (eds) Positron Emission Tomography. New York: Alan R Liss Inc, pp 1 - 42
82. Raichle M E, Larson K B, Phelps M E, Grubb R L, Welch M J, Ter-Pogossian M M (1975) Am J Physiol 228: 1936 - 1948
83. Raichle M E, Welch M J, Grubb R L, Higgins C S, Ter-Pogossian M M, Larson K B (1978) Science 199: 986 - 987
84. Neely J R, Morgan H E (1974) Annu Rev Physiol 36: 413 - 457
85. Phelps M E, Mazziotta J C, Huang S C (1982) J Cereb Blood Flow Metab 2: 113 - 62
86. Sokoloff L, Smith C B (1983) In: Levin S (ed) Tracer Kinetics and Physiologic Modeling. Berlin: Springer-Verlag, pp 202 - 235
87. Marshall R C, Tillisch J H, Phelps M E, Huang S-C, Carson R, Henze E, Schelbert H R (1983) Circulation 67: 766 - 778
88. Perloff J K, Henze E (1984) Schelbert H R. Circulation 69: 33 - 42
89. Schwaiger M, Schelbert H R, Ellison D, Hansen H, Yeatman L, Vinten-Johansen J, Selin C, Barrio J, Phelps M E (1985) J Am Coll Cardiol 6: 336 - 347
90. Schelbert H R, Henze E, Phelps M E, Kuhl D E (1982) Am Heart J 103: 588 - 597
91. Opie L H (1968) Am Heart J 76: 685 - 698
92. Most A S, Brachfield N, Gorlin R, Wahren J (1969) J Clin Invest 48: 1177 - 1188
93. Miller H I, Yum K Y, Durham B C (1971) Am J Physiol 220: 589 - 596
94. Neely J R, Rovetto M J, Oram J F (1972) Prog Cardiovasc Dis 15: 289 - 329
95. Evans J R, Gunton R W, Baker R G, Beanlands D S, Spears J C (1965) Circ Res 16: 1 - 10
96. Gunton R W, Evans J R, Baker R G, Spears J C, Beanlands D S (1965) Am J Cardiol 16: 482 - 487
97. Poe N D, Robinson G D, Zielinski F W, Cabeen W R, Smith J W, Gomes A S (1977) Radiology 124: 419 - 424
98. Poe N D, Robinson G D, Graham L S, MacDonald N S (1976) J Nucl Med 17: 1077 - 1082
99. Daus H J, Reske S N, Vyska K (1981) In: Schmidt H A E, Wolf F (eds) 18th Annual Meeting European Society of Nuclear Medicine 1980. Stuttgart: Schattauer Verlag, pp 108 - 111
100. Hoeck A, Freundlieb C, Vyska K, Loesse B, Erbel R, Feinendegen L E (1983) J Nucl Med 24: 22 - 28
101. Machulla H-J, Marsmann M, Dutschka K (1980) Eur J Nucl Med 5: 171 - 173
102. Rellas J S, Corbett J R, Kulkarni P, Morgan C, Devous M D, Buja M, Bush L, Parkey R W,

Willerson J T, Lewis S E (1983) Am J Cardiol 52: 1326 - 1332

103. Reske S N, Machulla H-J, Winkler C (1982) J Nucl Med 23: P10
104. Reske S N, Sauer W, Machulla H-J, Winkler C (1984) J Nucl Med 25: 1335 - 1342
105. Reske S N, Sauer W, Machulla H-J, Knust J, Winkler C (1985) Eur J Nucl Med 10: 228 - 234
106. Reske S N, Simon H, Machulla H-J, Biersack H J, Knopp R, Winkler C (1982) J Nucl Med 23: P34
107. Dudczak R, Hoefer R (1983) J Radioanal Chem 79: 329 - 336
108. Dudczak R, Schmoliner R, Kletter K, Frischauf H, Angelberger P (1983) J Nucl Med Allied Sci 27: 267 - 279
109. Dudczak R (1983) Wien Klin Wochenschr 95: 4 - 35
110. van der Wall E E, Westera G, Heidendal G A K, den Hollander W (1981) Eur J Nucl Med 6: 581 - 584
111. van der Wall E E, den Hollander W, Heidendal G A K, Westera G, Majid PA, Roos J P (1981) Eur J Nucl Med 6: 383 - 389
112. van der Wall E E, Heidendal G A K, den Hollander W, Westera G, Roos J P (1983) Postgrad Med J 59(Suppl 3): 38 - 40
113. Feinendegen L E, Vyska K, Freundlieb Chr, Hoeck A, Machulla H J, Kloster G, Stoekling G (1981) Eur J Nucl Med 6: 191 - 200
114. Freundlieb C, Hoeck A, Vyska K, Feinendegen L E, Machulla H-J, Stoecklin G (1980) J Nucl Med 21: 1043 - 1050
115. van der Wall E E (1985) Eur Heart J 6(Suppl B): 29 - 38
116. Dudczak R, Kletter K, Frischauf H, Losert U, Angelberger P, Schmoliner R (1984) Eur J Nucl Med 9: 81 - 85
117. Ercan M, Senekowitsch R, Bauer R, Reidel G, Kriegel H, Pabst H W (1983) Int J Appl Radiat Isot 34: 1519 - 1524
118. Coenen H H, Harmand M-F, Kloster G, Stoecklin G (1981) J Nucl Med 22: 891 - 896
119. Basmadjian G P, Parker G R, Magarian R A, Kirschner AS, Ice RD (1978) J Labelled Compd Radiopharm 16: 33 - 34
120. Basmadjian G P, Mills S L, Parker G R, Kirschner A S, Ice R D, Magarian R A (1978) J Nucl Med 19: 718
121. Knapp F F (1980) In: Spencer R P (ed) Radiopharmaceuticals Structure-Activity Relationships. New York: Grune & Stratton, pp 345 - 391
122. Goodman M M, Knapp F F, Callahan A P, Ferren L A (1982) J Med Chem 25: 613 - 618
123. Knapp F F, Ambrose K R, Callahan A P (1979) Radiopharmaceuticals II. Society of Nuclear Medicine, New York
124. Knapp F F, Ambrose K R, Callahan A P, Ferren L A, Grigsby R A, Irgolic K J (1981) J Nucl Med 22: 988 - 993
125. Knapp F F, Goodman M M, Callahan A P, Ferren L A, Kabalka G W, Sastry K A R (1983) J Med Chem 26: 1293 - 1300
126. Knapp F F, Srivastava P C, Callahan A P, Cunningham E B, Kabalka G W, Sastry K A R (1984) J Med Chem 27: 57 - 63
127. Goodman M M, Knapp F F (1982) J Org Chem 47: 3004 - 3006
128. Goodman M M, Knapp F F, Callahan A P, Ferren L A (1982) J Nucl Med 23: 904 - 908
129. Livni E, Elmaleh D R, Schluederberg J (1982) In: Nuclear Medicine & Biology Advances, Vol 2. New York: Pergamon Press, pp 1684 - 1686
130. Elmaleh D R, Livni E, Levy S, Schluederberg C J, Strauss H W (1982) J Nucl Med 23: P103 - P104
131. Elmaleh D R, Livni E, Okada R, Needham F-L, Schleuderberg J, Strauss H W (1985) Nucl Med Commun 6: 287 - 297
132. Goodman M M, Knapp F F, Elmaleh D R, Strauss H W (1984) J Org Chem 49: 2322 - 2325
133. Livni E, Elmaleh D R, Barlai-Kovach M M, Goodman M M, Knapp F F, Strauss H W (1985) Eur Heart J 6(Suppl B): 85 - 89

134. Yonekura Y, Brill A B, Som P, Yamamoto K, Srivastava S C, Iwai J, Elmalch D R, Livni E, Strauss H W, Goodman M M, Knapp F F (1985) Science 227: 1494 - 1496
135. Yonekura Y, Tamalki N, Torizuka K (1983) J Nucl Med 24: P24
136. Yamamato K, Som P, Brill A B (1984) J Nucl Med 25: P31
137. Knapp F F, Goodman M M, Kirsch G, Callahan A P (1985) J Nucl Med 26: P123
138. Antony G J, Landau B R (1968) J Lipid Res 9: 267 - 269
139. Machulla H-J, Kartje M, Vyska K, Mehdorn H M, Knust E J (1985) J Nucl Med 26: P123
140. Sobel B E (1979) Adv Cardiol 26: 15 - 29
141. Schelbert H R, Henze E, Phelps M E (1980) Semin Nucl Med 10: 355 - 373
142. Schelbert H R, Phelps M E, Hoffman E, Huang S-C, Kuhl D E (1980) Am J Cardiol 46: 1269 - 1277
143. Sobel B E, Ter-Pogossian M M, Geltman E M (1981) Hosp Pract 16: 93 - 97, 101 - 1903
144. Sobel B E (1982) Am Heart J 103: 673 - 681
145. Sobel B E, Bergman S R (1982) Int J Cardiol 2: 273 - 277
146. Geltman E M, Sobel B E (1983) Chest 83: 553 - 557
147. Phelps M E, Hoffman E J, Selin C, Huang S C, Robinson G, MacDonald N, Schelbert H, Kuhl D E (1978) J Nucl Med 19: 1311 - 1319
148. Schoen H R, Schelbert H R, Phelps M E (1983) Nuklearmedizin 22: 171 - 180
149. Budinger T F, Yano Y, Huesman R H, Derenzo S E, Moyer B R, Mathis C A, Ganz E, Knittel B (1983) Physiologist 26: 31 - 34
150. Rose C P, Goresky C A, Bach G G (1977) Circ Res 41: 515 - 533
151. Weiss E S, Hoffman E J, Phelps M E, Welch M J, Henry P D, Ter-Pogossian M M, Sobel B E (1976) Circ Res 39: 24 - 32
152. Weiss E S, Siegel B A, Sobel B E, Welch M J, Ter-Pogossian M M (1977) Prog Cardiovasc Dis 20: 191 - 206
153. Klein M S, Sobel B E (1979) In: Brest A N (ed) Cardiovascular Clinics. Philadelphia: Fa Davis Company,
154. Klein M S, Goldstein R A, Welch M J, Sobel B E (1979) Am J Physiol 237: H51 - H58
155. Hoffman E J, Phelps M E, Weiss E S, Welch M J, Coleman R E, Sobel B E, Ter-Pogossian M M (1977) J Nucl Med 18: 57 - 61
156. Ter-Pogossian M M, Klein M S, Markham J, Roberts R, Sobel B E (1980) Circulation 61: 242 - 255
157. Goldstein R A, Klein M S, Welch M J, Sobel B E (1980) J Nucl Med 21: 342 - 348
158. Weiss E S, Ahmed S A, Welch M J, Williamson J R, Ter-Pogossian M M, Sobel B E (1977) Circulation 55: 66 - 73
159. Geltman E M, Smith J L, Beecher D, Ludbrook P A, Ter-Pogossian M M, Sobel B E (1983) Am J Med 74: 773 - 785
160. Schoen H R, Schelbert H R, Robinson G, Najafi A, Huang S-C, Hansen H, Barrio J, Kuhl D E, Phelps M E (1982) Am Heart J 103: 532 - 547
161. Schoen H R, Schelbert H R, Najafi A, Hansen H, Huang H, Barrio J, Phelps M E (1982) Am Heart J 103: 548 - 561
162. Sobel B E, Geltman E M, Tiefenbrunn A J, Jaffe A S, Spadaro J J, Ter-Pogossian M M, Collen D, Ludbrook P A (1984) Circulation 69: 983 - 990
163. Livni E, Elmaleh D R, Levy S, Brownell G L, Strauss W H (1982) J Nucl Med 23: 169 - 175
164. Elmaleh D R, Livni E (1984) The 5th International Symposium on Radiopharmacology and Chemistry, Tokyo, pp 220 - 221
165. de Landsheere C, Wilson R, Shea M, Pike V, Elmaleh D, Levni E, Jones T, Maseri A, Selwyn A (1983) Circulation 68: III - 139
166. Henze E, Egbert J E, Barrio J R, Phelps M E, MacDonald N S, Schelbert H R (1982) J Nucl Med 23: P79
167. Knapp W H, Helus F, Ostertag H, Tillmanns H, Kuebler W (1982) Eur J Nucl Med 7: 211 -215

168. Myers W G, Bigler R E, Benua R S, Graham M C, Laughlin J S (1983) Eur J Nucl Med 8: 381 - 384
169. Pike V W, Eakins M N, Allan R M, Selwyn A P (1982) Int J Appl Radiat Isot 33: 505 - 512
170. Goldstein R A, Klein M S, Sobel B E (1980) J Nucl Med 21: 1101 - 1104
171. Buja L M, Parkey R W, Dees J H, Stokely E M, Harris R A, Bonte F J, Willerson J T (1975) Circulation 52: 596 - 607
172. Croft C H, Rude R E, Lewis S E, Parkey R W, Poole W K, Parker C, Fox N, Roberts R, Strauss H W, Thomas L J, Raabe D S, Sobel B E, Gold H K, Stone P H, Braunwald E, Willerson J T (1984) Am J Cardiol 53: 421 - 428
173. Willerson J T, Parkey R W, Bonte F J, Lewis S E, Corbett J, Buja M (1980) Semin Nucl Med 10: 54 - 69
174. Holman B L, Wynne J (1980) Radiol Clin North Am 18: 487 - 499
175. Pitt B, Thrall J H (1980) Am J Cardiol 46: 1215 - 1223
176. Mills S L, Basmadjian G P, Ice R D (1981) J Pharm Sci 70: 1 - 12
177. Bianco J A (1981) J Nucl Med 22: 739 - 742
178. Schelbert H R, Henze E, Wisenberg G (1981) CRC Crit Rev Diagn Imaging 16: 239 - 278
179. Williams B R (1981) Primary Care 8: 399 - 413
180. Willerson J T (1983) Cardiovasc Clin 13: 33 - 50
181. Wynne J, Holman B L (1980) Med Clin North Am 64: 119 - 144
182. Rossman D J, Strauss H W, Siegel M E, Pitt B (1975) J Nucl Med 16: 875 - 878
183. Cochavi S, Pohost G M, Elmaleh D R, Strauss H W (1979) J Nucl Med 20: 1013 - 1015
184. Gibson R E, Eckelman W C, Vieras F, Reba R C (1979) J Nucl Med 20: 865 - 870
185. Gibson R E, Weckstein D J, Jagoda E M, Rzeszotarski W J, Reba R C, Eckelman W C (1984) J Nucl Med 25: 214 - 222
186. Mazière M, Comar D, Godot J M, Collard Ph, Cepeda C, Naquet R (1981) Life Sci 29: 2391 - 2397
187. Sodoyez J C, Sodoyez-Goffaux F, Treves S, Kahn C R, von Frenkel R (1984) Diabetologia 26: 229 - 233
188. Bourgeois P, Fruehling J, Langohr M, Coel J, Verbist A, Ghanem G, Legros F (1983) J Endocrinol 98: 331 - 342
189. Khaw B A, Mattis J A, Melincoff G, Strauss H W, Gold H K, Haber E (1984) Hybridoma 3: 11 - 23
190. Katus H A, Yasuda T, Gold H K, Leinbach R C, Strauss H W, Waksmonski C, Haber E, Khaw B A (1984) Am J Cardiol 54: 964 - 970
191. Thakur M L, Gottschalk A, Zaret B L (1979) Circulation 60: 297 - 305
192. Wieland D M, Brownel L E, Rogers W L, Worthington K C, Wu J-L, Clinthorne N H, Otto C A, Swanson D P, Beierwaltes W H (1981) J Nucl Med 22: 22 - 31
193. Roberts A B, Lees A M, Lees A S *et al.* (1983) J Lipid Res 24: 1160-1167
194. Lees R S, Parkey R W, Graham K D *et al.* (1974) Radiology 110: 473-474
195. Lees R S, Lees A M, Strauss H W *et al.*(1985) J Nucl Med 26: 1056-1062

2. Myocardial imaging with radiolabeled free fatty acids: current views

E.E. van der WALL

Introduction

The regional, noninvasive assessment of myocardial functional integrity with the aim of identifying normal, ischemic and necrotic zones is highly desirable in patients with coronary artery disease (CAD). Therefore attempts have been made to determine the metabolic integrity of the myocardium quantitatively with radioactively labeled metabolic substrates. Since free fatty acids (FFA) are primary substrates of the normally perfused myocardium, it appears likely that radiolabeled FFA are suitable for the study of myocardial FFA metabolism.

Generally the following requirements for metabolic isotope tracers have to be met:

(a) they should be highly specific indicators of a given metabolic pathway;
(b) they must not alter the physiological behavior of metabolic substrates;
(c) they have to provide an adequate external detection by current imaging devices (gamma or positron camera);
(d) they must be clinically applicable.

These conditions are best fulfilled by radionuclides with chemical identities akin to physiological substrates such as carbon (C), nitrogen (N) and oxygen (O).

C-11, N-13, and O-15 are the isotopes of the constituents of most living matter and of most molecules involved in the majority of metabolic processes. Moreover they are positron-emitting radionuclides (Table 1) and the combined use with positron emission tomography (PET) offers potential advantages for the assessment of myocardial integrity. An added advantage of these radionuclides is their short half-lives, allowing repeated measurements at short intervals which can be of much importance in intervention procedures.

In spite of the advantages of C-11, N-13 and O-15, their use in the assessment of myocardial integrity has been documented only in a limited number of studies. This is due to several factors. Because of the short half-lives the production of these nuclides requires the availability of a cyclotron (or other

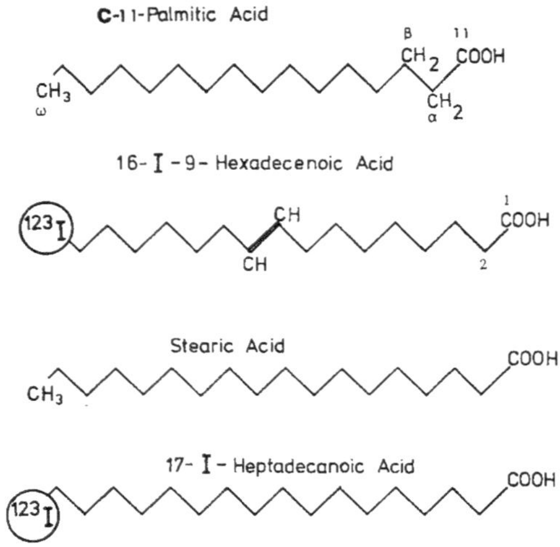

C-11-Palmitic Acid

16-I-9-Hexadecenoic Acid

Stearic Acid

17-I-Heptadecanoic Acid

Figure 1. General structure of C-11-palmitate, stearic acid and the most currently used iodinated free fatty acids.

particle accelerator) in the laboratory where they are to be used. Furthermore, the rapid incorporation of these nuclides into useful molecules is difficult, and the tomographic devices (special positron cameras) necessary for the imaging of these nuclides are complex and expensive. In the recent past, however, the usefulness of this approach has become generally accepted, and the scientific literature contains an increasing number of reports of the use of PET and physiological indicators in the study of the myocardium. Regarding FFA, it would be very convenient to use the isotopes of the natural elements of FFA, which are C, O and hydrogen (H), but only C-11 has proven to be adequate as a label to FFA.

Besides metabolic studies with PET, attention has been focused on gamma-emitting radionuclides labeled to FFA, because of potentially wider applicability and lower cost. Moreover, since most suitable gamma-emitting radionuclides have physical half-lives of more than several hours, no in-house cyclotron is required. For instance, iodine-123 (I-123, half-life 13.3 hours) may

Table 1. Positron- and gamma-emitting radionuclides potentially used for evaluation of cardiac metabolism

Radionuclide	Emission	Half-life	Production
0-15	positron (511 keV)	2.03 min	requires in-house cyclotron
N-13	positron (511 keV)	9.98 min	requires in-house cyclotron
C-11	positron (511 keV)	20.4 min	requires in-house cyclotron
I-123	gamma (159 keV)	13.3 h	cyclotron-produced
I-131	gamma (364 keV)	8.06 days	reactor-produced
Te-123m	gamma (159 keV)	120 days	cyclotron produced

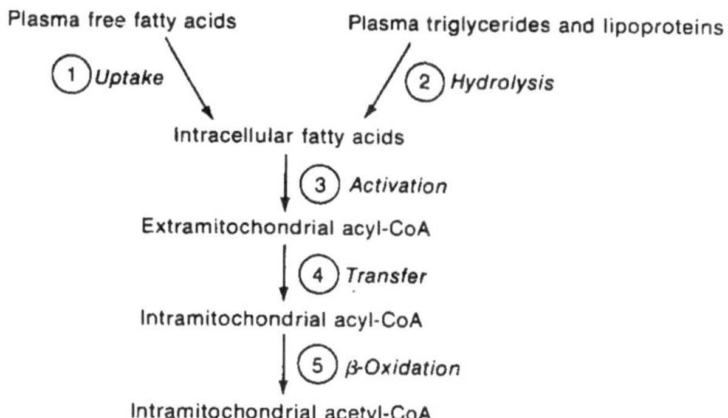

Figure 2. Overall scheme of fatty acid metabolism (From Katz A M, (1977) Physiology of the Heart, New York, Raven Press).

be very well tagged to FFA and can easily be detected with any commercially available gamma-camera.

Although many different labeled fatty acids have been studied, this review will mainly call attention to the most important investigations in this field, i.e. the study of FFA labeled with the physiological tracer C-11 and with I-123 (Figure 1).

We will firstly describe the myocardial FFA metabolism, then consider the metabolism and kinetics of radiolabeled FFA and finally discuss the potential clinical value of radiolabeled FFA.

Myocardial fatty acid metabolism

FFA are preferred myocardial substrates and fatty acid oxidation normally accounts for 60 to 80% of energy production by the heart. Even when moderate ischemia supervenes, FFA liberated from triglycerides are metabolized in preference to glucose. However, under conditions of marked ischemia or severe hypoxia (oxygen delivery less than 20% of normal), anaerobic metabolism provides a substantial proportion of energy via glycolytic mechanisms.

The metabolic pathway of fatty acid has been well clarified (Figure 2). Long-chain fatty acids are synthesized in the liver and adipose tissue, transported in blood bound primarily to albumin, and extracted by myocardium as a function of several factors including: chain length, molarity of both albumin and fatty acid, metabolic integrity of the cell, perfusion (since regional coronary flow determines residence time), and myocardial energy requirements. Both ischemia and hypoxia lead to decreased extraction.

Fatty acids in interstitial or intracellular fluid are bound to soluble proteins, and uptake of fatty acids into the cell appears to depend on competition between cellular binding sites and binding sites on albumin. Intracellular fatty

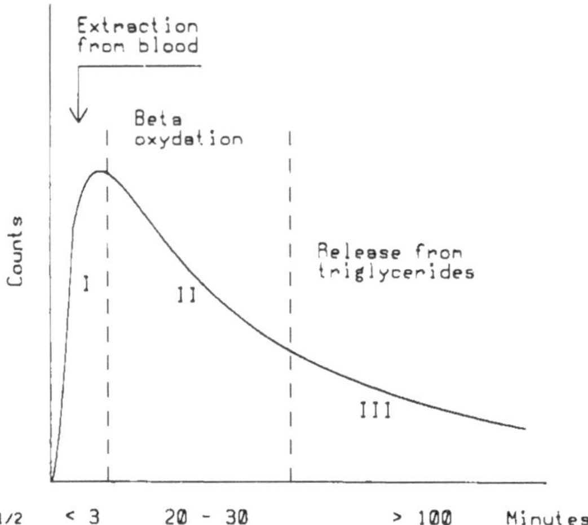

Figure 3. Schematic illustration of the characteristic time-activity curve of clinically used radiolabeled FFA in the myocardium. Three different phases are recognized.

acids are activated and converted to thioester derivatives in the cytosol in reactions requiring both coenzyme A (CoA) and ATP. Esterified fatty acids may undergo oxidation or incorporation into triglycerides.

Activated fatty acids in the cytosol cannot be oxidized directly. They are first transported across the mitochondrial membrane by acyl CoA carnitine transferases specific for chain length and intimately associated with mitochondrial membranes. Carnitine-dependent translocation facilitates ingress of acyl CoA into the mitochondrial matrix where beta-oxidation occurs. Acyl CoA is oxidized to produce acetyl CoA which is oxidized via the Krebs cycle with liberation of CO_2 and synthesis of intracellular ATP. The knowledge of altered fatty acid metabolism in myocardial ischemia stimulated labeling procedures with FFA for the detection of CAD.

Metabolism and pharmacokinetic behaviour of labeled FFA

The first efforts with radiolabeled FFA were mainly pointed at the search for myocardial imaging agents. It was only recently that the noninvasive study of regional metabolic turnover rates in the myocardium has become a potential issue. For quantification of metabolic rates, the pharmacokinetics of these tracers in the myocardium in terms of uptake and clearance and their relationship to the biochemical process must be known.

Previous experimental studies [1,2] have revealed a similar type of pharmacokinetics in the heart both for C-11-palmitic acid and for iodinated fatty acids (Figure 3). The kinetics exhibit a fast uptake which represents the extraction from blood (phase I). This first phase simply reflects perfusion as has been demonstrated by studies [3] comparing N-13-H3 and C-11-palmitic acid. Then, two elimination phases follow, a fast and a slow one. The fast elimination phase (phase II) is considered to represent beta-oxidation and is clinically the most relevant phase. The third phase can be attributed to release of fatty acids which has been stored before as triglycerides and phospholipids. Turnover rates of the labeled FFA can be expressed in terms of half-time values (minutes) calculated from the best-fit mono- or biexponential function of the different phases of the time-activity curve. For I-123 terminally labeled to heptadecanoic acid, the fast elimination phase has a half-time of about 25 min in man. Regarding C-11-palmitate, about similar half-time values have been clinically demonstrated [4]. The slow elimination (phase III) can hardly be seen in man and imaging is generally stopped 30 to 60 min after injection because the activity levels become too low for appropriate measurements.

The resemblance of the clearance curves of I-123-FFA and of C-11-palmitate suggests that clearance of I-123 reflects natural metabolism of FFA. Small differences in clearance pattern may still be expected since the C-11 label is removed from the fatty acid in the first step of beta-oxidation with subsequent degrading in the Krebs cycle and exhalation as C-11-02, while the radioiodine label at the terminal carbon atom is probably removed in the last step of beta-oxidation and released into the circulation before or in the Krebs cycle.

Accordingly, the kinetics of I-123-FFA may parallel metabolism of FFA in uptake of FFA and beta-oxidation pathway. Therefore, clearance of I-123-FFA has been regarded to reflect metabolic turnover of FFA in the myocardium. This view is partly supported by Dudczak *et al.* [5] and Comet *et al.* [6], who experimentally demonstrated that halothane anesthesia and cardiac drugs, such as verapamil and propanolol, considerably influenced the clearance rates. In contrast, doxorubicin did not change the elimination rates of I-123-HDA, obtained from dog hearts. As a result, considerable debate has nowadays arisen about the proper explanation for the elimination half-time in the second phase. It has been postulated that the measured half-times of iodinated FFA do not correlate with beta-oxidation but are due to the rate of diffusion of free iodide from the mitochondria into the coronary circulation [8]. Such non-specific deiodination would limit the use of iodinated FFA to evaluate oxidative FFA metabolism based on analysis of myocardial clearance curves. (See also chapters 5 and 6 on this particular subject).

On the other hand, with respect to C-11-palmitate, it remains to be proven that clearance of tracer is really due to oxidative metabolism with resultant formation of C-11-02 and not to washout of oxidation products, such as short-chain intermediates via the coronary circulation [9]. In experiments with C-14 palmitate in rabbit hearts [23] it was observed that at 5 min almost 40% of extracted myocardial activity was already in the aqueous phase, indicating the early presence of products of palmitate catabolism. These factors become of crucial importance during reduced oxidative metabolism induced either by the decreased coronary flow (ischemia) or diminished oxygen delivery (hypoxia).

Lerch *et al.* [10] demonstrated that clearance of C-11-palmitate was constantly depressed in regions with restricted oxygen supply regardless of concomitant reduction of flow, and they concluded that metabolism itself is the major determinant of reduced regional clearance. Schelbert *et al.* [11] suggested that results would be distorted because of altered residence time (i.e. duration of myocardial exposure to labeled substrates) or that altered washout would mask detection of impaired metabolism caused by ischemia or hypoxia. Later studies by his group indicated that measuring FFA oxidation rates is still possible in ischemia but probably with a lower accuracy than in normal myocardium [12].

The exact mechanism can only be clarified by experimentally studying the content of free I-123 or free C-11-02 per unit myocardial weight or from coronary venous blood when measured acutely after injection and under different pathophysiological circumstances.

Recent results obtained from canine studies by our group [13] and Kloster *et al.* [14], in which a rather high percentage of free iodide (40-60%) was found a few minutes after injection of I-123-heptadecanoic acid (I-123-HDA), suggest that the diffusion of iodide from the cell to the circulation is an important step in the description of myocardial clearance rates (See chapter 7).

Fox *et al.* (66) reported that under normal conditions about 45% of C-11-palmitate has metabolized while 6% showed back-diffusion in unaltered form. In contrast, with ischemia 17% was metabolized to C-11-O_2, while 16% (i.e. half of the amount cleared) evolved as C-11-palmitate. It was concluded that effects of nonmetabolized FFA must be taken into account when analyzing clearance curves (See chapter 10).

Further studies are therefore needed to unravel the intimate relationship between uptake and clearance of labeled FFA, and to prove whether they really represent oxidative myocardial FFA metabolism.

Experimental and clinical results

C-11-palmitate

C-11 provides a particularly suitable label for FFA imaging because of its property as a positron emitting radionuclide. C-11 labeled to palmitate was first used for the visualization of the myocardium by PET in 1976 [12]. C-11-palmitate was found to accumulate substantially in isolated perfused hearts under aerobic conditions, and since reduction of coronary flow is accompanied by decreased FFA extraction, C-11-palmitate was utilized to image normal, transiently ischemic, and irreversibly injured myocardium in intact dogs.

In later studies, Weiss *et al.* [16] determined the distribution of the tracer in the dog heart by positron emission transaxial tomography (PETT) and demonstrated that significant reversal of depressed C-11-palmitate accumulation in

Normal

Ischemia

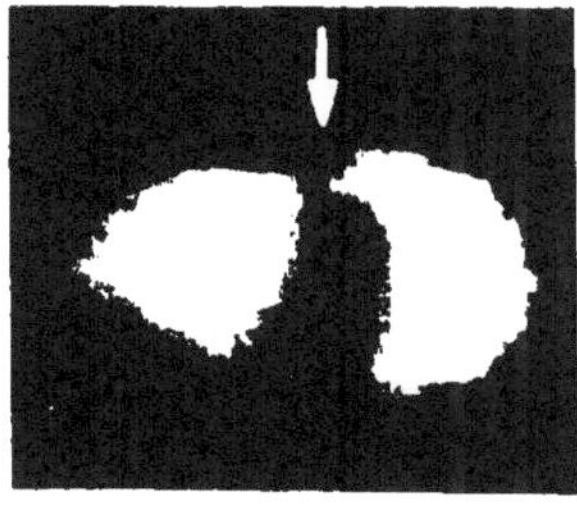

Reperfusion

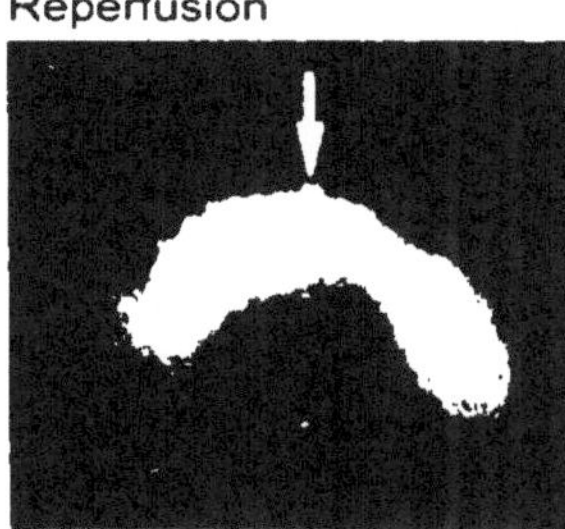

Figure 4. Positron-emission transaxial tomography after induction of transient myocardial ischemia by constriction of an exteriorized coronary artery occlusive cuff in an intact dog. Each image represents a reconstructed cross-sectional slice through the heart at the ventricular level. Anterior, posterior, left and right are indicated by the letters A, P, L, and R, respectively. In the top panel homogeneous accumulation of C-11-palmitate acid is evident in the normal left ventricular myocardium. The tomogram was obtained during a 20-min interval after intravenous injection of tracer. In the center panel, a transmural defect representing failure of accumulation (arrow) of C-11-palmitate is present anteriorly in an image obtained after 30 min of myocardial ischemia. The image shown in the lower panel was obtained during the 20-min interval immediately following release of the coronary artery occlusive cuff after an interval of ischemia of 30 min, hence insufficient to produce extensive infarction. As can be seen, after reperfusion, myocardial metabolic integrity is demonstrable in the area of the previous defect (arrow) and, in fact, the accumulation of tracer in this region exceeds that adjacent and presumably normal myocardium. (From E S Weiss *et al.*, Circ Res 39: 24 - 32, 1976. By permission of the American Heart Association Inc.)

the ischemic zone occurred when coronary artery occlusion was maintained for less than 20 min, but that an irreversibly reduced uptake pattern was observed when reperfusion was delayed for 60 min or more (Figure 4). In a clinical study, Sobel *et al.* [17] demonstrated with PETT that the distribution of C-11-palmitate in patients with remote myocardial infarction was analogous to the distribution observed in animals with experimentally-induced infarction. Subsequent studies in man have shown that infarct size determined by PET correlated with infarct size assessed by creatine kinase (MB) blood curves [18]. Geltman *et al.* [19] showed in 46 patients that both transmural and nontransmural infarctions could be detected with PET. All 22 patients with transmural infarctions had decreased C-11-palmitate uptake in the infarcted regions while in 23 out of 24 patients with nontransmural infarctions the area of diminished C-11-palmitate uptake was often nontransmural and a thin area of normal C-11 uptake was present. Moreover, a heterogeneous uptake pattern was observed in the adjacent myocardium, suggesting an admixture of normal cells in the surrounding area.

Regarding kinetics of C-11-palmitate Schoen *et al.* [20] showed that labeled palmitate cleared from the myocardium in a biexponential fashion, indicating tracer distribution between at least two pools with different turnover rates. This clearance pattern reflects the distribution of FFA between immediate oxidation (the rapid turnover phase) and the intermediate storage in the endogeneous lipid pool (the slow turnover phase).

Al these studies indicate a promising and practical application for C-11-palmitate, especially since the evaluation of the effectiveness of therapeutic intervention for the protection of ischemic myocardium requires the quantitative assessment of the distribution and extent of jeopardized and irreversibly injured myocardium. Bergmann *et al.* [22] experimentally demonstrated in 1982 (by measuring uptake of C-11-palmitate) that successful streptokinase treatment, when initiated within 4 h after occlusion, showed preservation of cardiac metabolism while later treatment did not result in significant salutary metabolic effects. Also Ludbrook *et al.* [22] studied 17 patients with C-11-palmitate after therapy with intracoronary streptokinase and demonstrated in the 8 patients with successful thrombolysis increased uptake of C-11-palmitate in the affected areas indicating improvement of regional metabolism and salvage of jeopardized myocardial tissue. Recently reported studies [4, 9, 10, 20, 23] by the groups of Schelbert *et al.* and Sobel *et al.* have delineated the myocardial kinetics under normal and ischemic conditions, and the rate of clearance of C-11 activity from the myocardium was considered as an index of the oxidation rate of C-11-palmitate. It was shown in dogs and also in patients with exercise-induced ischemia that clearance of C-11-palmitate from ischemic regions was decreased compared to normal regions. Henze *et al.* [4] demonstrated in patients with pacemaker-induced ischemia that clearance from the ischemic regions was substantially decreased compared to normal myocardial regions. On the other hand, increases in cardiac work and myocardial oxygen consump-

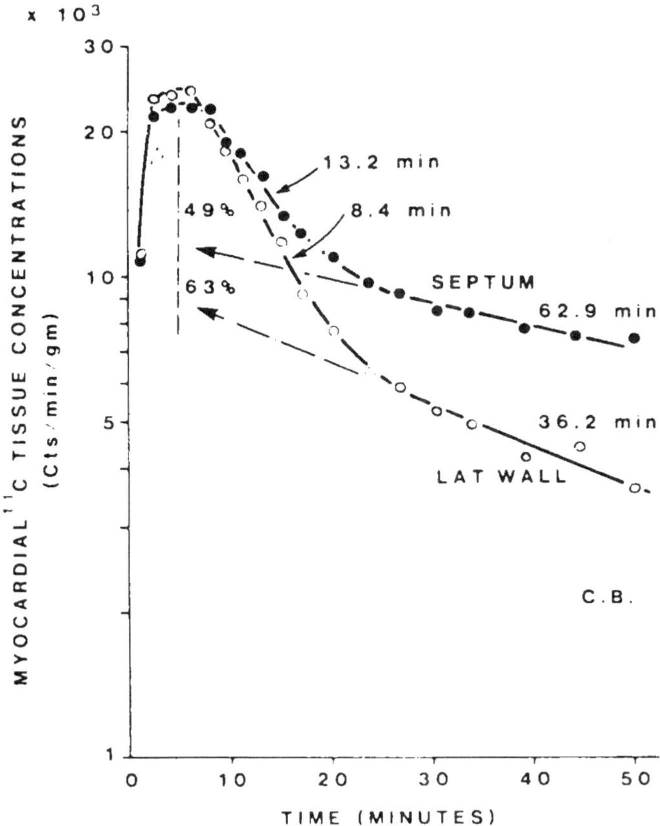

Figure 5. Time-activity curves obtained during pacing-induced ischemia, derived from a region of interest over the nonischemic septum and the ischemic lateral wall. C-11 activity increases in both normal (open circles) and ischemic (closed circles) myocardium. Subsequent clearance of C-11 activity from ischemic and normal myocardium is biexponential. By back-extrapolation of the slow clearance phase, the relative sizes of the early rapid components can be estimated. In ischemic compared with normal myocardium, the relative size of the early curve component is smaller (49% vs 63%), and the half-time of the early clearance phase is slower (8.4 min vs 13.2 min). (From M Grover and H R Schelbert, Positron emission computed tomography. In: Digital Cardiac Imaging, Eds. A J Buda and E J Delp, 1985, Martinus Nijhoff Publishers, with permission)

tion raise the fraction of tracer entering the rapid turnover pool and accelerate the clearance rate of C-11 activity from myocardial tissue, which reflects enhanced FFA oxidation as a response to higher energy demands (Figure 5).

Table 2 shows the clearance rates of the most currently used labeled FFA expressed in minutes half-time. Chapter 10 gives an extensive evaluation of recent studies with C-11-palmitate.

Radioiodinated FFA

One of the earliest attempts at cardiac imaging was performed with FFA labeled with iodine (I-131, half-life 8.06 days). In 1965, Evans *et al.* [24] iodinated oleic acid across the double bond and demonstrated that this could be used to visualize the myocardium and to detect myocardial infarction. This substance never became clinically useful because of its low specific activity, poor imaging quality and limitations in administered activity, dictated by radiation dosimetry. Moreover, iodination of FFA at the double bond strongly influenced extraction and elimination of the labeled compound.

In 1975, Robinson *et al.* [25] made considerable progress by introducing radioiodine into the terminal (omega) position of a fatty acid (hexadecenoic acid) without altering its extraction efficiency compared to the naturally occurring compound. Poe *et al.* [26] postulated that the iodine atom in the terminal position maintains a configuration similar to a methyl group (both with an

Table 2. Metabolic clearance rates of various labeled FFA from normal and ischemic myocardial regions (in minutes).

FFA	Species	Clearance rates (Phase II) in minutes half-time		Reference number
		normal	ischemia (I)[f]	
C-11-palmitate	dog	8.8 ± 3.5	14.9 ± 7.0	[62]
	dog	11.6	> 12[g]	[9]
	man	22.6 ± 5.6	> 23[g]	[4]
I-131-HA[a]	dog	20.0 ± 2.3	[h]	[2]
	dog	14.2 ± 1.4	22.6 ± 1.8	[36]
I-123-HA[b]	dog	14.0 ± 6.7	[h]	[6]
	man	25	> 48[g]	[29]
	man	[h]	(18.5 ± 2.5, AMI)[e]	[33]
I-123-HDA[c]	man	25.0 ± 5.0	31.8 ± 19.6[i]	[30]
	man	24	46	[34]
	man	20-30	35-50	[63]
	man	27.5 ± 3.0	46 ± 7.1 (16.8 ± 3.5, AMI)[e]	[33,35]
I-123-PPA[d]	dog	42	202, AMI[e]	[50]
	man	50-60	80-150	[53]
	man	46	61	[48]
	man	> 60[g]	[h]	[51]

[a] I-131-hexadecenoic acid.
[b] I-123-hexadecenoic acid.
[c] I-123-heptadecanoic acid.
[d] I-123-phenyl-pentadecanoic acid.
[e] Acute myocardial infarction.
[f] Transient ischemia, unless otherwise noted.
[g] No exact values mentioned.
[h] Not studied.
[i] Obtained from the entire myocardium.

atomic radius of 2 Angstrom) and that the resultant molecule behaves as though it possesses an extra carbon atom. In this context 16-iodo-hexadecenoic acid would behave like heptadecanoic acid. Furthermore, it was shown that a chain length of 15 to 21 carbon atoms had the most optimal myocardial extraction [27], indicating that for metabolic studies a chain length of 16 or 17 carbon atoms appears to be very suitable (See also chapter 3).

Terminally labeled hexadecenoic acid demonstrated an initial myocardial distribution proportional to blood flow and, when labeled with I-123, its myocardial extraction of 78% and blood clearance half-time of 1.7 min closely resembled K-43 and Tl-201 distribution [2,28] (See also chapter 4). From these studies it was inferred that I-123-FFA are distributed according to myocardial blood flow and subsequently metabolized by known metabolic pathways. Compared to I-123, Tl-201 has a low photon-energy of 80 keV resulting in important tissue absorption, and moreover a rather long physical (72 h) and myocardial half-life (7 h) which gives a total body exposure of 210 mrads/mCi and precludes rapid sequential imaging. I-123 is a gamma-emitter with suitable photon-energy (159 keV) for the currently available gamma-cameras, it has a favourable physical half-life of 13.3 h and offers a relatively low whole body radiation dose to the patient (30 mrads/mCi). Table 3 shows the most important radiophysical proporties of Tl-201 and I-123-FFA.

In 1977, Poe *et al.* [29] injected 5 mCi I-123-HA intravenously in patients with CAD and images containing about one million net counts from the total myocardium could be obtained within 10 min. In 1978, Machulla *et al.* [1] experimentally used various radiolabeled FFA and showed that terminally labeled I-123-HDA had a myocardial uptake and elimination almost the same as that of C-11-palmitate. This study has been clinically extended in 1980 by the group of Feinendegen *et al.* [30] and demonstrated reduced tracer uptake in ischemic myocardial zones using I-123-HDA. Not only high quality images were obtained, but also elimination of I-123 from the myocardium could be followed by calculating clearance half-times of I-123-HDA from distinct myocardial regions. All these investigative studies emphasized the potential value of I-123-FFA (hexadecenoic and heptadecanoic acid) for myocardial scintigraphy not only for myocardial imaging purposes, but also to evaluate myocardial metabolism in patients with CAD.

So far, clinical studies have been hampered by restricted commercial supply

Table 3. Radiophysical properties of Tl-201 and of I-123-FFA

	Tl-201	I-123-FFA
Gamma camera detection efficiency (keV)	80	159
Myocardial extraction (%)	87	78
Physical half-life (hours)	72	13
Biological half-life (hours)	7	0.5
Body exposure (mrads/mCi)	210	30

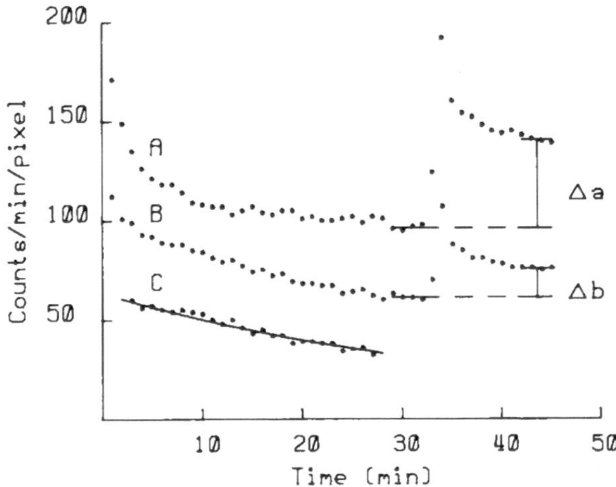

Regions of interest (ROI) are made over lung tissue and a distinct part of the myocardium, resulting in curve A, resp. B. After administration of 123-I-iodide, 30 min after injection of 123-I-FFA, in both regions an increase is found proportional to the amount of circulating blood in the ROI (Δa, resp. Δb).

Consequently the count-rate (CR) in lung tissue is proportional to the concentration of circulating in the blood i.e. CR (I-total, A) = CR (I^-, A). Furthermore the CR in the myocardium will be proportional to the amount of circulating blood iodide plus the amount of "bound" fatty acid, CR (I-FFA, B). Therefore the following equation is valid:

$$\mathrm{CR\ (I\text{-}FFA,\ B} = \mathrm{CR\ (I\text{-}total,\ B)} - \frac{\Delta b}{\Delta a} \cdot \mathrm{CR\ (I\text{-}total,\ A)}.$$

If CR (I-FFA, B) is plotted versus time, the blood background corrected curve is found, which represents the net turnover of 123-I-FFA in the myocardium. So for every point (t)* in the corrected curve C holds:

$$C(t) = B(t) - \frac{\Delta b}{\Delta a} \,.\, A(t).$$

* every fifth point plotted

Figure 6. Schematic illustration of the correction method.

and the technical problem of a rapidly increasing background radioactivity due to release of free radioiodide into circulation after administration of I-123-FFA. It has been shown that within 15 min after intravenous administration of I-123-HDA, about 50% of the radioactivity in the blood consists of free iodide, which implies that only within this time-limit (preferably within 10 min after administration) good analogue images can be obtained [31]. Roesler *et al.* [32] studied patients with CAD, using a 7-pinhole collimator and compared the imaging quality of I-123-HDA with that of Tl-201. Similar images were observed and I-123-HDA proved to have no advantages over Tl-201 with respect to imaging quality.

The background problem has been met by a specially designed computer-aided correction procedure, thoroughly described by Van der Wall *et al.* [33].

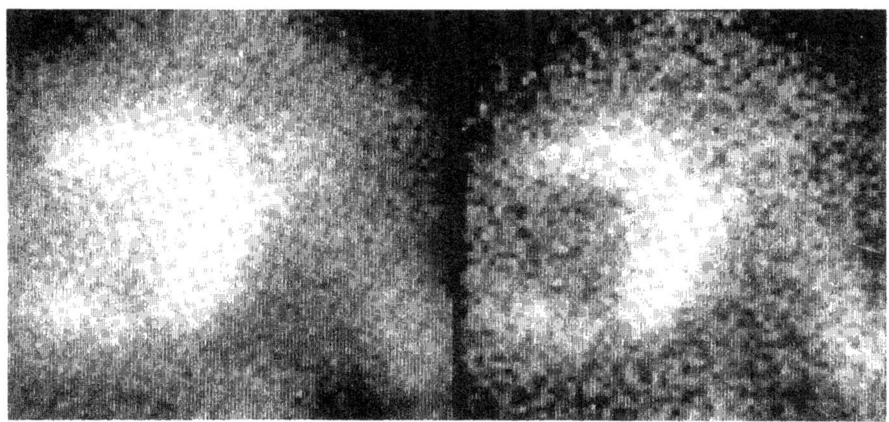

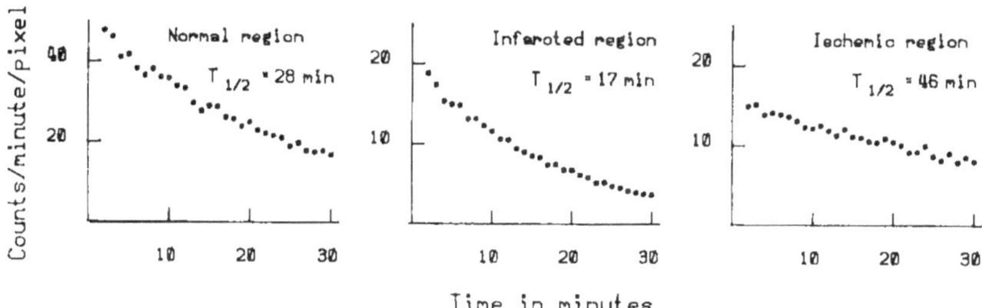

Figure 7. Myocardial I-123-heptadecanoic acid scintigram before (left) and after correction in a patient with anteroseptal infarction.

Figure 8. Time-activity curves derived from normal, ischemic and infarcted myocardial region.

The correction method must be used to correct the serial images for background activity from the I-123 in the blood pool i.e. for iodide not bound to the myocardial cells. The procedure is based on the quantitative evaluation of the contribution of inorganic I-123 to the image. Its principle is schematically presented in Figure 6.

The correction procedure results in good quality scintigrams which provide a better contrast between myocardial and surrounding tissue (Figure 7), and this procedure enables the calculation of time-activity curves which may serve as a parameter for the metabolic turnover of FFA in the myocardium. A drawback of turnover rate measurements is the long imaging period of 45 min and the acquisition of one single view per study which may underdiagnose the presence of CAD. The single view problem can of course be obviated by employment of a biplanar collimator [34].

We studied the kinetics of I-123-FFA in patients with stable and unstable angina pectoris, and patients with acute myocardial infarction (AMI) and we observed different turnover rates of normally perfused, transient ischemic and acutely infarcted areas [33,35]. With reference to half-time values measured in apparently normal regions (20-30 min), we demonstrated increased values in ischemic zones (>40 min) and decreased values (<20 min) in infarcted zones, suggesting a slow and a fast metabolic turnover of I-123-FFA respectively. Figure 8 gives schematically the observed turnover rates from different myocardial regions. Based on our results, it was postulated that I-123-FFA offer the diagnostic potential to distinguish *reversible* from *irreversible* ischemia. Although clinically interesting, and supported by animal experiments [36] and other clinical studies [37], these findings have to be confirmed by studies in much larger populations. Another application of I-123-HDA is its use in patients after successful thrombolysis. Two clinical studies [38,39] reported the value of I-123-HDA in assessing the metabolic integrity of reperfused myocardium within 1 week after AMI, based on the reduction of defect size and normalization of half-time values. Also in patients with congestive cardiomyopathy (COCM), it has been shown that the determination of clearance rates could be of significant value [40]. All patients with COCM showed inhomogeneous tracer distribution and slow clearance rates of I-123-HDA,suggesting altered FFA metabolism in diseased myocardial regions. In a recent study by Rabinowitz *et al.* [41] it was reported that scintigraphy with I-123-HDA should be of interest as a screening test for carnitine deficiency in patients with a variety of cardiomyopathies.

Classification of primary cardiomyopathies is currently based on anatomic and functional abnormalities regardless of the underlying etiology. Biochemical studies will not only enhance our understanding of these disorders as well as their detection and characterization but will also aid in the development of effective treatment [65].

Also results of venous bypass surgery and the effect of cardiac rehabilitation have been assessed with I-123-HDA by the measurement of myocardial clearance rates [42,43].

Future prospects

Recently, new biochemical concepts have been proposed to avoid the high background activity in imaging studies of the myocardium [44]. Attaching the iodine label to a benzene ring located in the terminal position of a fatty acid (I-123-phenyl-pentadecanoic acid; I-123-PPA) results in a radiopharmaceutical which shows essentially no release of free radioiodide into the circulation (Figure 9). The final catabolite of I-123-PPA consists of benzoic acid, which is fastly detoxificated and so obviates background problems.

Uptake of I-123-PPA parallels regional myocardial flow in both normal and ischemic myocardium [45], and I-123-PPA can therefore be employed for imaging purposes [46]. Since the breakdown products of phenyl-fatty acids will reside much longer in the cells, myocardial clearance will be considerably

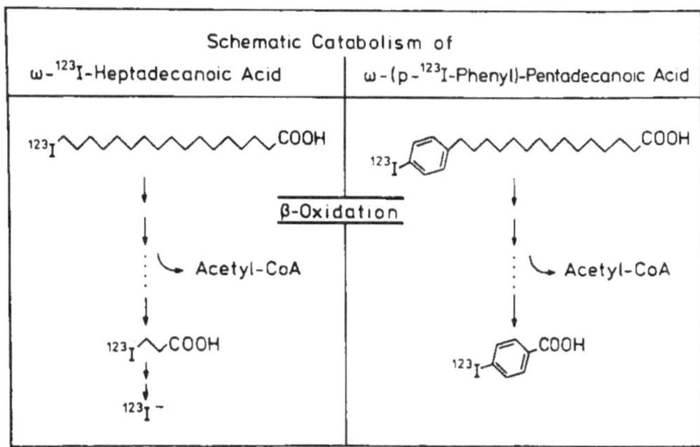

Figure 9. Final products from I-123-heptadecanoic acid (free radioiodide) and from I-123-phenyl-pentadecanoic acid (benzoic acid). Reproduced from Machulla [44].

delayed and makes proper metabolic studies very complicated [47], although recent papers have reported the value of clearance rates of I-123-PPA for the detection of CAD and the evaluation of cardiomyopathies [48-51]. Reske *et al.*[52] compared quantitatively the uptake and metabolism of I-PPA with C-14-palmitate in rats, and observed a very similar pattern for both tracers. Moreover they showed in canine studies that initial uptake of I-PPA was related to myocardial uptake both under control conditions and in ischemia. In clinical studies, patients with significant CAD and with myocardial infarction were accurately detected and localized with I-123-PPA. In our institution, elimination half-times of much more than 60 min from normal human hearts have been calculated [51], which probably excludes measurement of oxidative metabolism and will only reflect turnover of triglycerides [53]. Chapter 8 reports the most recent results with I-PPA.

A next labeled fatty acid that recently [54] has been proposed is tellurium-123m-9-telluraheptadecanoic acid (Te-123m-THDA). This radiopharmaceutical gives a reasonable imaging quality in dog hearts. However, the physical and myocardial biological half-lives of Te-123m are respectively 120 and 7 days, which precludes metabolic clearance studies. In addition, and apart from high radiation doses, experimental studies [55] showed toxic effects in rats, and further toxicity studies are necessary before considering Te-123m-THDA as a myocardial imaging agent in man.

An other new metabolic tracer is C-11-beta-methyl-heptadecanoic acid (C-11-BMHDA) [56]. This compound is obtained by inserting a methyl radical in the beta-position and so inhibits beta-oxidation. It is therefore trapped in the myocardium and can not further be metabolized (nearly constant level of activity in the dog myocardium for 60 min). Therefore, the beta-methyl branched FFA are very suitable for studies of regional distribution and can be used to study myocardial perfusion, but more importantly, can be used to study aberrations in FFA metabolism under normal flow conditions where regional FFA uptake may be correlated with several aspects of regional metabolism. In a recent study [57] by our group, we evaluated the uptake and kinetics of 15-p-(I-125)-iodophenyl-3-beta-methyl-pentadecanoic acid (I-125-BMPPA) in diabetic rats. It was shown that myocardial uptake in diabetic rats was higher than in normal rats despite increased plasma FFA. Furthermore, washout over 60 min was slower in the diabetic hearts compared to the normal hearts.

It was concluded that radiolabeled I-BMPPA handling is different in diabetic myocardium compared to nondiabetic myocardium, which may have important implications for myocardial imaging. In chapter 9 the value of the methyl-branched I-FFA will be extensively discussed.

Newer developments concern with different biochemical steps in the metabolism of FFA such as studies with C-11 labeled acetate and pyruvate. These labeled metabolic products may provide insight into the overall metabolism of the heart under various conditions. Moreover, enzyme deficiencies (for instance lack of carnitine) can be detected with these labeled metabolic products and the therapeutic effectiveness can be evaluated.

Conclusion

Cardiac disease, in particular CAD, is at present most frequently diagnosed and treated in its final stage, after structural or anatomic derangements are already present.

However, disease begins at the biochemical level and therapies are designed to halt or reverse abnormal biochemical processes, restore delivery of biochemical nutrients, or supplement depleted ones. Any technique that provides biochemically specific information about the myocardium could play a vital role in the early diagnosis and effective management of human cardiac disease [65].

Until now, clinical studies have been scarce mainly due to restricted availability of radiopharmaceuticals and to limited equipment facilities.

Positron emission tomography

The PET technique potentially provides a unique tool to investigate regional myocardial metabolism noninvasively, although the initial as well as the operational costs of positron emission tomography have been major limitations for widespread application and the number of positron cameras throughout the world is still very small. In addition, one might legitimately question the usefulness of an imaging technique limited to the small number of positron-emitting radionuclides as compared to the considerably greater number of gamma-emitters, particularly in light of the fact that positron emission tomographs are expensive and complex devices which cannot be used for the imaging of the more common gamma-ray emitters. However, dedicated and reliable medical minicyclotrons with less technical requirements and lower costs are currently developed, combined with automated synthesis techniques.

A substantial problem is the proper interpretation of clearance curves because of back-diffusion of nonmetabolized substrates.

At present, clinical studies with C-11-palmitate are limited and its interest is still of investigational value. In a recent experimental study by Schwaiger *et al.* [58], it was reported that C-11-palmitate in conjunction with PET may be helpful to identify reversibly injured myocardium. This finding stimulates continuation of metabolic studies with C-11-palmitate. Further studies will be needed to demonstrate the clinical utility of the PET technique for detection of cardiac disease prior to irreversible damage and to design therapeutic regimens more precisely.

Radioiodinated FFA

Radioiodinated FFA have become commercially available and can therefore be used on a routine basis in clinical practice [59-61, 67].

Regarding clinical use, we think it wise to make a clear distinction between studies for imaging purposes and for metabolic investigations. As for imaging in patients with CAD, excellent images can be obtained. Similar to C-11-palmitate, however, the value of the kinetics remain to be established. The study of myocardial FFA metabolism by the noninvasive measurement of turnover rates is still in the experimental phase and its understanding needs the combined efforts of both nuclear medicine and myocardial biochemistry. Adequate application of I-FFA will give more information of cardiac function than just the scintigraphic pictures do. Valid questions with respect to analysis of metabolic clearance rates are

1) how long after injection should we measure,
2) is the correction method really necessary,
3) which part of the curve has to be considered,
4) do we have to apply a mono- or biexponential curve fitting, and lastly
5) do we really measure FFA degradation or are other mechanisms responsible for the observed phenomenon.

Still controversies exist, whether deiodination of I-123-FFA is a nonspecific process or is related to oxidative FFA metabolism. An urgent problem that has to be solved is the understanding of the coupling of flow and metabolism i.e. the relation between uptake and elimination of metabolic tracers especially under conditions of myocardial exercise and ischemia. Unless the exact mechanism of the metabolic kinetics has been elucidated, the clinical value of labeled FFA as metabolic tracers will be limited. Well-controlled experimental studies have to be carried out to make the labeled FFA clinically useful and "this general class" of studies will represent the next stratum of nuclear cardiology investigations.

Acknowledgements

Secretarial help by M. Koelemay is gratefully acknowledged.

References

1. Machulla H J, Stoecklin G, Kupfernagel C *et al.* (1978) Comparative evaluation of fatty acids labeled with C-11, Cl-34m, Br-77 and I-123 for metabolic studies of the myocardium: concise communication. J Nucl Med 19: 298 - 302
2. Poe N D, Robinson jr G D, Graham L S, MacDonald N S (1976) Experimental basis for myocardial imaging with I-123-labeled hexadecenoic acid. J Nucl Med 17: 1077 - 82
3. Schelbert H R, Henze E, Huang S C, Phelps M E (1981) Relationship between myocardial blood flow and uptake and utilization of free fatty acids (FFA) J Nucl Med 22: p10
4. Henze E, Guzy P, Schelbert H (1983) Metabolic effects of cardiac work on normal and ischemic myocardum in man measured noninvasively with C-11-palmitate and positron emission tomography (PET). Eur Soc Cardiol Working Group on Use of Isotopes in Cardiol, Rotterdam (abstract)
5. Dudczak R, Kletter K, Frischauf H, Losert U, Angelberger P, Schmoliner R (1984) The use of I-123-labeled heptadecanoic acid (HDA) as metabolic tracer: Preliminary report. Eur J Nucl Med 9: 81 - 85
6. Comet M, Wolf J E, Pilichowski P, Mathieu J P, Dubois F, Riche F, Busquet G, Lidal M, Godart J, Pernin C, Gaudy M. (1982) Influence du propranolol sur l'activite myocardique apres injection i.v. d'acide 16 I(123) hexadecene 9 oique. In: Faivre G, Bertrand A, Cherrier F, Amor M, Neimann J L (eds) Noninvasive methods in ischemic heart disease. Nancy, Specia, pp 295 - 99
7. Styles C B, Noujaim A A, Jugdutt B I *et al.* (1983) Effect of doxorubicin on (omega-I-131) heptadecanoic acid myocardial scintigraphy and echocardiography in dogs. J Nucl Med 24: 1012 - 18
8. Stoecklin G (1981) Evaluation of radiohalogen labelled fatty acids for heart studies. Nuklearmedizin (Suppl) 19: 1 - 6.
9. Lerch R A, Ambos H D, Bergmann S R, Welch M J, Ter-Pogossian M M, Sobel B E (1981) Localization of viable, ischemic myocardium by positron- emission tomography with C-11-palmitate. Circulation 64: 689 - 99
10. Lerch R A, Bergmann S R, Ambos H D, Welch M J, Ter-Pogossian M M, Sobel B E (1982) Effect of flow-independent reduction of metabolism on regional myocardial clearance of C-11-palmitate. Circulation 65: 731 - 38
11. Schelbert H R, Phelps M E, Hoffman E, Huang S C, Kuhl D E (1980) Regional myocardial blood flow, metabolism and function assessed noninvasively with positron emission tomography. Am J Cardiol 46: 1269 - 77
12. Schoen H R, Schelbert H R, Najafi A *et al.* (1982) C-11 labeled palmitic acid for the noninvasive evaluation of regional myocardial fatty acid metabolism with positron-computed tomography. II. Kinetics of C-11-palmitic acid in acutely ischemic myocardium. Am Heart J 103: 548 - 61
13. Visser F C, Westera G, Eenige van M J, van der Wall E E, den Hollander W, Roos J P (1985) The myocardial elimination rate of radioiodinated heptadecanoic acid. Eur J Nucl Med 10: 118 - 22

14. Kloster G, Stoecklin G, Smith E F, Schroer K (1984) Omega-halofatty acids: A probe for mitochondrial membrane integrity. In vitro investigations in normal and ischaemic myocardium. Eur J Nucl Med 9: 305 - 11
15. Weiss E S, Hoffman E J, Phelps M E *et al.* (1976) External detection and visualization of myocardial ischemia with C-11-substrates in vitro and in vivo. Circ Res 39: 24 - 32
16. Weiss E S, Ahmed S A, Welch M J, Williamson J R, Ter-Pogossian M M, Sobel B E (1977) Quantification of infarction in cross sections of canine myocardium in vivo with positron emission transaxial tomography and C-11-palmitate. Circulation 55: 66 - 73
17. Sobel B E, Weiss E S, Welch M J, Siegel B A, Ter-Pogossian M M (1977) Detection of remote myocardial infarction in patients with positron emission transaxial tomography and intravenous C-11-palmitate. Circulation 55: 853 - 57
18. Ter-Pogossian M M, Klein M S, Markham J, Roberts R, Sobel B E (1980) Regional assessment of myocardial metabolic integrity in vivo by positron-emission tomography with C-11-labeled palmitate. Circulation 61: 242 - 55
19. Geltman E M, Biello D, Welch M J, Ter-Pogossian M M, Roberts R, Sobel B E (1982) Characterization of nontransmural myocardial infarction by positron-emission tomography. Circulation 65: 747 - 55
20. Schoen H R, Schelbert H R, Robinson G, Najafi A, Huang S C, Hansen H *et al.* C-11-labeled palmitate acid for the noninvasive evaluation of regional myocardial fatty acid metabolism with positron-computed tomography. I. Kinetics of C-11-palmitic acid in normal myocardium. Am Heart J 103: 532 - 47
21. Bergmann S R, Lerch R A, Fox K A A *et al.* (1982) Temporal dependence of beneficial effects of coronary thrombolysis characterized by positron tomography. Am J Med 73: 573 - 81
22. Ludbrook P A, Geltman E M, Tiefenbrunn A J, Jaffe A S, Sobel B E (1983) Restoration of regional myocardial metabolism by coronary thrombolysis in patients. Circulation (abstract) 68: III, 325
23. Goldstein R A, Klein M S, Welch M J, Sobel B E (1980) External assessment of myocardial metabolism with C-11-palmitate in vivo. J Nucl Med 21: 342 - 48
24. Evans J R, Phil D, Gunton R W, Baker R G, Spears J C, Beanlands D S. (1965) Use of radioiodinated fatty acid for photoscans of the heart. Circ Res 16: 1 - 10
25. Robinson jr G D, Lee A W (1975) Radioiodinated fatty acids for heart imaging: iodine monochloride addition compared with iodide replacement labeling. J Nucl Med 16: 17 - 21
26. Poe N D, Robinson jr G D, MacDonald N S (1975) Myocardial extraction of labeled long-chain fatty acid analogs. Proc Soc Exp Biol Med 148: 215 - 18
27. Otto C A, Brown L E, Wieland D M, Beierwaltes W H (1981) Radioiodinated fatty acid for myocardial imaging: Effects of chain length. J Nucl Med 22: 613 - 18
28. Westera G, van der Wall E E, Heidendal G A K, van den Bos G C (1980) A comparison between terminally radioiodinated hexadecenoic acid (I-HA) and Tl-201-thallium chloride in the dog heart. Implications for the use of I-HA for myocardial imaging. Eur J Nucl Med 5: 339 - 43
29. Poe N D, Robinson jr G D, Zielinski F W, Cabeen jr W R, Smith J W, Gomes A S (1977) Myocardial imaging with I-123-hexadecenoic acid. Radiology 124: 419 - 24
30. Freundlieb C, Hoeck A, Vyska K, Feinendegen L E, Machulla H J, Stoecklin G (1980) Myocardial imaging and metabolic studies with (17-I-123)iodoheptadecanoic acid. J Nucl Med 21: 1043 - 50
31. Van der Wall E E, Heidendal G A K, den Hollander W, Westera G, Roos J P (1980) I-123 labeled hexadecenoic acid in comparison with thallium-201 for myocardial imaging in coronary heart disease. A preliminary study. Eur J Nucl Med 5: 401 - 05
32, Roesler H, Hess T, Weiss M *et al.* (1983) Tomoscintigraphic assessment of myocardial metabolic heterogenity. J Nucl Med 24: 285 - 96
33. Van der Wall E E, den Hollander W, Heidendal G A K, Westera G, Majid P A, Roos J P (1981)

Dynamic myocardial scintigraphy with I-123 labeled free fatty acids in patients with myocardial infarction. Eur J Nucl Med 6: 383 - 89

34. Aurich D, Reske S N, Biersack H J *et al.* (1982) Biplanar sequential scintigraphy of the myocardium by means of 123-I-heptadecanoic acid. In: Raynaud C (ed) Nucl Med Biol, Proc third World Congr Nucl Med Biol Paris II Pergamon Press, pp 1389 - 91
35. van der Wall E E, Heidendal G A K, den Hollander W, Westera G, Roos J P (1981) Metabolic myocardial imaging with I-123 labeled heptadecanoic acid in patients with angina pectoris. Eur J Nucl Med 6: 391 - 96
36. van der Wall E E, Westera G, den Hollander W, Visser F C (1981) External detection of regional myocardial metabolism with radioiodinated hexadecenoic acid in the dog heart. Eur J Nucl Med 6: 147 - 51
37. Huckell V F, Lyster D M, Morrison R T (1980) The potential role of 123 iodine-hexadecenoic acid in assessing normal and abnormal myocardial metabolism. J Nucl Med 21: p57
38. Pachinger O, Sochor H, Ogris E, Probst P, Klicpera M, Kaindl F (1982) Salvage of ischemic myocardium by intracoronary streptokinase therapy? In: Faivre G, Bertrand A, Cherrier F, Amor M, Neimann J L (eds) Non invasive methods in ischemic heart disease. Nancy, Specia, pp 410 - 414
39. Visser F C, Westera G, van der Wall E E, Roos J P (1985) Dynamic free fatty acid scintigraphy in patients with successful thrombolysis after acute myocardial infarction. Clin Nucl Med 10: 35 - 39
40. Hoeck A, Freundlieb C, Vyska K, Loesse B, Erbel R, Feinendegen L E (1983) Myocardial imaging and metabolic studies with (17-I-123)iodoheptadecanoic acid in patients with idiopathic congestive cardiomyopathy. J Nucl Med 24: 22 - 28
41. Rabinovitch M A, Kalff V, Allen R *et al.* (1985) 123-I-Hexadecanoic acid metabolic probe of cardiomyopathy. Eur J Nucl Med 10: 222 - 27
42. Freundlieb C, Hoeck A, Vyska K, Erbel R, Feinendegen L E (1982) Fatty acid uptake and turnover rate in the ischemic heart before and after bypass surgery. In: Raynaud (ed) Nucl Med Biol, Proc third World Congr Nucl Med Biol Paris II Pergamon Press pp 1392 - 95
43. Hoeck A, Freundlieb C, Vyska K *et al.* (1982) The influence of rehabilitation training on fatty acid metabolism in patients with myocardial infarction. In: Faivre G, Bertrand A, Cherrier F, Amor M, Neimann J L (eds) Non invasive methods in ischemic heart disease. Nancy, Specia, pp 300 - 303
44. Machulla H J, Marsmann M, Dutschka K (1980) Biochemical concept and synthesis of a radioiodinated phenylfatty acid for in vivo metabolic studies of the myocardium. Eur J Nucl Med 5: 171 - 73
45. Reske S N, Schoen S, Knust E J, Machulla H J, Eichelkrant W, Halm N, Winkler C. (1984) Relation of myocardial blood flow and initial cardiac uptake of 15-(p-I-123-phenyl)-pentadecanoic acid in the canine heart. Nucl Med 23: 83 - 85
46. Sun Q X, Zhang J, Ji Q M, Wang Y C, Xie D F, Hua R L, He W Y, Shi X C, Li Y J, Jiang C J. (1984) Pharmacology of radioiodinated hexadecenoic acid. A myocardial imaging agent. Nucl Med 23: 73 - 74
47. Coenen H H, Harmand M F, Kloster G, Stoecklin G (1981) 15-(p-(Br-75)bromophenyl)-pentadecanoic acid: Pharmacokinetics and potential as heart agent. J Nucl Med 22: 891 - 96
48. Dudczak R, Schmoliner R, Kletter K, Frischauf H, Angelberger P (1983) Clinical evaluation of I-123-labeled p-phenylpentadecanoic acid (p-IPPA) for myocardial scintigraphy. J Nucl Med All Sci 27: 267 - 79
49. Rellas J S, Corbett J R, Kulkarni P *et al.* (1983) Iodine-123 -phenylpentadecanoic acid: Detection of acute myocardial infarction and injury in dogs using an iodinated fatty acid and single-photon emission tomography. Am J Cardiol 52: 1326 - 32
50. Reske S N, Biersack H J, Lackner K *et al.* (1982) Assessment of regional myocardial uptake and metabolism of omega-(p-I-123-phenyl)-pentadecanoic acid with serial single-photon emission tomography. Nucl Med 21: 249 - 53

51. Visser F C, van der Wall E E, Eenige van M J. Elimination rates of I-123-labeled phenylpentadecanoic acid in patients after acute myocardial infarction. Preliminary results
52. Reske S N (1985) 123-I-Phenylpentadecanoic acid as a tracer of cardiac free fatty acid metabolism. Experimental and clinical results. Eur Heart J (suppl B) 6: 39 - 47
53. Reske S N, Machulla H J, Biersack H J, Simon H, Knopp R, Winkler C (1982) Metabolic turnover of P-I-123-phenylpentadecanoic acid in the myocardium. In: Raynaud C (ed) Nucl Med Biol, Proc third World Congr Nucl Med Biol Paris III Pergamon Press, pp 2522 - 25
54. Okada R D, Knapp jr F F, Elmaleh D R, Yasuda T, Boucher C A, Strauss H W (1982) Tellurium-123m-labeled-9-telluraheptadecanoic acid: A possible cardiac imaging agent. Circulation 65: 305 - 10
55. Elmaleh D R, Knapp jr F F, Yasuda T *et al.* (1981) Myocardial imaging with 9-(Te-123m)telluraheptadecanoic acid. J Nucl Med 22: 994 - 99
56. Livni E, Elmaleh D R, Levy S, Brownell G L, Strauss W H (1982) Beta-methyl(1-C-11)heptadecanoic acid: A new myocardial metabolic tracer for positron emission tomography. J Nucl Med 23: 169 - 75
57. van der Wall E E, Barrett E, Strauss H W *et al.* (1985) Altered uptake and kinetics of radioiodinated 15-P-(I-125)-iodophenyl-3-methylpentadecanoic acid in diabetic myocardium. Circulation (abstract) 72(suppl III): 424
58. Schwaiger M, Schelbert H R, Keen R *et al.* (1985) Retention and clearance of C-11-palmitic acid in ischemic and reperfused canine myocardium. J Am Coll Cardiol 6: 311 - 20
59. Machulla H J, Knust E J (1984) Recent developments in the field of I-123-radiopharmaceuticals. Nucl Med 23: 111 - 18
60. van der Wall E E (1984) Myocardial imaging with radiolabeled free fatty acids. In: Simoons M L, Reiber J H C (eds) Nuclear imaging in clinical cardiology. The Hague: Martinus Nijhoff, pp 83 - 102
61. van der Wall E E (1985) Myocardial imaging with radiolabeled free fatty acids: A critical review. Eur Heart J (suppl B) 6: 29 - 38
62. Schelbert H R, Henze E, Keen R, Huang H, Barrio J, Phelps M (1982) Regional fatty acid metabolism in acute myocardial ischemia demonstrated noninvasively by C-11-palmitate (CPA) and positron tomography (PET). Circulation (abstract) 66(suppl II): 126
63. Vyska K, Hoeck A, Freundlieb C *et al.* (1979) Myocardial imaging and measurement of myocardial fatty acid metabolism using omega-I-123-heptadecanoic acid. J Nucl Med (abstract) 20: 650
64. Grover M, Schelbert H R (1985) Assessment of regional myocardial substrate metabolism with positron emission tomography. In: G Pohost (Ed) New concepts in cardiac imaging 1985 Boston. Hall Medical Publishers.
65. Schelbert H R, Phelps M E, Shine K I (1983) Imaging metabolism and biochemistry: a new look at the heart. Am Heart J 105: 552 - 526
66. Fox K A A, Abendschein D R, Ambos H D, Sobel B E, Bergmann S R (1985) Efflux of metabolized and nonmetabolized fatty acid from canine myocardium tomographically. Circ Res 57: 232 - 243.
67. van der Wall EE (1986). Myocardial imaging with radiolabeled free fatty acids: Applications and limitations. Eur J Nucl Med 12: S11 - S15.

3. Chain-modified radioiodinated fatty acids

C.A. OTTO

Introduction

Myocardial perfusion has been experimentally and clinically evaluated by intravenously administered gamma-emitting radiopharmaceuticals such as thallium-201 (^{201}Tl). Evaluation of myocardial metabolism using radiopharmaceuticals as an alternative to and/or a complement of perfusion is desirable. Metabolic studies could have clinical applications in early detection of heart disease and serial monitoring of the effects of therapy. Since fatty acids constitute the major energy source of heart tissue through β-oxidation catabolism and since they are efficiently extracted from the blood by the heart, efforts have been made to radiolabel these acids and to evaluate them in normal and damaged heart tissue. Although the myocardium extracts and metabolizes both odd and even numbered carbon chain lengths as well as both saturated and unsaturated fatty acids, the acids primarily metabolized are the 16-carbon saturated palmitic acid (x=14 in the formula below), the 18-carbon saturated stearic acid (x=16) and the 18-carbon unsaturated oleic acid (x=y=7).

saturated fatty acid general formula:
$CH_3(CH_2)_xCO_2H$
unsaturated fatty acid general formula:
$CH_3(CH_2)_xCH = CH(CH_2)_yCO_2H$

Because of the attractive radionuclide properties of ^{123}I (159 keV gamma emission energy and 13.2 h half-life) and the ease of labeling alkyl fatty acids by radioiodide exchange, radioiodinated straight-chain 16 to 18 carbon alkyl fatty acids were the first of the radiolabeled acids to be studied.

Overview of fatty acid metabolism

A brief review of fatty acid metabolism is appropriate for an understanding of

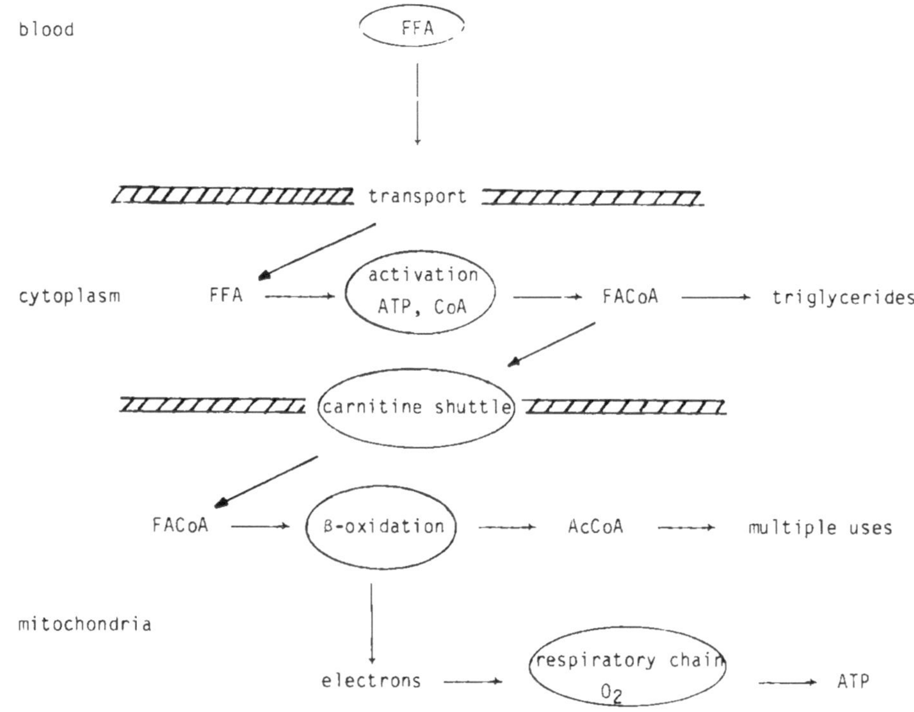

Figure 1. Schematic of FFA metabolism. The most important steps are encircled.

the role of radioiodinated fatty acids. Figure 1 is a schematic highlighting the most important steps. Free fatty acids (FFA) are found in blood plasma usually complexed to serum albumin but occasionally as triglycerides and less frequently as FFA. They diffuse through the capillary wall into the interstitial space where they may be temporarily complexed to proteins. A second diffusion of the FFA through the cellular membrane into the cytoplasm occurs, thus completing FFA transport. Once in the cytoplasm, FFA are activated to acyl-CoA esters (FACoA) by an ATP requiring esterification with coenzyme A (CoA). FACoA undergoes either the principal metabolic steps of FA catabolism or is interconverted (reversibly) to other cellular constituents. Normally, less than 50% of the FACoA is interconverted to triglycerides, phospholipids or cholesterol esters. More than 50% is transported into the mitochondria via the carnitine shuttle operating in the mitochondrial membrane. The primary catabolism of FACoA is called β-oxidation and is located within the mitochondrial matrix.

Figure 2 is a schematic of β-oxidation. As can be seen the process involves successive dehydrogenation, hydration and dehydrogenation followed by cleavage into two fragments: a two-carbon catabolite, acetyl-CoA (AcCoA) and the remainder of the fatty acid also as a CoA ester. This shorter fatty acid

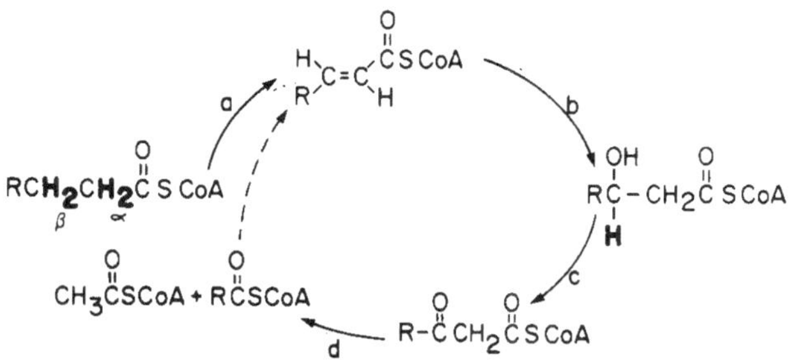

Figure 2. Scheme for β-oxidation of fatty acids: (A) acyl-CoA dehydrogenase; (B) enoyl-CoA hydrase; (C) 3-L-hydroxyacyl-CoA dehydrogenase; (D) β-ketoacyl-CoA thiolase. (Reprinted by permission from J Nucl Med 1984, 25: 75 - 80)

CoA ester cycles through β-oxidation losing two carbons as AcCoA per cycle until the final passage yields two molecules of AcCoA for even carbon fatty acids or one molecule of AcCoA and one molecule of a three carbon CoA ester, propyl-CoA, for odd carbon fatty acids.

Although only four enzymatic steps are shown, there are more than four enzymes used in total FACoA catabolism. There are various enzymes for each step which are specific for different chain lengths. For example, long (~C_{16}), medium (~C_{10}) and short (~C_4) chain β-hydroxyacyl dehydrogenases are present in the mitochondrial matrix.

There are actually two catabolites of β-oxidation: AcCoA and electrons. Electrons are produced in the two dehydrogenation steps and are carried via NADH and $FADH_2$ to the respiratory chain. They are ultimately involved in the reduction of oxygen and in the synthesis of ATP. AcCoA can be metabolized via the Krebs cycle which yields more electrons for the respiratory chain and CO_2. AcCoA can also be returned to the cytoplasm where it is used in fatty acid and steroid synthesis, as an acetylating agent or in gluconeogenesis.

Evident from this brief summary is the fact that there are a number of critical steps or requirements in fatty acid metabolism. An intact, fully functional mitochondrial matrix is of course necessary. In addition to this, a functioning carnitine shuttle within the mitochondrial membrane is essential. In the cytoplasm, FACoA is synthesized in a reaction requiring FFA, CoA and ATP. ATP is synthesized in the mitochondria in a process dependent on oxygen availability as an acceptor of electrons. Finally, the entire scheme is dependent on the intracellular availability of FFA which will vary with FFA blood concentrations.

The difficulty in using nuclear medicine techniques to assess specific reactions or aspects in fatty acid metbolism is readily apparent in face of the number of steps involved from transport into the cell through catabolism. The initial goal in using radioiodinated fatty acids as imaging agents was to obtain information on the efficiency or functioning of the total process and then to determine if this could be diagnostically useful.

Radioiodinated fatty acid development

The potential utility of radioiodinated fatty acids as myocardial imaging agents was first demonstrated in 1964 by Evans *et al.* [1]. An ^{131}I-oleic acid derivative prepared by ^{131}ICl addition across the carbon-carbon double bond of oleic acid, see equation (1), was used to detect areas of myocardial infarction in dog

(1)

$$CH_3(CH_2)_7CH = CH(CH_2)_7CO_2H \xrightarrow{^{131}ICl} CH_3(CH_2)_7\underset{}{\overset{Cl\,(*I)}{CH}} - \underset{*I(Cl)}{CH}(CH_2)_7CO_2H$$

hearts. There are two disadvantages to the use of this iodinated fatty acid: 1) iodine monochloride (ICl) addition presumably yields two isomeric products (a 9-iodo-10-chloro and a 9-chloro-10-iodo derivative) in about equal proportions and 2) it has been shown that ICl addition sharply reduces myocardial extraction [2,3] possibly due to steric changes induced by the bulky I and Cl atoms on adjacent carbons. Although this fatty acid was further evaluated in dogs [4] and in humans [5], no new studies have appeared due to the development of other radioiodinated fatty acids with myocardial extraction efficiencies similar to those found for naturally occurring fatty acids.

Two studies have shown that terminally iodinated alkyl and alkenyl fatty

$$*I\text{-}(CH_2)_x\text{-}CO_2H$$

acids (ω-iodo fatty acids), are extracted as efficiently as the parent ^{11}C acids. Poe *et al.* [2] found that myocardial extraction efficiency of an alkenyl acid, ^{131}I-ω-iodo-hexadecenoic acid ($77 \pm 11.0\%$, $N = 7$) was similar to the extraction efficiency of ^{11}C-oleic acid ($61 \pm 7.8\%$, $N = 3$). A definitive study by Machulla *et al.* [6] compared position of radiohalogen attachment (α and ω) and radiohalogen (^{34m}Cl, ^{77}Br and ^{123}I) with the parent ^{11}C fatty acids. In mice the myocardial extraction of ω-halo fatty acids was higher than α-halo acids. Of the radiohalogens studied, ^{123}I-ω-labeled fatty acid was comparable in extraction to the parent ^{11}C fatty acid whereas ^{77}Br and ^{34m}Cl ω-labeled acids were extracted about 50% less efficiently. The similarity in extraction between ω-iodo alkanoic acids and their parent acids is probably due to the similarity in size and location between ω-iodine atom and an ω-methyl ($-CH_3$) group. The iodine atom has a diameter of 2.15 Å vs. 2.0 Å for a $-CH_3$ group.

The most extensively evaluated ω-iodo alkyl fatty acid is ω-iodoheptadecanoic acid (17 carbons) [7,8], but ω-iodo-9-hexadecenioc acid (16 carbons) [9-11], has also been studied. These acids bearing ^{123}I or ^{131}I isotopes have been studied in animals and humans with both normal and diseased hearts. Details of clinical studies will be presented in other chapters.

A major limitation to the use of radioiodinated alkyl fatty acids is the significant amount of *in vivo* deiodination which degrades image quality and increases blood activity levels. Early reports suggested that deiodination resulted from active metabolism rather than simple hydrolysis [9]. Robinson *et al.* [9,10] were among the first to suggest that changes in the structure of the ω-iodo fatty acid might alter the rate of deiodination. Two changes suggested included the substitution of a fluorine atom for a hydrogen and the use of a longer (⩾C20) fatty acid.

Studies evaluating the effect of structural changes on myocardial localization and deiodination were initiated. These experiments included fatty acids modified in chain length, by branching, by unsaturation and by carbon-iodine bond stabilization. The rationale and results for each series of experiments is discussed as follows.

Effects of chain length

One means of reducing myocardial turnover rates (increase $t_{1/2}$) is to promote myocardial storage of fatty acids as triglycerides, phospholipids or cholesterol esters.

One of the effects of rapeseed oil in the diet is formation of cardiac lipidoses which have since been attributed to a component of rapeseed oil: erucic acid, a 22-carbon fatty acid with one double bond [12-15]. Since this relationship was established, the metabolism of erucic acid has been thoroughly studied. At least two studies reported lower rates of acyl-CoA activation and lower rates of β-oxidation [16-18]. Other effects such as changes in phospholipid metabolism [19] have been reported.

Two studies using *in vivo* techniques offer clear support for the storage of erucic acid in triglycerides. Vasdev and Kako [20] injected rats with ^{14}C-erucic acid and determined the percent distribution of radioactivity in various tissue lipid fractions. At t = 5 min, more than 50% of the radioactivity present in the myocardium was recovered in the triglyceride fraction. Labeled erucic acid was also recovered (<20%) in both the FFA and phospholipid fraction. Ong *et al.* [21] performed tissue distribution studies using 1-^{14}C labeled erucic acid. They determined that most erucic acid was taken up by the liver. Their data indicate rapid metabolic transformations in all organs except the heart. Analysis of different lipid classes in the heart showed that >80% of erucic acid was in the form of triglycerides at all time intervals studied from 2 to 30 min.

Thus, >50% (and possibly >80%) of a 22-carbon fatty acid is stored in the heart in the form of triglycerides as opposed to <50% of a normal substrate

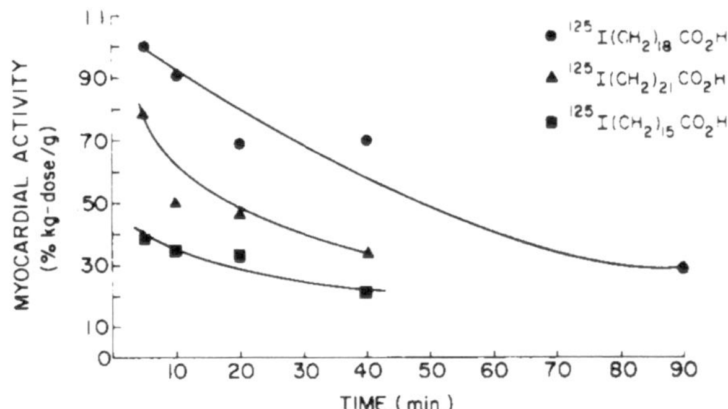

Figure 3. Myocardial activity of iodofatty acids against time. Each data point represents three animals. (Reprinted by permission from J Nucl Med 1981, 22: 613 - 618)

fatty acid of 16 to 18 carbons. In addition, it has been shown that longer chain fatty acids are also extracted efficiently from the blood and can be metabolized, albeit slowly.

Based on the above information, six terminally radioiodinated, fully saturated fatty acids of molecular structure $^{125}I(CH_2)_nCO_2H$ where n = 10, 12, 15, 18, 21 and 26 were synthesized and evaluated in rats [22].

Clearance of radioactivity from the rat myocardium for n = 10, 12 and 15 is dependent on chain length as expected [9]. Generally, at time intervals longer than 5 min, longer chain lengths correlated with higher myocardial radioactivity values. Clearance of radioactivity for n = 15, 18 and 21 is shown in Figure 3. The excellent myocardial extraction of the n = 18 and 21 ω-iodo acids is also shown. For n = 18, the myocardial activity value at t = 5 min is about 3-fold higher than that for n = 15 while the saturated ω-iodo analog of erucic acid was 2-fold higher. That a longer myocardial residence time was achieved by lengthening the fatty acid carbon chain is illustrated by the fact that radioactivity levels fall 30% from t = 5 min to t = 40 min for n = 18 but over the same time frame, there is a 46% reduction in activity levels for n = 15. Therefore, not only are activity levels higher for n = 18 compared to the more natural length n = 15, but retention is also longer.

The longer retention and higher activity levels observed in the myocardium for n = 18 relative to n = 15 prompted an analysis of the form of radioactivity in the heart for these two acids. Figure 4 shows the cellular distribution of radioactivity in an organic extraction of heart homogenates (for details see [22]). Analysis was performed at 5 and 20 min for n = 15 and at 5 and 40 min for n = 18. Only these two acids were analyzed, as the shorter chain acids (n = 10 and 12) had short myocardial residence times and were expected to behave similarly to n = 15. Likewise, the longer chain acid, n = 21 was expected to behave similar to n = 18.

A large difference in the cellular distribution of radioactivity between the n = 15 and n = 18 acids was observed. About 65% of the recovered

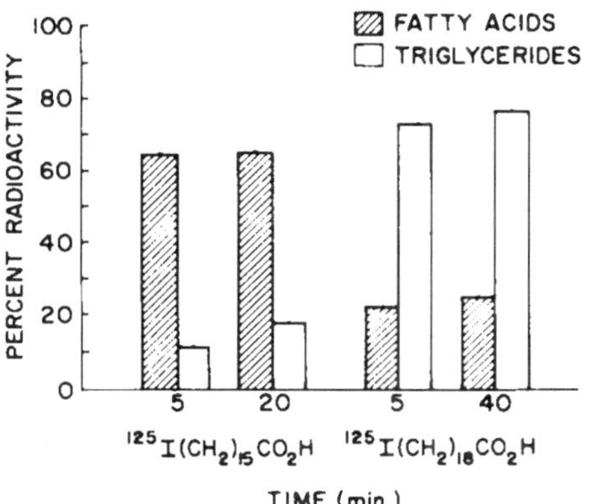

Figure 4. Distribution of radioactivity between free fatty acids and triglycerides. Each bar represents three samples from each of three animals. Data for each time are calculated assuming initial activity in sample was 100%. (Reprinted by permission from J Nucl Med 1981, 22: 613 - 618)

radioactivity was associated with the FFA band for n = 15 in contrast to about 22% for n = 18. The triglyceride fraction contained about 15% of the activity for n = 15 but 74% for n = 18 [22].

The longer myocardial residence time of radioactivity for both n = 18 and 21 may be related to storage of these ω-iodo fatty acids as triglycerides although this is not clear at present. For ω-iodo fatty acids which approximate the naturally occurring fatty acids in chain length, the rate-limiting step for decreasing radioactivity levels in the heart is apparently the diffusion of free radioiodide into the blood [23,24]. The mechanism of radioiodide release from the labeled acid is unknown. However, for the n = 18 ω-iodo acid, less than 10% of the radioactivity is as free radioiodide. In addition, the rate of accumulation of radioactivity in the thyroid, which is an indicator of free radioiodide in the blood, is lower for the longer chain fatty acids [22]. Apparently, the rate-limiting step for the longer acids is not diffusion of radioiodide. It may be that incorporation into triglycerides decreases the rate(s) of free radioiodide formation and leads to increased myocardial residence time.

In summary, this study on effect of chain length has shown that increasing carbon numbers relative to naturally occurring chain lengths of 16 and 18 carbons significantly increases myocardial radioactivity values at $t \geqslant 5$ min post injection. Residence time in the myocardium has also increased as has the percentage of radioactivity incorporated into triglycerides. The data suggest that an ω-iodo alkanoic acid of 19 carbons has potential for myocardial imaging, possibly as a probe of storage function.

Effects of unsaturation

Since the longer chain ω-iodo acids appear to probe a process other than β-oxidation, efforts to assess active metabolism should use fatty acids of natural lengths. If free radioiodide is released from the final catabolite of β-oxidation, iodoacetyl CoA (IAcCoA), then inhibition or prevention of β--oxidation should prolong myocardial residence time. In order to evaluate this possibility, the desired ω-iodo acid is one which behaves as a naturally occurring fatty acid through the steps of diffusion in the cell, activation by CoA ester formation and carnitine-mediated transport into the mitochondria but which inhibits or is not a substrate for the enzymatic reactions of β-oxidation. Several types of fatty acids may meet these requirements: unsaturated acids (both double and triple bonds), branched-chain acids and telluro acids (discussed in chapter 9). In this and the following section, results of studies using the former two classes will be discussed.

Inhibition of β-oxidation may be achieved by the judicious placement of unsaturated carbon-carbon bonds within the fatty acid. Two different types of unsaturation are possible: carbon-carbon triple bonds and carbon-carbon double bonds.

triple bond (alkyne)	$-C\equiv C-$
double bond (alkene)	$-HC=CH-$

The synthesis and evaluation of an ω-iodo alkynoic fatty acid, $^{125}I(CH_2)_4C\equiv C(CH_2)_7CO_2H$ [25] was accomplished because of the potential for mechanism based irreversible inhibition (suicide inhibition). Bloch [26] has shown such inhibition of *E. coli* dehydrase with 3-decynoic acid. The mechanism of this inhibition involves enzymatic conversion of the triple bond to a reactive allene which bonds covalently to histidine at the active site of the enzyme [27]. In the myocardium enoyl-CoA isomerase has the potential to generate a reactive allene during normal β-oxidation. Allenes could be expected from a triple bond at a 3-, 5-, or other odd-numbered carbon atom.

Evaluation of the ω-iodo alkynoic acid was first performed in rats. The myocardial radioactivity values were low; only 20-25% of the activity of a comparable length straight-chain saturated fatty acid at 5 min was observed. Previous data suggested that the rat heart might be more sensitive to carbon chain manipulation so the alkynoic acid was also evaluated in dogs. The data obtained showed that myocardial activity for the alkynoic acid was experimentally equivalent to a comparable alkanoic acid at both 5 and 20 min post injection [25]. Blood values for the alkynoic acid were higher than the straight-chain analog. Based on the data obtained from the ω-iodo alkynoic acid, it is apparent that inclusion of a triple bond did not alter the rate of deiodination. It is not clear whether deiodination is due to a process unrelated to β-oxidation or whether the alkynoic acid did not act as a suicide inhibitor but instead underwent β-oxidation. Testing this type of inhibition will require synthesis of an alkynoic acid with a stable carbon-iodine bond (see later discussion).

Inhibition of β-oxidation may also be achieved by the inclusion of carbon-carbon double bonds at appropriate locations within the fatty acid (alkenoic acids). Hypoglycin and its straight chain fatty acid analog 4-pentenoic acid (4-PA) (structure below) have long been known to inhibit long chain fatty acid oxidation *in vivo*. Studies of 4-PA [28,29] have shown that a metabolite of 4-PA acts to inhibit one or more enzymes of β-oxidation. One metabolite proposed to be responsible for inhibition is 2,4-pentadienoyl-CoA (structure below) a conjugated alkenoic acid ester. One study presents evidence for inhibition of the first dehydrogenation [30] but two other studies report strong inhibition of the 3-ketoacyl-CoA thiolase [31-33], the cleavage step of β-oxidation producing AcCoA and a new, shorter acyl-CoA. However, another metabolite, 3-keto-4-pentenoic acid, appears to inhibit the thiolase both reversibly and irreversibly [34].

4-pentenoic acid	$CH_2=CHCH_2CH_2CO_2H$
2,4-pentadienoyl-CoA	$CH_2=CHCH=CH-\overset{O}{\overset{\Vert}{C}}-CoA$
3-keto-4-pentenoic acid	$CH_2=CH-\overset{O}{\overset{\Vert}{C}}-CH_2CO_2H$

Long chain fatty acids containing double bonds at even numbered positions (4-, 6-, etc.) should inhibit β-oxidation as longchain analogs of either 2, 4-dienoyl-CoA esters or 3-keto-4-pentenoyl-CoA esters, would arise from normal β-oxidation processes. Studies by Lippel *et al.* [35,36] Reitz *et al.* [37] and others [38-40] utilizing positional isomers of octadecenoic acid have shown alternating patterns of behavior in activation and in storage as triglycerides, phospholipids and cholesterol esters. Thus, metabolic properties appear to be governed by the position of the double bond. It may be that formation of conjugated bonds versus formation of nonconjugated bonds during β-oxidation accounts for the observed alternating patterns. A report [41] has appeared which suggests that β-oxidation was inhibited by octadecenoic acid with double bonds at even positions. There was evidence for the formation of new enoic acids (unidentified) of shorter length corresponding to those predicted if a conjugated diene was formed and acted an inhibitor.

The presence of an odd-even effect for double-bond position coupled with the evidence for β-oxidation inhibition by even position double bonds prompted evaluation of an even (double bond at carbon 4) and an odd position (double bond at carbon 9) ω-iodohexadecenoic acid.

Even position	$^{125}I(CH_2)_{11}CH=CH(CH_2)_2CO_2H$
Odd postion	$^{125}I(CH_2)_6CH=CH(CH_2)_7CO_2H$

For the even position acid, heart values decreased from 0.23 ± 0.01% kg dose/g

(N = 5) at t = 5 min to 0.14 ± 0.01 at t = 20 min, a decrease of 40%. At t = 40 min, the value was 0.15 ± 0.01% kg dose/g (N = 5). For the odd position acid, heart values were 0.57 ± 0.06% kg dose/g (N = 5) at 5 min and 0.16 ± 0.01 at 20 min, a decrease of 70%. Liver and blood values for both even and odd position acids were experimentally equivalent. The thyroid values were quite different. The odd position double bond may be expected to behave as a saturated ω-iodo acid; that is, β-oxidation should not be inhibited; however, the thyroid values rose rapidly from 2.98 ± 0.36% kg dose/g at 5 min to 10.1 ± 0.9 at 20 min, a faster accumulation than observed for the saturated acid [22]. The thyroid values for the even position alkenoic acid rose more slowly; at t = 20 min the thyroid value was half that observed for the odd position acid.

Incorporation of a double bond at an even position resulted in: 1) a reduction of myocardial activity levels at t = 5 min, 2) a slower rate of decreasing myocardial activity relative to the odd position acid, and 3) a slower rate of thyroid activity increase. The reduction of activity levels in the heart may reflect the sensitivity of the rat heart to carbon chain manipulations. It cannot be said that β-oxidation inhibition has been achieved. The rate of myocardial activity decrease and thyroid activity increase for the even acid closely parallels results obtained with the long chain ω-iodo fatty acids which were shown to be stored as triglycerides. Further work is needed to determine whether inhibition or storage has occurred.

Effects of branched-chain acids

Alteration of the normal, straight-chain, saturated acids by introducing alkyl branching is the second approach to inhibition of β-oxidation to be discusssed in this chapter.

An examination of the essential steps of β-oxidation (Figure 2) reveals several sites for interference in the process by mono- or dialkylation. Interference can occur in two ways: a) the acid is a potential substrate but acts as an inhibitor, and b) the acid is theoretically not a substrate and acts as an anti-metabolite. Of the various alkyl groups which could be substituted for hydrogen, the best is expected to be the methyl, $-CH_3$, group. It is the smallest alkyl group and would provide the least steric hindrance to transport and activation. Since β-oxidation consists of repeated passages through four enzymatic reactions, branching could occur at the α or β carbon of the original acid or at incipient α or β carbons. For example, a methyl group at carbon 5 should have the same inhibitory or anti-metabolite activity as a methyl at carbon 3. Carbon 5 becomes a β carbon after one cycle through β-oxidation.

The first step of β-oxidation, catalyzed by acyl-CoA dehydrogenase, requires minimally one hydrogen atom on both α and β carbons (indicated in bold face in Figure 2 and labeled in Figure 5 below). Dialkylation at either the α or β

Potential inhibition by dimethylation

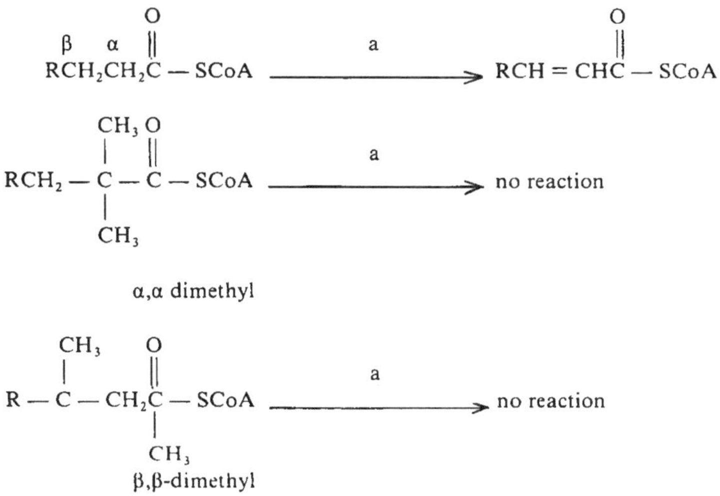

$$\underset{\beta\ \ \alpha}{RCH_2CH_2}\overset{O}{\overset{\|}{C}}-SCoA \xrightarrow{a} RCH=CH\overset{O}{\overset{\|}{C}}-SCoA$$

$$RCH_2-\underset{CH_3}{\overset{CH_3}{\overset{|}{\underset{|}{C}}}}-\overset{O}{\overset{\|}{C}}-SCoA \xrightarrow{a} \text{no reaction}$$

α,α dimethyl

$$R-\underset{CH_3}{\overset{CH_3}{\overset{|}{\underset{|}{C}}}}-CH_2\overset{O}{\overset{\|}{C}}-SCoA \xrightarrow{a} \text{no reaction}$$

β,β-dimethyl

Figure 5. Inhibition by dimethyl-substituted fatty acids:
a = acyl-CoA dehydrogenase.

carbon would theoretically yield a fatty acid which would be an anti-metabolite. There is in fact experimental evidence that neither α,α-dimethyl nor β,β-dimethyl fatty acids undergo β-oxidation. Bergström *et al.* [42] and Tryding and Westöö [43] have demonstrated that β-oxidation of 2,2-dimethylstearic acid (an α,α-dimethyl acid) does not occur. Goodman and Steinberg [44] studied 3,3-dimethylphenylmyristic acid (a β,β-dimethyl acid) and concluded that *in vivo* oxidation proceeds slowly or not at all. Monoalkylation at either the α or β carbon would yield a fatty acid which may function as an inhibitor of acyl-CoA dehydrogenase.

The third step of β-oxidation, the second dehydrogenation to yield a β-ketoacyl-CoA ester, requires the presence of a β-hydrogen. Monoalkylation at the β carbon should yield an anti-metabolite, see Figure 6. Monoalkylation at the α carbon would yield an acid capable of reaction but one which may act as an inhibitor. In addition, the second and fourth steps, hydration and thiolase cleavage, respectively, may be inhibited by α or β monoalkylation.

A preliminary evaluation of branching at the β position was reported by our laboratory [45]. The compound evaluated was 13-(^{125}I)iodo-3-methyltridecanoic acid, a β-methyl 13 carbon chain acid, x = 10 in the structure below.

$$^{*}I(CH_2)_x\underset{CH_3}{CH}CH_2CO_2H$$

The results were not promising as myocardial radioactivity levels at t = 5 min

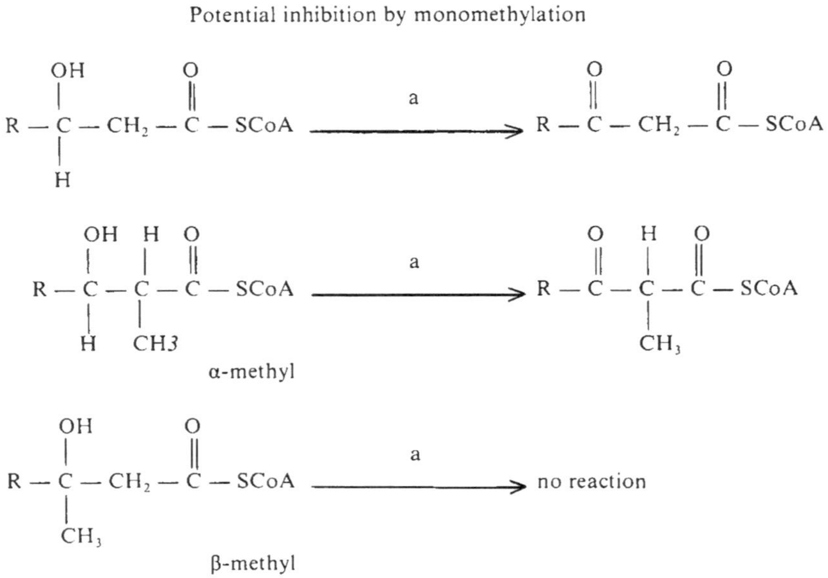

Potential inhibition by monomethylation

$$R-CH(OH)-CH_2-C(=O)-SCoA \xrightarrow{a} R-C(=O)-CH_2-C(=O)-SCoA$$

$$R-CH(OH)-CH(CH_3)-C(=O)-SCoA \xrightarrow{a} R-C(=O)-CH(CH_3)-C(=O)-SCoA$$

α-methyl

$$R-C(OH)(CH_3)-CH_2-C(=O)-SCoA \xrightarrow{a} \text{no reaction}$$

β-methyl

Figure 6. Inhibition by α or β monomethyl-substituted fatty acids: a = 3-L-hydroxyacyl-CoA dehydrogenase

were low and residence time short. Furthermore, blood and thyroid activity values were high, suggestive of extensive deiodination. Myocardial radioactivity values for β-methyl ^{11}C fatty acids have been obtained and are reported to be high and essentially constant over 1 h [46,47]. These acids behaved as expected for an anti-metabolite and gave support to the hypothesis that interference of normal β-oxidation by branching would increase myocardial residence time.

A more detailed evaluation of the effects of alkylation and chain length was completed and the results published [48]. As observed previously for unbranched acids, chain length of the β-methyl fatty acids also affected myocardial activity levels. The natural-length, 16-carbon acid ($x = 13$ in structure above) had myocardial radioactivity values 2.5-fold greater at $t = 5$ min than the 13-carbon β-methyl acid. The value at 5 min for the 16-carbon β-methyl acid, $0.34 \pm 0.04\%$ kg dose/g, is experimentally equivalent to the value for the straight-chain 16-carbon acid [22]. This suggests that the presence of the β-methyl substituent does not significantly alter myocardial concentration for alkyl fatty acids. Thus, monoalkylation at the β-carbon apparently does not interfere with transport into the myocardial cell for alkyl fatty acids.

Dialkylation at the β-carbon virtually eliminated myocardial extraction. Activity levels are reduced by a factor of ten for a β,β-dimethyl acid in comparison with either the 16-carbon straight-chain or 16-carbon β-methyl acids. Liver concentration for the β,β-dimethyl acid was 3-fold greater at $t = 5$ min than for the β-methyl acid.

If the β-methyl alkyl fatty acids are not substrates for the second dehydrogenation step of β-oxidation, then a linear or slowly decreasing relationship between radioactivity level and time is expected. This type of relationship was observed by Livni *et al.* [46] for the ^{11}C β-methyl acid. F F Knapp, Jr *et al.* [49] observed extensive deiodination of 17-(^{131}I)iodo-9-telluroheptadecanoic acid (17-iodo-9-THDA). Degradation of 17-iodo-9-THDA by β-oxidation is not expected to continue beyond the tellurium atom; thus, this acid is also expected to function as an anti-metabolite of β-oxidation. The difference in behavior between the ω-iodo β-methyl acid, 17-iodo-9-THDA, and the ^{11}C β-methyl acid, all of which are theoretical anti-metabolites, strongly suggests chemical or enzymatic deiodination of the ω-iodo branched chain alkanoic acids independent of β-oxidation. This deiodination presumably can occur for the ω-iodo straight-chain fatty acids as well.

The assumptions that radioiodide is released from IAcCoA, the final catabolite of β-oxidation, and that inhibition or prevention of β-oxidation would prolong myocardial residence time of ω-iodo alkyl acids, are clearly not supported by the data presented in this and the preceding section. Although rapid deiodination occurs both for ω-iodo acids designed to inhibit or prevent β-oxidation and for straight-chain acids, it cannot be concluded that all deiodination is unrelated to β-oxidation. The mechanism of radioiodide release from ω-iodo acids is still unknown but the evidence presented here, together with data from the ω-iodo aryl acids (see following discussion), suggests that hydrolysis may be a major contributor to free radioiodide.

Stabilization of carbon-iodine bond

Deiodination of the ω-iodo alkanoic acids may result from direct cleavage of the carbon-iodine bond by hydrolysis or enzymatic activity acting on the injected radiolabeled acid. Loss of iodide from the postulated final catabolites, iodoacetyl- or iodopropyl-CoA is also possible but evidence presented in this chapter suggests that only a small amount of deiodination is related to the process of β-oxidation. Iodine attached to a -CH_2- group (ICH_2-) is known to be easily displaced by other molecules such as water. The length of the carbon to iodine bond reflects the strength of this bond. If the length of the bond could be reduced, bond strength would increase and the rate of deiodination by displacement should decrease. Increasing bond strength can be referred to as bond stabilization. For iodine, this stabilization can be achieved by using vinylic or aryl carbons as illustrated below instead of alkyl carbons as used previously. Both types of stabilization have been evaluated.

vinylic stabilization I — C = C —

aryl stabilization I—⟨◯⟩—

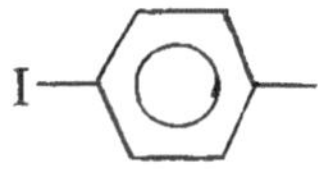

An ω-iodo vinylic acid, ^{125}I-11-iodo-10-undecenoic acid, was prepared using a

$$^{125}ICH = CH(CH_2)_8CO_2H$$

precursor prepared by Dr G.W. Kabalka of the University of Tennessee and evaluated in rats [50]. Heart values at t = 5 min were lower than observed for the saturated ω-iodo analog: 0.17 ± 0.01% kg dose/g vs 0.35 ± 0.02% [22]. Liver, lung and thyroid values were comparable for both acids. Blood values were considerably elevated for the ω-iodo vinylic acid (0.34 ± 0.01% kg dose/g at t = 5 min) than for the saturated analog (0.21 ± 0.02% [22]). The low myocardial values coupled with high blood values were not promising in terms of imaging. Further efforts using vinyl stabilization have not been pursued.

Machulla, in 1980, coupled Knoop's demonstration of the mechanism of β-oxidation using ω-phenyl fatty acids with the greater stability of aryl carbon-iodine bonds towards hydrolysis and proposed ω-iodophenyl fatty acids as

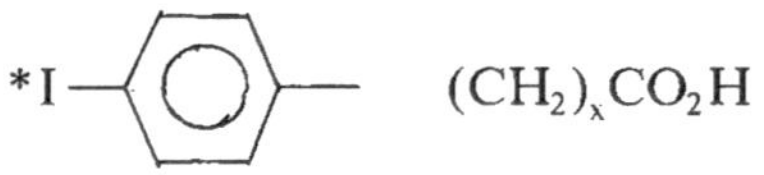

*I—⟨◯⟩— $(CH_2)_xCO_2H$

candidates for metabolic probes of the myocardium [51]. Further work established that ω-bromophenyl fatty acids [52,53] are also useful as myocardial imaging agents. Dehalogenation is not observed with either ω-halophenyl fatty acid [51,52]; thus, the problems of hydrolysis found for the ω-iodo alkyl acids are avoided. The decreasing radioactivity levels in the heart are now related to the diffusion out of the heart of the observed catabolites, p-halobenzoic acid and p-halophenylpropanoic acid [52], rather than to diffusion of free radioiodine. It remains to be firmly established that the rates of decreasing myocardial radioactivity levels are quantitatively correlated to the rate of β-oxidation.

As Machulla had previously studied the dependence of uptake and elimination on chain length and had determined that the 15 carbon length (x = 14 in structure above) was optimal [54], the combined effects of chain branching and chain length within the ω-iodophenyl fatty acids were studied.

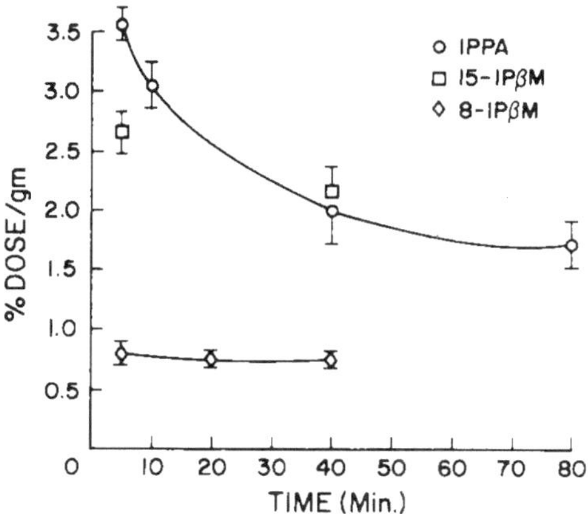

Figure 7. Time course of radioactivity in myocardium of rats after i.v. injection of IPPA and 8-IPβM. (Reprinted by permission from J Nucl Med 1984, 25: 75 - 80)

Myocardial activity levels for the iodide-stabilized ω-iodophenyl β-methyl fatty acids were found to be dependent on chain length [48]. For example, at

$$*I - C_6H_4 - (CH_2)_x - \underset{\displaystyle CH_3}{CH} - CH_2CO_2H$$

t = 5 min the activity in the heart for 15-(p-[^{125}I]iodophenyl)-3-methylpentadecanoic acid (15-IPβM) (x = 12 in structure above) was 2.66 ± 0.18% dose/g whereas the value for 8-(p-[^{125}I]iodophenyl)-3-methyloctanoic acid (8-IPβM) was 0.80 ± 0.10. In contrast to another study comparing straight-chain with branched chain ω-iodophenyl acids [55], it was found that branching reduced myocardial activity levels as the value for the straight-chain acid, 15-(p-[^{125}I]-iodophenyl)pentadecanoic acid (IPPA), was 3.56 ± 0.14% dose/g, about 33% higher than observed for 15-IPβM. This is also in contrast to the effects of branching in the ω-iodo alkyl fatty acids where myocardial activity values at t = 5 min were not significantly affected by branching for a 16-carbon acid.

Figure 7 illustrates the time course of activity for IPPA and 8-IPβM. Data at 5 and 40 min from 15-IPβM are included for purposes of comparison. The difference in the time course between straight-chain and branched chain ω-iodo-phenyl acids is clear. IPPA is expected to behave as 15-(p-[^{75}Br]bromophenyl)-pentadecanoic acid (BPPA) [52], which has been shown to undergo β-oxidation. The activity of IPPA in the heart decreases with time as was observed for BPPA. Both aryl branched-chain acids remain in the heart at experimentally constant levels from 5 to 40 min. These results parallel data obtained with a β-methyl-^{11}C alkyl fatty acid [46]. The slower rate (or lack) of metabolism of the branched chain acids suggested by the data can be explained by assuming that these acids are not substrates for β-oxidation.

In an effort to probe the means of myocardial retention of the ω-phenyl β-methyl branched acids, subcellular distribution studies using a centrifugation procedure of both 8- and 15-IPβM and IPPA were performed. The theoretical product of dehydrogenation and hydration, the first two steps of β-oxidation, is a β-hydroxy, β-methyl acid which should be an anti-metabolite for the second dehydrogenation. One could postulate that the anti-metabolite would be trapped in the mitochondria and that radioactivity in the mitochondria would increase with time as the fatty acid extracted from the blood underwent β-oxidation.

Although significant differences in the distribution of subcellular radioactivity was found [56] for the three acids evaluated, the distribution does not support trapping of the aryl β-methyl acids in the mitochondria. For both 8- and 15-IPβM approximately constant levels of radioactivity were found in the mitochondria at both time intervals studied. Due to possible differences in lipophilicity between aryl and alkyl fatty acids, the distribution of radioactivity for the β-methyl fatty acid may be different and may show evidence for mitochondrial trapping.

The chain length of the aryl β-methyl fatty acids affected the location of radioactivity within the cell. The longer chain 15-IPβM and IPPA were both associated largely with the nuclear/membrane fraction whereas the shorter 8-IPβM was largely found in the cytosol [56].

Summary

Several carbon chain manipulations have been studied in terms of their effects on myocardial activity levels and residence time. The manipulations examined included: chain length, chain branching, chain unsaturation, and carbon--iodine bond stabilization. It was found that chain length affects myocardial activity levels for both straight-chain alkyl acids and branched chain alkyl and aryl acids. Similar results have been reported for the straight-chain aryl acids [54]. Generally, the longer chain lengths correlated with higher myocardial activity levels and longer residence times. This behavior is attributed to storage as triglycerides. Branched chain acids are designed to be anti-metabolites but only the aryl β-methyl acids possessed the expected time course of constant or very slowly decreasing activity levels. The alkyl β-methyl acids underwent rapid deiodination — a process apparently independent of β-oxidation. Inhibition of β-oxidation by incorporation of carbon-carbon double and triple bonds was studied. A double bond at an even carbon position (carbon four) resulted in increased residence time but was accompanied by reduced myocardial activity.

Deiodination of ω-iodo alkyl fatty acids prevented an assessment of suicide inhibition using an unsaturated alkynoic acid.

Stabilization of the carbon-iodine bond by attachment of iodine to a vinylic or aryl carbon was studied. The low myocardial values and high blood values observed for an eleven carbon ω-iodo vinylic fatty acid were not encouraging but ω-iodo aryl fatty acids appear to avoid the problems of rapid deiodination.

Future developments

Basic research is still needed in order to clearly understand and interpret the human myocardial images obtained using radioiodinated fatty acids. Two areas of research include chemical and biochemical studies. Future chemical research efforts may include the synthesis and radiolabeling of several types of fatty acids not yet thoroughly examined. For example, since chain length has been shown to be important, vinylic stabilization of the carbon-iodine bond should be studied using chain lengths of 16 or 17 carbons. Alkynyl stabilization (*I — C = C —) has not been examined in detail. In light of the rapid deiodination experienced with the ω-iodo alkyl acids, inhibition by incorporation of double or triple bonds needs to be reevaluated using stable carbon-iodine bonds. Biochemical analysis of *in vivo* enzymatic rates of all steps of fatty acid catabolism is needed. Changes in subcellular location with time in normal and diseased heart tissue is also needed.

Perhaps one of the most promising areas of research in terms of imaging is the combined usage of several different metabolic probes. For example, a recent report uses both a glucose and a fatty acid probe to determine the effects of hypertension on global and regional substrate uptake in rat heart [57]. Use of combinations of fatty acids which inhibit different steps of β-oxidation or which are primarily stored may permit an accurate metabolic assessment of fatty acid utilization and may therefore be useful in diagnosis of cardiac disease.

References

1. Evans J R, Gunton R W, Baker R G *et al.* (1965) Use of radioiodinated fatty acid for photoscans of the heart. Circ Res 16: 1 - 10
2. Poe N D, Robinson G D Jr, MacDonald N S (1975) Myocardial extraction of labelled long-chain fatty acid analogs. Proc Soc Exp Biol Med 148: 215 - 218
3. Robinson G D Jr, Lee A W (1975) Radioiodinated fatty acids for heart imaging: iodine monochloride addition compared with iodide replacement labeling. J Nucl Med 16: 17 - 21
4. Bonte F J, Graham K D, Moore J G (1973) Experimental myocardial imaging with ^{131}I-labeled oleic acid. Radiology 108: 195 - 196
5. Gunton R W, Evans J R, Baker R G *et al.* (1965) Demonstration of myocardial infarction by photoscans of the heart in man. Am J Cardiol 16: 482 - 487

6. Machulla H-J, Stöcklin G, Kupfernagel C *et al.* (1978) Comparative evaluation of fatty acids labeled with C-11, Cl-34m, Br-77, and I-123 for metabolic studies of the myocardium: concise communication. J Nucl Med 19: 298 - 302
7. Höck A, Freundlieb C, Vyska K *et al.* (1983) Myocardial imaging and studies with (17-123I)iodoheptadecanoic acid in patients with idiopathic congestive cardiomyopathy. J Nucl Med 24: 22 - 28
8. van der Wall E E, Heidendal G A, den Hollander W *et al.* (1983) Myocardial scintigraphy with 123I-labelled heptadecanoic acid in patients with unstable angina pectoris. Postgrad Med J 59,(Suppl 3): 38 - 40
9. Robinson G D Jr (1977) Synthesis of ^{123}I-16-iodo-9-hexadecenoic acid and derivatives for use as myocardial perfusion imaging agents. Int J Appl Rad Isot 28: 149 - 155
10. Poe N D, Robinson G D Jr, Graham L S *et al.* (1976) Experimental basis for myocardial imaging with ^{123}I-labeled hexadecenoic acid. J Nucl Med 17: 1077 - 1082
11. Poe N D, Robinson G D Jr, Zielinski F W *et al.* (1977) Myocardial imaging with ^{123}I-hexadecenoic acid. Radiology 124: 419 - 424
12. Rocquelin G, Sergiel J P, Martin B *et al.* (1971) Nutritive value of refined rapeseed oils: Review. J Am Oil Chem Soc 48: 728 - 732
13. Beare-Rogers J L, Nera E A (1972) Cardiac fatty acids and histopathology of rats, pigs, monkeys and gerbils fed rapeseed oil. Comp Biochem Physiol 41B: 793 - 800
14. Beare-Rogers J L, Nera E A, Craig B M (1972) Accumulation of cardiac fatty acids in rats fed synthesized oils containing C_{22} fatty acids. Lipids 7: 46 - 50
15. Engfelt B (ed) (1976) Morphological and biochemical effects of orally administered rapeseed oil in rat myocardium. Acta Med Scand. (Suppl) 585: 1 - 86
16. Christiansen R Z, Christophersen B O, Bremer J (1977) Monoethylenic C_{20} and C_{22} fatty acids in marine oil and rapeseed oil. Studies on their oxidation and on their relative ability to inhibit palmitate oxidation in heart and liver mitochondria. Biochim Biophys Acta 487: 28 - 36
17. Cheng C-K, Pande S V (1975) Erucic acid metabolism by rat heart preparations. Lipids 10: 335 - 339
18. Christophersen B O, Christiansen R Z (1975) Studies on the mechanism of the inhibitory effects of erucylcarnitine in rat heart mitochondria. Biochim Biophys Acta 388: 402 - 412
19. Ishinaga M, Sato J, Kitigawa Y *et al.* (1982) Perturbation of phospholipid metabolism by erucic acid in male Sprague-Dawley rat heart. J Biochem (Tokyo) 92: 253 - 263
20. Vasdev S C, Kako K J (1977) Incorporation of fatty acids into rat heart lipids. *In vivo* and *in vitro* studies. J Mol Cell Cardiol 9: 617 - 631
21. Ong N, Bezard J, LeCerf J (1977) Incorporation and metabolic conversion of erucic acid in various tissue of the rat in short term experiments. Lipids 12: 563 - 569
22. Otto C A, Brown L E, Wieland D M *et al.* (1981) Radioiodinated fatty acid for myocardial imaging: effects of chain length. J Nucl Med 22: 613 - 618
23. Kloster G, Stöcklin G (1982) Determination of the rate-determining step in halofatty acid turnover in the heart. Radioakt Isot Klin Forsch 15: 235 - 241
24. Stöcklin G (1982) Evaluation of radiohalogen labelled fatty acids for heart studies. Nuklearmedizin (Suppl) 19: 229 - 304
25. Otto C A, Brown L E, Wieland D M *et al.* (1981) Synthesis of ^{125}I-labeled 14-iodo-9-tetradecynoic acid. J Labeled Compd Radiopharm 18: 1347 - 1355
26. Helmkamp G M Jr, Rando R R, Brock D J H *et al.* (1968) β-Hydroxydecanoyl thioester dehydrase. J Biol Chem 243: 3229 - 3231
27. Endo K, Helmkamp G M Jr, Bloch K (1970) Mode of inhibition of β-hydrocydecanoyl thioester dehydrase by 3-decynoyl-N-acetylcysteamine. J Biol Chem 245: 4293 - 4296
28. Sherratt H S A, Holland P C, Osmundsen H *et al.* (1975) On the mechanism of inhibition of fatty acid oxidation by hypoglycin and by pent-4-enoic acid. In: Kean E A (ed) Hypoglycin: Proceedings of a Symposium, Kingston, Jamaica, Vol. 3. New York: Academic Press, p 127

29. Sherratt H S A, Osmundsen H (1976) Commentary on the mechanisms of some pharmacological actions of the hypoglycaemic toxins hypoglycin and pent-4-enoic acid. A way out of the present confusion. Biochem Pharm 25: 743 - 750
30. Osmundsen H (1978) Effects of pent-4-enoate on flux through acyl-CoA dehydrogenases of β-oxidation in intact rat liver mitochondria. FEBS Lett 88: 219 - 222
31. Fong J C, Schulz H (1978) On the rate-determining step of fatty acid oxidation in heart. J Biol Chem 253: 6917 - 6922
32. Holland P C, Senior A E, Sherratt H S A (1973) Biochemical effects of the hypoglycaemic compound pent-4-enoic acid and related non-hypoglycaemic fatty acids. Biochem J 136: 173 -184
33. Holland P C, Sherratt H S A (1973) Biochemical effects of the hypoglycaemic compound pent-4-enoic acid and related non-hypoglycaemic fatty acids. Biochem J 136: 157 - 171
34. Schulz H (1983) Metabolism of 4-pentenoic acid and inhibition of thiolase by metabolites of 4-pentenoic acid. Biochemistry 22: 1827 - 1832
35. Lippel K, Carpenter D, Gunstone F D. (1973) Activation of long chain fatty acids by subcellular fractions of rat liver. III. Effect of ethylenic bond position on acyl-CoA formation of *cis*-octadecenoates. Lipids 8: 124 - 128
36. Lippel K. Gunsone F D, Barve J A (1973) Activation of long chain fatty acids by subcellular fractions of rat liver. II. Effect of ethylenic bond position on acyl-CoA formation of *trans*-octadecenoates. Lipids 8: 119 - 123
37. Reitz R C, El-Sheikh M, Lands W E M *et al.* (1969) Effects of ethylenic bond position upon acyltransferase activity with isomeric *cis*-octadecenoyl coenzyme A thiol esters. Biochim Biophys Acta 176: 480 - 490
38. Sgoutas D, Jones R, Befanis P. (1976) In vitro incorporation of isomeric cis-octadecanoic acids by rat liver mitochondria. Biochim Biophys Acta 441: 14 - 24
39. Sgoutas D S (1971) Comparative studies on the hydrolysis of odd-chain and even-chain fatty acid cholesterol esters by rat liver sterol-ester hydrolase. Biochim Biophys Acta 239: 469 - 474
40. Goller H J, Sgoutas D S (1970) Further studies on the fatty acid specificity of rat liver sterol-ester hydrolase. Biochem 9: 4801 - 4806
41. Willebrands A F, van der Veen K J (1966) The metabolism of elaidic acid in the perfused rat heart. Biochim Biophys Acta 116: 583 - 585
42. Bergström S, Borgström B, Tryding N. (1954) Intestinal absorption and metabolism of 2,2-dimethylstearic acid in the rat. Biochem J 58: 604 - 608
43. Tryding N, Westöö G (1956) Synthesis and metabolism of 2,2-dimethylnonadecanoic acid. Acta Chem Scand 10: 1234 - 1242
44. Goodman D S, Steinberg D (1958) Studies in the metabolism of 3,3-dimethyl phenylmyristic acid, a nonoxidizable fatty acid analogue. J Biol Chem 233: 1066 - 1071
45. Otto C A, Brown L E, Wieland D M *et al* (1981) Structure-distribution study of I-125-ω-iodo-fatty acids. J Labelled Compd Radiopharm 18: 43 - 44
46. Livni E, Elmaleh D R, Levy S *et al.* (1982) Beta-methyl(1-^{11}C)heptadecanoic acid: a new myocardial metabolic tracer for positron emission tomography. J Nucl Med 23: 169 - 175
47. Elmaleh D R, Livni E, Levy S *et al.* (1983) Comparison of ^{11}C and ^{14}C-labeled fatty acids and their β-methyl analogs. Int J Nucl Med Biol 10: 181 - 187
48. Otto C A, Brown L E, Scott A M (1984) Radioiodinated branched chain fatty acids: substrates for beta oxidation? Concise communication. J Nucl Med 25: 75 - 80
49. Goodman M M, Knapp F F Jr, Callahan A P *et al.* (1982) Synthesis and biological evaluation of 17-(^{131}I)iodo-9-telluraheptadecanoic acid, a potential new myocardial imaging agent. J Med Chem 25: 613 - 618
50. Otto C A, unpublished data
51. Machulla H-J, Marsmann M, Dutschka K (1980) Biochemical concept and synthesis of a radioiodinated phenylfatty acid for *in vivo* metabolic studies of the myocardium. Eur J Nucl Med 5: 171 - 173

52. Coenen H H, Harmand M-F, Kloster G *et al.* (1981) 15(p-(^{75}Br)bromophenyl)pentadecanoic acid: pharmacokinetics and potential as heart agent. J Nucl Med 22: 891 - 896
53. Machulla H-J, Marsmann, Dutschka K *et al.* (1980) Radiopharmaceuticals. II. Radiobromination of phenylpentadecanoic acid and biodistribution in mice. Radiochem Radional Lett 42: 243 - 250
54. Machulla H J, Dutschka K, van Beuningen D *et al.* (1981) Development of 15-(p-iodine-123-pehyl)-pentadecanoic acid for *in vivo* diagnosis of the myocardium. J Radioanal Chem 65: 279 - 286
55. Goodman M M, Kirsch G, Knapp F F Jr (1984) Synthesis and evaluation of radioiodinated terminal P-iodophenyl-substituted α- and β-methyl-branched fatty acids. J Med Chem 27: 390 - 397
56. Otto C A, Brown L E, Lee H: Subcellular distribution of (^{125}I)iodoaryl beta-methyl fatty acids. Accepted for publication by Int J Nucl Med Biol
57. Yonekura Y, Brill A B, Som P *et al.* (1985) Regional myocardial substrate uptake in hypertensive rats: a quantitative autoradiographic measurement. Science 227: 1494 - 1496

4. Uptake and distribution of radioiodinated free fatty acids in the dog heart

G. WESTERA, F.C. VISSER and E.E. van der WALL

Introduction

The heart may be considered as a machine which continuously performs a substantial amount of work. The energy required for that work is (under normal circumstances) to a large extent (60-70%) supplied by the oxidation of free (unesterified) fatty acids [1]. This makes such compounds attractive targets in the search for a tracer to follow myocardial energy metabolism. When labeled with a gamma radiation emitting isotope, such substances may be observed with a gamma-camera and eventually their time course in the heart can be studied *in vivo* and differences in metabolic behaviour between normal and pathological heart tissue may be noticed.

Free fatty acids consist of atoms of the elements carbon (C), hydrogen and oxygen. The only gamma-emitting isotope of one of these elements which can reasonably be used for labeling free fatty acids and subsequent biological studies is carbon-11 (^{11}C). The 20 min half-life of ^{11}C obviously limits its applicability: one has to prepare the isotope "in house", for which a suitable particle accelerator (cyclotron or Van der Graaf-generator) is needed and only short-time studies can be performed. Furthermore ^{11}C is a positron emitter and for its detection one essentially needs a positron emission tomographic system. This combination of technical facilities is very expensive and available in only a few institutes.

A lot of effort has therefore been spent on the design, synthesis and evaluation of free fatty acids labeled with suitable, gamma-emitting heteroisotopes (halogens, mainly iodine, tellurium). We have recently reviewed this subject, with respect to the aspect of free fatty acids uptake in the heart [2], which is of course the first feature of importance after application of a radiopharmaceutical.

In this chapter we shall describe our work on the uptake of several iodinated free fatty acids in the heart, their regional distribution and the influence of coronary artery occlusion and medication with beta-blocking pharmaceuticals on both uptake and regional distribution.

Total uptake of free fatty acids in the left ventricle of the dog heart

The iodinated free fatty acids studied by us were 17-iodoheptadecanoic acid (I-HDA), 16-iodo-9-hexadecenoic acid (I-HA) and 15-(4-iodophenyl)-pentadecanoic acid (I-PPA). These have been thoroughly evaluated in experimental and clinical studies [2]. Free fatty acids with a chain length of 16 or 18 C-atoms are most abundant in nature and their uptake by the myocardium is highest.

The iodine in the used iodinated free fatty acids is attached to the end of the carbon chain (omega position); in this way its nature of hetero-atom is disguised: the iodine has about the size of a methyl-group and the biological properties of omega-iodinated free fatty acids resemble very closely those of the analogous normal free fatty acids with a chain one C-atom longer [3]. In our animal studies we used I-125 and I-131 as radiotracer. The feature of the phenyl-group in 15-(4-iodophenyl)-pentadecanoic acid was added because this was supposed to prolong myocardial retention, to reduce blood background levels and to prevent the iodine from finding its way to the thyroid [4], because the final catabolyte will be iodobenzoic acid instead of iodide.

The uptake of these compounds in the left ventricle of the dog heart for normal myocardium and for hearts made ischemic by occlusion of a branch of the left anterior descending coronary artery (LAD) is given in Table 1. The data are presented as a percentage of the injected dose (% i.d.) (not per unit weight), because we did not find a relationship between uptake and weight of the myocardium [5,6]. This stands to reason, while the energy requirements of the heart and not the weight of myocardial tissue will determine the demand for its major fuel [7]. Values for the uptake of ^{201}Tl-thallium-chloride have been

Table 1. Uptake of iodinated free fatty acids in the left ventricle of the dog heart[a] (mean ± S.D.)

	Normal myocardium		Occluded myocardium[b]	
	n[c]	% i.d.[d]	n[c]	% i.d.
I-HDA	4	4.2 ± 0.6	6	2.6 ± 0.6
I-HA	4	2.4 ± 0.6	7	2.4 ± 0.6
I-PPA	1	4.5	5	2.8 ± 0.8
^{201}Tl	4	4.6 ± 0.6	6	3.4 ± 0.6

The following will apply throughout this chapter:

[a] Uptake was measured 2-5 min after injection.

[b] Occluded myocardium: of these dogs a branch of the left anterior descending coronary artery was occluded.

[c] n = number of dogs.

[d] % i.d. = percentage of injected dose.

For other abbreviations see Text.

added, because ^{201}Tl is known (except under conditions of extremely low or high flow) to delineate regional perfusion [8].

For the uptake in normal myocardium, no difference was found between 17-iodoheptadecanoic acid (which is similar to that of naturally occurring free fatty acids [3]) and 15-(4-iodophenyl)-pentadecanoic acid. The length of the carbon + I-chain will be about the same for 17-iodoheptadecanoic acid and 15-(4-iodophenyl)-pentadecanoic acid, but the presence of the phenyl-group makes the end of the carbon-chain more rigid. Nevertheless this does not seem to influence the uptake significantly.

On the contrary, the uptake of 16-iodo-9-hexadecenoic acid was significantly lower than for 17-iodo-heptadecanoic acid. 16-iodo-9-hexadecenoic acid is an analogue of a fatty acid with a 17-carbon chain and 17-iodoheptadecanoic acid of an 18-carbon chain. Obviously the presence of an even number of "C-atoms" (like in naturally occurring free fatty acids) is essential for efficient myocardial uptake. We do not think the unsaturated double bond in 16-iodo-9-hexadecenoic acid to be an important factor, because a double bond has been shown not to influence myocardial uptake [9].

Passive diffusion has been postulated to be the mechanism of free fatty acid uptake. Nevertheless, it is hard to see how such a mechanism could discriminate between a 17- or 18-carbon chain, as it would only reflect differences in the lipophilicity of the carbon chain. An elegant hypothesis, which can be used to explain the known facts about myocardial uptake is the "dual uptake mechanism" idea: uptake is supposed to be governed by two mechanisms. Besides the *passive diffusion* there exists a *carrier mediated proces*, responsible for part of the myocardial free fatty acid uptake [10].

Earlier *in vitro* free fatty acid uptake experiments with cultured cardiac cells from chicken embryo [11] led to the same postulate and recently it was shown, that there may be an albumin receptor on the heart cell surface which mediates free fatty acid uptake [12].

Table 2. Uptake of radioiodinated free fatty acids in the left ventricle of the dog heart, when injected as a mixture.[a] (mean ± S.D.)

	Normal myocardium		Occluded myocardium	
Mixture	n	% i.d.	n	% i.d.
I-HDA + I-HA	1		5	
I-HDA		2.7		2.0 ± 0.5
I-HA		1.0		1.2 ± 0.3
I-HDA + I-PPA	1		5	
I-HDA		1.9		1.6 ± 0.6
I-PPA		2.3		1.9 ± 0.7

[a] The notes of Table 1 apply.
For abbreviations see Text.

Our results with the iodinated free fatty acid uptake when two iodinated free fatty acids were injected as a mixture point in the same direction (Table 2). The data indicate a diminished uptake for the individual iodinated free fatty acids. This competitive uptake is indicative for a dual uptake mechanism [10]. The similar affinity of myocardial cells for 16-iodo-9-hexadecenoic acid and 15-(4-iodophenyl)-pentadecanoic acid, higher as compared to 16-iodo-9-hexadecenoic acid, is also confirmed by these experiments.

Influence of ischemia

The influence of ischemia on myocardial uptake is clear (Tables 1 and 2): 17-iodoheptadecanoic acid and 15-(4-iodophenyl)-pentadecanoic acid uptake is diminished; 16-iodo-9-hexadecenoic acid uptake remains similar for ischemic myocardium. Again the hypothesis of a dual uptake mechanism i.e.

- *passive diffusion,* determined by the lipophilicity of the free fatty acids involved, and
- *a "carrier mediated"* mechanism favouring "natural" fatty acids with 18 (or 16) C-atoms

gives an attractive explanation. Ischemia requires the reduction of the supply of free fatty acids to myocardial cells: the heart changes its fuel for oxydation to carbohydrates [13] because they use less oxygen. This happens also in tissue adjacent to ischemic tissue [14]. For that purpose its carrier mediated mechanism is switched off, whereas this is not possible for passive diffusion. 16-iodo-9-hexadecenoic acid uptake remains the same (only passive diffusion), while 17-iodoheptadecanoic acid and 15-(4-iodophenyl)-pentadecanoic acid uptake is reduced.

The data from studies where a mixture of iodinated free fatty acids was injected in occluded dog myocardium (Table 2) confirm the above-mentioned conclusions. The decrease in free fatty acid uptake was accompanied by a decrease in myocardial blood flow, as indicated by the decrease in ^{201}Tl uptake. It seems (although the difference is not statistically significant) that 17-iodoheptadecanoic acid and 15-(4-iodophenyl)-pentadecanoic acid uptake is diminished more than flow [15], which may be explained by the shift from free fatty acids to carbohydrate metabolism [13,14].

Influence of beta-blocking agents

We also studied the influence of beta-blocking agents on the uptake of iodinated free fatty acids and ^{201}Tl in the heart [16], because of the obvious interest from the side of nuclear medicine to know about the influence of medication on uptake and distribution of a radiopharmaceutical. Besides, high myocardial free fatty acid concentrations may result in larger injury during and more arrhythmias after myocardial infarction [17,18].

Beta-sympatholitica act by the following mechanism of action: the beta-blocking agent occupies the catecholamine receptors (beta-receptors) and therefore the activating influence of the catecholamines is impaired. We have studied four beta-blocking agents with different properties [19]:

Table 3. Myocardial uptake (mean ± S.D.) of 17-iodoheptadecanoic acid (I-HDA) and ^{201}Tl under beta-blockade.[a]

	n[b]	I-HDA	^{201}Tl
Normal myocardium			
Control	4	4.2 ± 0.6	4.6 ± 0.6
Pindolol	4	2.5 ± 0.6	3.4 ± 0.6
Metoprolol	4	2.4 ± 0.2	3.0 ± 0.3
Timolol	4	2.7 ± 0.2	2.9 ± 0.4
Propranolol	4	3.8 ± 1.0	4.2 ± 1.7
Occluded myocardium			
Control	6	2.6 ± 0.3	3.4 ± 0.6
Pindolol	6	2.0 ±0.4	2.8 ± 0.6
Metoprolol	6	2.5 ± 0.9	3.0 ± 0.5
Timolol	6	2.2 ± 0.4	3.3 ± 0.7
Propranolol	6	3.4 ± 0.7	3.2 ± 0.3

[a] Equipotent doses of the beta-blockers were used.
[b] n = number of dogs.

Table 4. Plasma free fatty acid concentrations (mMol/l) before and after administration of beta-blocking agents[a]

Normal myocardium (n = 4)		After beta-blockade
0.70 ± 0.58	Pindolol	0.94 ± 0.41
0.35 ± 0.21	Metoprolol	0.35 ± 0.22
0.36 ± 0.24	Timolol	0.21 ± 0.11
0.30 ± 0.15	Propranolol	0.30 ± 0.16
Occluded myocardium (n = 6)		**After beta-blockade**
0.25 ± 0.09	Pindolol	0.41 ± 0.10
0.15 ± 0.10	Metoprolol	0.14 ± 0.09
0.38 ± 0.08	Timolol	0.27 ± 0.05
0.41 ± 0.16	Propranolol	0.28 ± 0.10

[a] The administration of ^{131}I-HDA did not change plasma free fatty acid concentration.

(1) pindolol, which has intrinsic sympathicomimetic activity (ISA), thus a partial stimulating influence of its own;
(2) metoprolol, which is cardioselective and blocks only beta-l receptors;
(3) propranolol, which shows membrane stabilizing activity (MSA); and
(4) timolol, without any outspoken special properties.

Besides the myocardial 17-iodoheptadecanoic acid uptake, we also measured the plasma free fatty acid concentrations (Table 4), because beta-blockers influence this parameter [19,23] and obviously the plasma free fatty acid concentration may in turn determine or at least influence the uptake of free fatty acids.

In the normal myocardium the percentage uptake was diminished after beta-blockade in accord with previous findings [24,26]except for blocking with propranolol. The absolute uptake, which can be estimated if the plasma free fatty acid concentration is also taken into account, is lower too, even where for pindolol the plasma concentration is increased.

After occlusion of a coronary artery diminished uptake was already expected (Table 1) and "treatment" with beta-blocking agents exerted little additional influence. In fact propranolol even caused an increase in percentage uptake, but as this is accompanied by a drop in plasma free fatty acids, the absolute amount of free fatty acids extracted by the heart may not have changed much. The same is probably true for pindolol, where the opposite situation exists: lower percentage uptake at higher plasma concentrations. Metoprolol did neither influence plasma concentration nor percentage uptake [21,22]. Timolol did not influence the percentage uptake, but with the lower plasma free fatty acid concentration, total uptake must have been diminished.

If it may be thought likely, that beta-blocking agents influence the "carrier mediated" uptake mechanism, the diminished uptake in normal myocardium can be understood. In occluded myocardium the carrier mediated mechanism has already been switched off, and it may depend on the individual properties of the beta-blocking agents, if any further effect may be noted. To verify if the metabolic consequences are linked with the special properties of the compounds (ISA, MSA, beta-l selectivity) more experiments are needed.

Regional distribution of myocardial iodinated free fatty acids

The iodinated free fatty acid uptake experiments were also designed to measure regional distribution of these compounds. After sacrificing the animals a few minutes after injection of the iodinated free fatty acids the heart was excised and cut into pieces according to a fixed pattern and the iodinated free fatty acid activity in the various pieces was determined. Thus a regional distribution was found, which we expressed as the endocardial/epicardial ratio: the ratio between uptake in the endocardium and the epicardium and, where appropriate, as the ratio between uptake in the nonischemic and the ischemic myocardium (Tables 5,6).

The endo-/epi-ratio was the same for all tracers studied and the same value was also found in normal parts of occluded myocardium. The value of ~1.2 indicates a higher uptake in the subendocardium. As can be seen from the equivalent ^{201}Tl-value, the distribution was according to flow. The higher iodinated free fatty acid uptake in the subendocardium parallels the flow-distribution and indicates that the subendocardium also performs most of the myocardial work.

In the ischemic part of occluded myocardium the endo-/epi-ratio was much lower (Table 5) than in normal tissue. This may be expected, because it is well

Table 5. The ratio of uptake of iodinated free fatty acids in the endocardium over the epicardium (endo-/epi-ratio), when injected with ^{201}Tl (A), or as a mixture (B)

		Normal myocardium		Occluded myocardium		
		n		n	Nonischemic	Ischemic
A	I-HA	4	1.29 ± 0.06	7	1.13 ± 0.12	0.83 ± 0.18
	I-HDA	4	1.21 ± 0.03	6	1.17 ± 0.09	0.57 ± 0.24
	I-PPA	1	1.12	5	1.14 ± 0.13	0.56 ± 0.18
	^{201}Tl	4	1.19 ± 0.02	6	1.16 ± 0.07	0.81 ± 0.19
B	I-HDA + I-HA					
	I-HA	1	1.27	5	1.17 ± 0.13	0.52 ± 0.08
	I-HDA	1	1.30	5	1.20 ± 0.12	0.48 ± 0.07
	I-HDA + I-PPA					
	I-HDA	1	1.08	5	1.17 ± 0.12	0.60 ± 0.11
	I-PPA	1	1.05	5	1.15 ± 0.11	0.55 ± 0.21

Table 6. The ratio between the uptake of iodinated free fatty acids in normal and ischemic myocardium, when injected with ^{201}Tl (A), or as a mixture (B)

		n	Ratio
A	I-HA	7	5.2 ± 3.1
	I-HDA	6	3.9 ± 0.9
	I-PPA	5	4.5 ± 1.2
	^{201}Tl	6	3.6 ± 0.7
B	I-HDA + I-HA		
	I-HA	5	3.4 ± 1.2
	I-HDA	5	4.1 ± 1.3
	I-HDA + I-PPA		
	I-HDA	5	4.4 ± 0.7
	I-PPA	5	5.3 ± 1.0

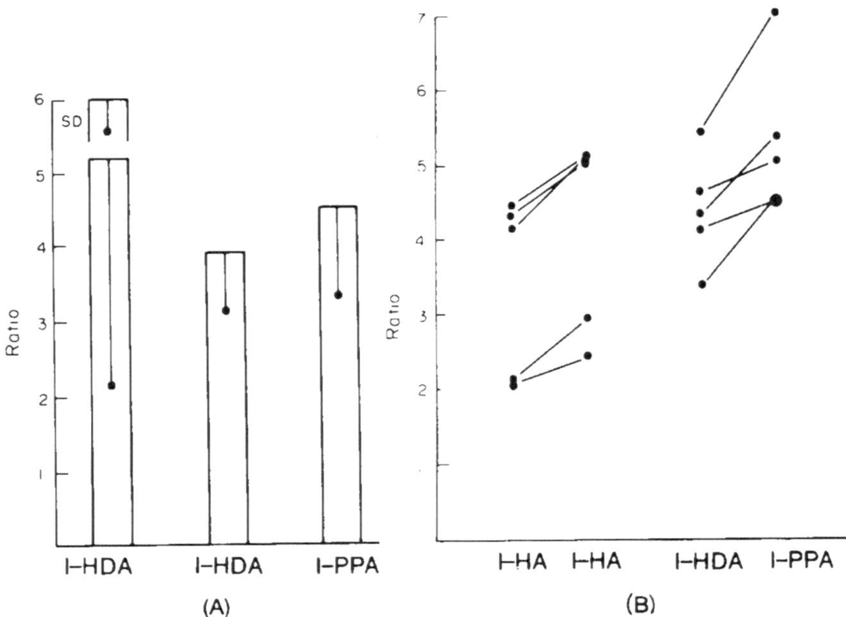

Figure 1. Ratio between uptake in nonischemic and ischemic part of occluded dog myocardium. (A) When one tracer FFA was administered; (B) For mixture of two acids. The connecting lines between the dots have no physical meaning. They just connect values found for the different acids in the same dog. For abbreviations see Text.

known [27] that myocardial ischemia starts from the endocardium to penetrate epicardial layers later on.

Although there is no statistically significant difference in uptake between the various tracers, it is interesting to notice that the two more "physiological" free fatty acids (17-iodoheptadecanoic acid and 15-(4-iodophenyl)-pentadecanoic acid) show a lower endo-/epi-ratio than the "flow tracer" ^{201}Tl and I-HA. This may be understood because the endocardium, more ischemic than the epicardium, will have to make the greater effort to shift its mechanism from free fatty acids to carbohydrates as the major fuel.

The residual uptake of iodinated free fatty acids in the ischemic area of occluded myocardium, is presented as the ratio uptake in normal over ischemic tissue. The data indicate that after occlusion still 15-20% is extracted by ischemic myocardial tissue. The residual flow seems a bit higher (though again the difference is not significant) fitting in with the picture of relatively diminished free fatty acid uptake.

Differences between the three free fatty acids can be seen (Figure 1) from the data obtained after injection of a mixture of two acids: the less "physiological" 16-iodo-9-hexadecanoic acid has been taken up relatively more by the ischemic myocardium.

The influence of beta-blockade on regional distribution

As treatment with beta-blockers is known to heavily influence the hemodynamic parameters of the heart, it is to be expected that it may also influence the metabolic processes which provide the energy for it.

The regional distribution of 17-iodoheptadecanoic acid (and ^{201}Tl) is given in Tables 7 and 8.

The expected drop in heart rate and systolic blood pressure was observed in all beta-blocked hearts. In the normal dog heart the distribution of 17-iodoheptadecanoic acid over endo- and epicardium was only altered in the case of metoprolol, where a relatively higher endocardial value was found. Relatively

Table 7. The ratio of uptake of 17-iodoheptadecanoic acid and ^{201}Tl in the endocardium over the epicardium under beta-blockade

	n	I-HDA	^{201}Tl
Normal myocardium			
Control	4	1.21 ± 0.03	1.20 ± 0.02
Pindolol	6	1.18 ± 0.05	1.19 ± 0.01
Metoprolol	6	1.38 ± 0.07	1.34 ± 0.10
Timolol	6	1.24 ± 0.08	1.32 ± 0.07
Propranolol	6	1.28 ± 0.06	1.33 ± 0.07
Occluded myocardium, normal part			
Control		1.18 ± 0.08	1.19 ± 0.07
Pindolol		1.26 ± 0.05	1.22 ± 0.09
Metoprolol		1.38 ± 0.09	1.29 ± 0.10
Timolol		1.33 ± 0.21	1.24 ± 0.23
Propranolol		1.24 ± 0.16	1.24 ± 0.17
Occluded myocardium, ischemic part			
Control		0.67 ± 0.30	0.85 ± 0.20
Pindolol		0.57 ± 0.24	0.81 ± 0.33
Metoprolol		0.94[a]	0.95 ± 0.30
Timolol		1.02 ± 0.42	0.98 ± 0.28
Propranolol		0.72 ± 0.07	0.87 ± 0.03

[a] In only one dog enough endocardial tissue was ischemic to calculate the endo-/epi-ratio.

Table 8. The ratio between the uptake of 17-iodoheptadecanoic acid (I-HDA) and $^{201}TlCl$ in normal and ischemic myocardium under beta-blockade.

	I-HDA	^{201}Tl
Control	3.9 ± 0.9	3.7 ± 1.1.
Pindolol	4.4 ± 1.2	4.1 ± 1.4
Metoprolol	2.8 ± 0.7	2.7 ± 0.8
Timolol	3.1 ± 1.0	3.3 ± 1.4
Propranolol	3.2 ± 1.1	3.0 ± 0.8

increased flow was observed in the endocardium for metoprolol, timolol and propranolol. Pindolol exerts no such action: the ISA keeps things going just like the normal catecholamines would do. The relative increase of 17-iodo-heptadecanoic acid uptake in normal endocardial tissue after metoprolol was also seen in occluded dog hearts, although it was not accompanied here by a concomitant flow redistribution.

In ischemic heart muscle some interesting observations seem tentatively possible:

- pindolol and propranolol do not influence the endo-/epi-ratio for 17-iodo-heptadecanoic acid nor $^{201}TlCl$, indicating lack of specific influence on the more severely ischemic endocardium;
- metoprolol and timolol both induced a relatively higher uptake of 17-iodo-heptadecanoic acid (and of ^{201}Tl) in the endocardium.

In both cases the ischemic lesions after occlusion of the left anterior descendens coronary artery branch were only large enough in one or two cases to allow the measurement of the endo-/epi-ratio. Thus these beta-blockers seem to enable occluded myocardium to better maintain oxidative free fatty acid metabolism.

From the ratio of uptake in normal and ischemic tissue (Table 8) it seems to be (although the differences are not statistically significant) that beta-blockade (except with pindolol) favours higher flow (^{201}Tl) through the ischemic part accompanied by higher uptake of 17-iodoheptadecanoic acid (25% residual uptake compared to 15-20%, again with the exception of pindolol). This also indicates more persistence of free fatty acid metabolism in the ischemic areas after beta-blockade.

Conclusions

- The 17-C-free fatty acid analog 16-iodo-9-hexadecenoic acid shows lower uptake in the heart than its "18-C"-counterparts 17-iodoheptadecanoic acid and 15-(4-iodophenyl)-pentadecanoic acid.
- This supports the hypothesis of a dual mechanism for free fatty acid uptake:
  - *passive diffusion,* plus
  - *a carrier mediated mechanism.*
- Occluded myocardium takes up less iodinated free fatty acids (except 16-iodo-9-hexadecanoic acid).
- Administration of beta-blocking agents reduces free fatty acid uptake in the normal heart; in the occluded heart various effects are found for the different beta-blockers.
- Plasma free fatty acid levels are influenced differently by the individual beta-blocking agents.
- The ratio of uptake of iodinated free fatty acids and ^{201}Tl in the normal heart is > 1 (~1.2) indicating higher flow and more active energy producing metabolism in the endocardium.

- In the normal part of occluded myocardium this ratio is similar to control hearts.
- The endo-/epi-ratio is < 1 in the ischemic part of occluded myocardium, showing relatively less flow and metabolism in the normally more active endocardium.
- Residual 17-iodoheptadecanoic extraction in the ischemic area of occluded heart is ~ 15% (similar for ^{201}Tl).
- Endo-/epi-ratios for 17-iodoheptadecanoic acid are influenced differently by beta-blockade. 17-iodoheptadecanoic acid uptake is increased only by metoprolol. Flow is increased by metoprolol, timolol and propranolol in the normal heart.
- In the normal part of the occluded heart the flow-redistribution is absent and only metoprolol increases the endo-/epi-ratio for 17-iodoheptadecanoic acid.
- The endo-/epi-ratio (17-iodoheptadecanoic acid and ^{201}Tl) in the ischemic part of occluded myocardium is not influenced by pindolol and propranolol. Metoprolol and timolol cause a relatively higher endocardial uptake.
- Under metoprolol, timolol and propranolol the residual 17-iodoheptadecanoic acid and ^{201}Tl uptake in the ischemic tissue is increased (25%).

The implications of the above mentioned data for the use of iodinated free fatty acids as radiopharmaceuticals are not too many.
- There seems to be no reason to prefer iodinated free fatty acids to ^{201}Tl for the delineation of myocardial ischemia, since uptake and distribution are similar. Iodinated free fatty acids must be used because of their energy metabolism related properties.
- The 17-C-analog 16-iodo-9-hexadecanoic acid will in this respect behave inferior to 17-iodoheptadecanoic acid and (15-(4-iodophenyl)-pentadecanoic acid. From the point of view of uptake and regional distribution of the radiopharmaceutical no differences were seen between 17-iodoheptadecanoic acid and 15-(4-iodophenyl)-pentadecanoic acid. The dynamic behaviour will be treated elsewhere in this book (Chapters 2 and 7).
- Medication with beta-blocking agents does not greatly influence uptake in the ischemic heart, but it tends to reduce the target/nontarget ratio, which might make it more difficult to delineate the extent of ischemia.

Also is has been shown [28] that beta-blockade slows down myocardial elimination of iodinated free fatty acids, which has implications for the evaluation of dynamic scintigraphic studies with these compounds.

References

1. Neely J R, Rovetto M J, Oram J F (1972) Myocardial utilization of carbohydrate and lipids. Prog Cardiovasc Dis 15: 289 - 329
2. Westera G, Visser F C (1986) Myocardial uptake of radioactively labeled free fatty acids. Eur Heart J 6(Suppl B): 3 - 12

3. Poe N D, Robinson G D, MacDonald N S (1975) Myocardial extraction of labeled long chain fatty acid analogs. Proc Soc Exp Biol Med 148: 215 - 218
4. Machulla H-J, Marsmann M, Dutschka K, van Beuningen D (1980) Radiopharmaceuticals. II. Radiobromination of phenylpentadecanoic acid and biodistribution in mice. Radiochem Radioanal Letters 42: 243 - 250
5. Westera G, van der Wall E E, Heidendal G A K, van den Bos G C (1980) A comparison between terminally radio iodinated hexadecenoic acid and ^{201}Tl-thalliumchloride in the dog heart. Implications for the use of I-HA for myocardial imaging. Eur J Nucl Med 5: 339 - 343
6. van der Wall E E, Westera G, Heidendal G A K, Roos J P (1981) Comparison of radioiodinated 16-I-9-hexadecenoic acid and 17-I-heptadecanoic acid as radiopharmaceuticals for the study of myocardial metabolism. Eur J Nucl Med 6: 581 - 584
7. Schlant G R (1978) Metabolism of the heart. In: Hurst J W (ed) The Heart, New York: Mc Graw Hill Co, pp 107 - 118
8. Strauss H W, Harrison K, Langan J K, Lebowitz E, Pitt B (1975) Thallium- 201 for myocardial imaging. Relation of Tl-201 to regional myocardial perfusion. Circulation 51: 641 - 645
9. Riche F, Mathieu J P, Busquet G (1983) Etude biologique d'acides gras en C-16 marqués par un atome radioactif. J Biophys Med Nucl 7: 87 - 95
10. Westera G, van der Wall E E, Visser F C, den Hollander W, Heidendal G A K, Roos J P (1983) The uptake of iodinated free fatty acids in the (ischemic) dog heart. Indications for a dual uptake mechanism. Int J Nucl Med Biol 10: 231 - 236
11. Paris S, Samuel D, Ailhaud G (1979) Uptake of fatty acids by cultured cardiac cells from chicken embryo: evidence for a facilitation process without energy dependence. Biochimie 61: 361 - 367
12. Huetter J F, Piper H M, Spiekermann P G (1984) Myocardial fatty acid oxidation: evidence for an albumin-receptor mediated membrane transfer of fatty acids. Basic Res Cardiol 79: 274 - 282
13. Opie L H (1975) Metabolism of FFA, glucose and catecholamines in acute myocardial infarction. Relation to myocardial ischemia and infarct size. Am J Cardiol 36: 938 - 953
14. Liedtke A J, Nellis S H, Whitesell L F (1982) Effects of regional ischemia on metabolic function in adjacent aerobic myocardium. J Mol Cell Cardiol 14: 195 - 205
15. Westera G, van der Wall E E, Visser F C, Scholtalbers A S, van Eenige M J, Roos J P (1984) Myocardial uptake of iodinated free fatty acids and thallium-201 in experimental ischemia. Nucl Med 23: 321 - 325
16. Westera G, van der Wall E E, van Eenige M J, Scholtalbers A S, den Hollander W, Visser F C, Roos J P (1984) Metabolic consequences of beta-adrenergic receptor blockade for the acutely ischemic dog myocardium. Nucl Med 23: 35 - 40
17. Simonsen S, Kjekshus J K (1978) The effect of free fatty acids on myocardial oxygen consumption during atrial pacing and catecholamine infusion in man. Circulation 58: 484 - 491
18. Oliver M F (1978) Metabolism of the normal and ischemic myocardium. In: Dickinson C J, Marks J (eds) Developments in cardiovascular medicine, Baltimore: University Press, pp 145 - 164
19. Szekeres L (ed) (1980) Adrenergic Activators and Inhibitors, Handbook of Experimental Pharmacology, Vol 54/I. Berlin, Heidelberg: Spinger-Verlag
20. Blum J W, Froehli D, Kunz P (1982) Effects of catecholamines on plasma free fatty acids in fed and fasted cattle. Endocrinology 110: 452 - 460
21. Newman R J (1977) Comparison of the antilipolytic effect of metoprolol, acebutolol and propranolol in man. Br Med J II: 601 - 603
22. Raptis S J, Rosenthal J, Welzel D, Moulopoulos S (1981) Effects of cardioselective and non selective beta-blockade on adrenaline induced metabolic and cardiovascular responses in man. Eur J Clin Pharmacol 20: 17 - 22

23. Vik-Mo H, Mjos O D (1981) Influence of free fatty acids on myocardial oxygen consumption and ischemic injury. Am J Cardiol 48: 361 - 365
24. Glaviano V V, Masters T N (1967) The effect of intracoronary norepinephrine on cardiac metabolism before and after beta-adrenergic blockade. Fed Proc 26: 771 - 779
25. Marchetti G, Merlo L, Noseda V (1968) Myocardial uptake of free fatty acids and carbohydrates after beta-adrenergic blockade. Am J Cardiol 22: 370 - 374
26. Opie L H, Thomas M (1976) Propranolol and experimental myocardial infarction: Substrate effects. Postgrad Med J 52(Suppl 4): 124 - 133
27. Reimer K A, Lowe J E, Rasmussen M M, Jennings R B (1977) The wavefront phenomenon of ischemic cell death. 1. Myocardial infarct size vs. duration of coronary artery occlusion in dog. Circulation 56: 786 - 794
28. Comet M, Wolf J E, Pilichowsky P, Mathieu J P, Dubois F, Riché F, Busquet G, Vidal M, Godart F, Pernin C, Gaudy M (1982) Influence du propranolol sur l'activité myocardique après injection i.v. d'acide 16-I(123)-hexadecene-9-ioque. In: Faivre G, Bertrand A, Cherrier F, Amor M, Neimann J L (eds) Noninvasive methods in ischemic heart disease. Nancy: Specia, pp 295 - 299

5. Iodinated free fatty acids: reappraisal of methodology

M.J. van EENIGE, F.C. VISSER, C.M.B. DUWEL and J.P. ROOS

Introduction

Study of the metabolic processes in myocardial tissue is of great importance in exploring pathophysiological conditions of the heart. In normal physiological conditions the heart tissue uses free fatty acids (FFA) for about 70% of its energy production [1]. Thus, radiolabeled FFA are potential tracers for cardiac metabolism. In this chapter we will confine the discussion to the radiolabel I-123, with a gamma-energy at 159 keV, a physical half-life of 13.3 h and a low body exposure. Heptadecanoic acid labeled with I-123 (I-123-HDA) in the omega-position is structurally almost identical to the naturally occurring FFA [2] and will be the FFA of choice for the studies mentioned in this chapter.

After intravenous injection, I-123-HDA is rapidly extracted from the blood by the heart and other organs (Figure 1). In a few minutes almost all the heptadecanoic acid is extracted, half-time of heptadecanoic acid in blood amounts to 2-3 min [3]. In the heart a substantial part of the extracted heptadecanoic acid enters the oxidation process and the remaining heptadecanoic acid is stored in lipid pools [4]. As a result of beta-oxidation, radioiodide is split off and leaves the cardiac cell. Probably by passive diffusion, the radioiodide enters the circulation blood. Similar processes take place in other organs. As a consequence a high level of radioactivity is built up in the blood.

The clearance of radioactivity can be registered with a gammacamera and from these registration time-activity curves of myocardial regions may be calculated. Two main problems have arisen in the interpretation of time-activity curves. The first problem is concerned with the analysis of these curves and the second problem is related to the correction for background activity. Although our description of the very complicated metabolic process is simple, we will use it as the starting point to discuss the analysis of myocardial time-activity curves and the correction procedures for background activity.

There are two different ways to approach the problem of background activity. The first way is to correct for the background activity. Two of these

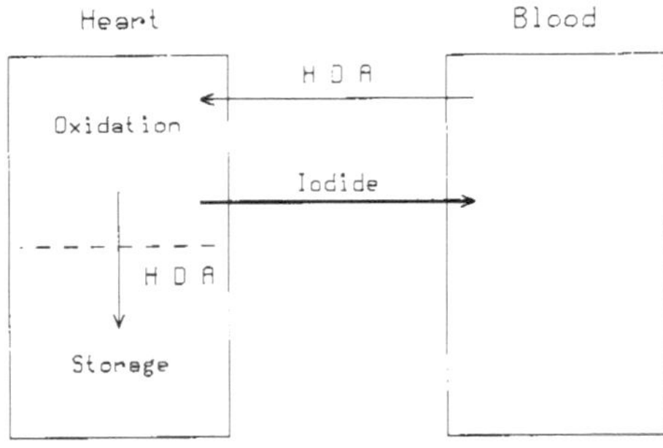

Figure 1. Simplified outline of the fate of 123-I-HDA: both stored heptadecanoic acid and free iodide in blood and tissue contribute to the background activity. HDA =heptadecanoic acid.

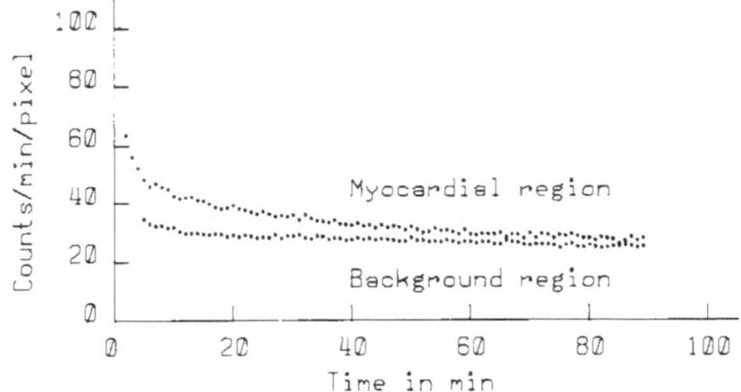

Figure 2. Example of time-acitivity curves derived from a myocardial region and a background region.

correction procedures will be discussed. The second way consists of analysis of the uncorrected time-activity curve.

Analysis of time-activity curves

To construct time-activity curves scintigrams of 1-min duration are registered. The 1-min frames are summed up and displayed on a video screen. Regions of interest are drawn and from the countrates in these regions time-activity curves are constructed. For the purpose of comparison the count rates are divided by the number of pixels of the region of interest, thus radioactivity is expressed in counts/min/pixel. An example of a myocardial time-activity curve, together with one derived from a background region, is given in Figure 2.

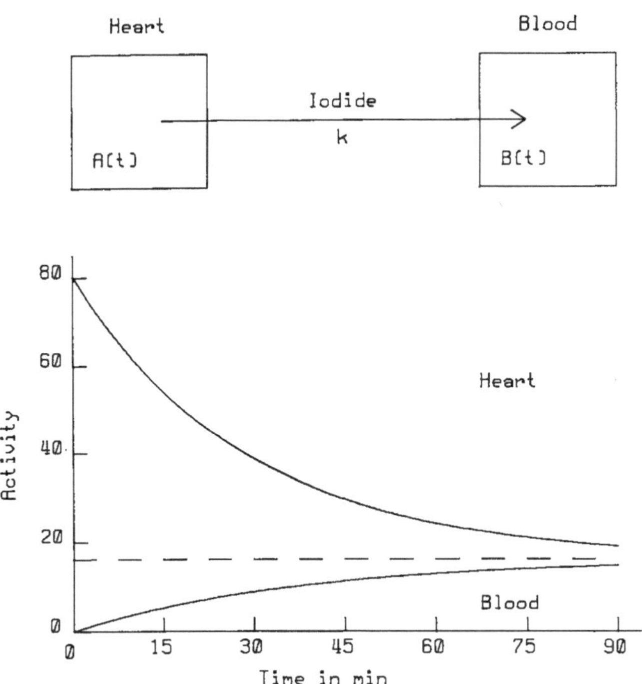

Figure 3. A simple model. Upper panel: clearance of iodide governed by rate constant k. Lower panel: resulting activity curves in heart and blood. After some time both reach the same constant level. A(t) = radioactivity in the heart at time t; B(t) = radioactivity in the blood at time t.

The model

Time-activity curves have the appearance of exponential curves with a negative exponent.

The curve is a very simple one and can be described with only a few parameters. Based on the simple description of the metabolic process in the heart, a simple model will be presented, the one-compartment model. The results of this model agree very well with the time-activity curves found in myocardial regions. The model is shown in the upper panel of Figure 3. Only the clearance of iodide from the heart is taken into account. A(t) is the activity in the heart at time t and B(t) the activity in blood. For a diffusion process the flow of iodode from heart to blood is proportional to the difference A(t) - B(t), with a rate constant k. After solving the differential equation governing this process we find:

$$A(t) = k1 + k2 \cdot e^{-k.t}$$

$A(t)$ = activity in heart at time t
$k1$ = constant value, depending on the capacity of heart and blood for iodide
$k2$ = constant

Both k1 and k2 depend on the injected dose of radioactivity.

$$k = \frac{\ln[2]}{T_{1/2}}$$

$T_{1/2}$ = half-time value.

In the lower panel of Figure 3 the time-activity curves in heart and blood are given.

With the help of the model we find a monoexponential behaviour of A(t). Derived from the above equation, A(t) will not approach zero with time, but will approach a constant value. This model is far from complete. In practice, radioactivity measured from a myocardial region originates not only from the iodide in the heart tissue, but also from the activity of stored heptadecanoic acid in the lipid pools and the radioactivity in blood. These activities are more or less constant and result in an increase of constant k1. The level of activity in blood is not only determined by the diffusion of iodide from the heart but comes also from metabolic processes in other organs. Again the result will be an increase of k1. The model is a simplification of the real and poorly understood processes which govern fatty acid metabolism in myocardium. As will be shown, the results of this model agree very well with the measured myocardial time-activity curves.

Monoexponential curves

Time-activity curves are often described as monoexponential curves. In most cases background correction is applied before curve fitting [3, 5-7]. The monoexponential curve is the simplest exponential curve. In formula:

$$A(t) = A(0) \cdot e^{\frac{-t.\ln(2)}{T_{1/2}}}$$

$A(t)$ = activity at time t
$A(0)$ = activity at time t=0
t = time in minutes
$T_{1/2}$ = half-time value in minutes

Thus, a monoexponential curve is completely determined by only two parameters, the amplitude at t=0 A(0) and the half-time value $T_{1/2}$.

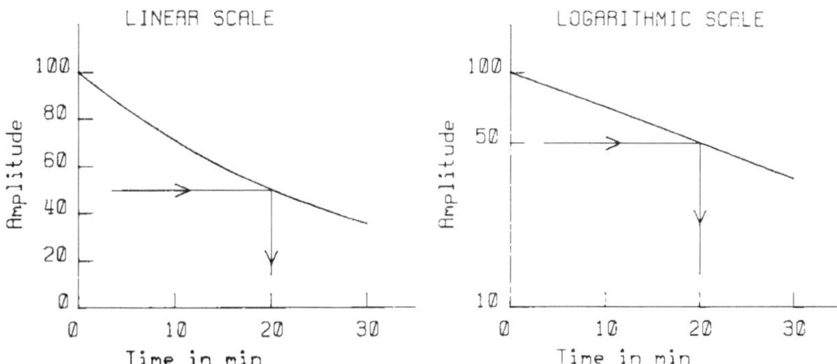

Figure 4. Example of a monoexponential curve. The half-time is the time the amplitude has decreased by a factor 2. Left panel: amplitude on a linear scale. Right panel: amplitude on a logarithmic scale.

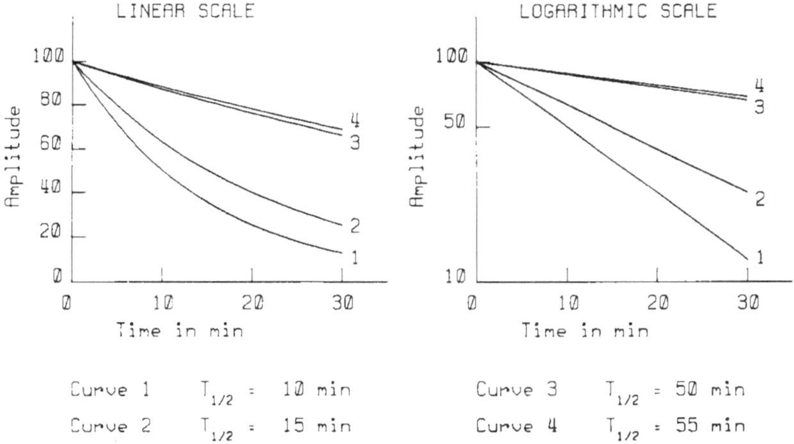

Figure 5. Monoexponential curves with different half-time values. On a scale of 0-30 min the difference between half-time values of 50 and 55 min is almost negligible.

So the monoexponential curve is defined by the same number of parameters as a straight line, representing a simple curve. In the case of a myocardial time-activity curve, A(0) depends on the regional extraction of heptadecanoic acid from blood and the injected dose of radioactivity, and $T\frac{1}{2}$ is supposed to be a parameter of myocardial metabolism.

From the formula of a monoexponential curve it follows:

$$\ln A(t) = \ln C(0) - \frac{t.\ln(2)}{T\frac{1}{2}}$$

which is the formula of a straight line.

A monoexponential curve results, in a straight line by drawing the activity along a logarithmic scale and the time along a linear scale (Figure 4). Left panel activity is shown on a linear scale and right panel activity on a logarithmic scale resulting in a straight line. From the formula it follows that the half-time is the time during which the amplitude of an exponential curve has decreased to half its value. This is illustrated in Figure 4 as well.

In Figure 5, on a time scale from 0-30 minutes, two sets of exponentials are shown with a difference in half-time value of 5 minutes, the first set with half-times of 10 and 15 minutes and the second with 50 and 55 minutes. The difference between two curves becomes rapidly negligible if, compared to the registration time, the half-time increases. From Figure 5 we conclude that in interpreting the difference between two half-times, the absolute values of the half-times must be taken into account.

Analysis of a monoexponential curve can be accomplished by fitting a straight line through the logarithms of the count rates by the method of least squares. Because of the logarithmic transformation low count rates will have more influence on the fitting procedure. This will become important if very low count rates are involved in the fitting process.

Biexponential curves

Registering scintigrams for more than about 30 min yields time-acitivity curves which cannot be fit adequately by monoexponential curves. Therefore biexponential curve fitting is applied in these cases [8-10]. A biexponential curve is the sum of two different monoexponential curves. Hence, a biexponential curve is completely defined by four parameters: two amplitudes and two half-time values. In Figure 6 an example of a biexponential curve is shown. On a logarithmic scale the curve is not simply composed of two straight lines.

Only when a biexponential curve consists of two monoexponential curves with very different half-time values, a simple curve fitting procedure, curve peeling, is applicable. In that case the last part of the biexponential curve is almost completely determined by the monoexponential curve having the highest half-time value. Thus, through the last part of the biexponential curve a monoexponential curve can be fitted, as described before. After subtraction of the found monoexponential curve from the original curve, again monoexponential fitting is applied to the remaining curve.

If for some reason curve fitting by applying the least squares method through the logarithms of the count rates is not adequate, curve fitting must be applied based on interpolation techniques. The latter requires more computer time, is apt to errors and is hardly necessary in the case of myocardial time-activity curves.

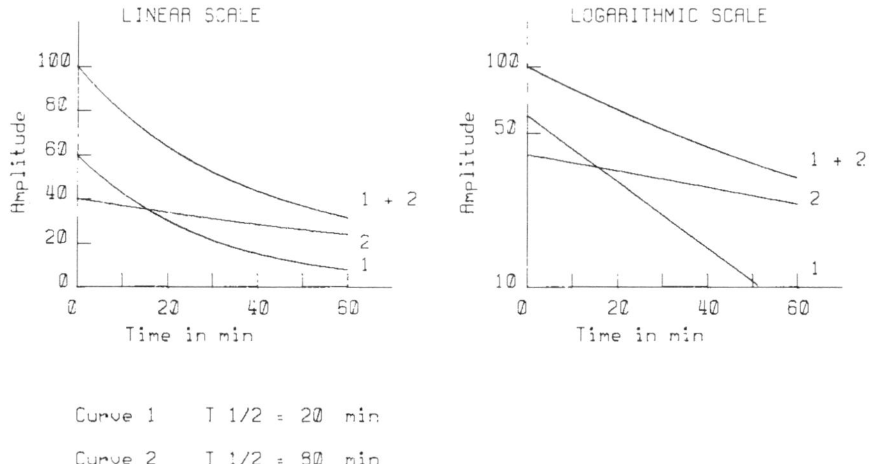

Figure 6. Example of biexponential curve consisting of two monoexponential curves (1 and 2) with different half-time values.

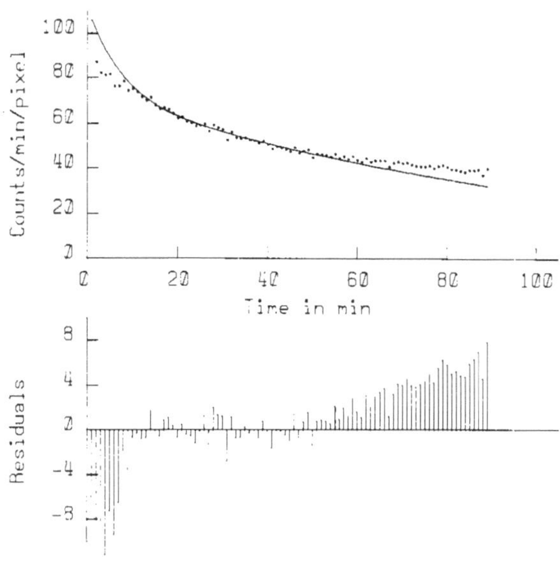

Figure 7. Upper panel: myocardial time-activity curve and the fitted curve. Lower panel: residuals = difference between time-activity curve and fitted value. Trends in residuals indicate a less satisfactory fit.

Reliability of parameters

The reliability of parameters of curve fitting, for instance amplitudes and half-time values, depends on the noise present in the time-activity curve, the choice of the start point for analysis, the registration time and last but not least on the choice of the type of curve to fit the measured time-activity curve. We will discuss these items briefly.

Noise

Besides the Poisson noise, inherent to the applied nuclear technique, many sources of noise contribute to the total noise found in a time-activity curve. Noise not only stems from cosmic sources, scatter in the region of interest and so forth, but also from movement artefacts of heart, lungs and total body and in part from the electronics between the crystal of the gamma camera and the final count rates stored on disc.

In Figure 7 a time-activity curve, together with a fitted curve, is shown in the upper panel. The differences between the time-activity curve and the fitted curve are called the residuals and are shown in the lower panel of Figure 7. The mean difference can be calculated from:

$$\sqrt{\frac{\Sigma \text{ residuals}^2}{n - 2}}$$

We will call the mean difference, expressed as a percentage of the mean count rate, the "residual coefficient of variation." The magnitude of the residual coefficient of variation depends on the noise present in the time-activity curve and on the correctness of the fit of this curve. Thus the residual coefficient of variation is not only a measure for the noise, but can also be used to compare fittings with different types of curves. In the latter case attention has to be paid to trends in the residuals indicating unsatisfactory fits. The correlation coefficient, often used to express the quality of a fit, is less adequate because of its dependence on the half-time value.

Startpoint of analysis

In the first few minutes after injection the radioactivity in a myocardial region not only stems from the activity originating from myocardium and from radioiodide in blood but also from heptadecanoic acid in blood. To avoid this complicating factor, the start of the analysis is chosen somewhere between 5 and 10 minutes.

Registration time

It is also evident that within certain limits the reliability of the parameters of curve fitting will increase with increasing registration time. Also misfits will become more clear, indicated by trends in the residuals, with increasing registration time.

Type of fitted curve

The choice of the type of curve to fit, with monoexponential, biexponential, etc., is very important in the analysis of time-activity curves. If the process governing the time-activity curve is basically monoexponential, fitting with a biexponential curve leads to too many parameters. These parameters will be interdependent and will have no value of their own. If the origin of the time-activity curve has a biexponential behaviour, fitting with a monoexponential curve will lead to parameter values far apart from the real parameters. Not only the residual coefficient of variation will be useful to choose the correct curve to fit with, but also an inspection of the residuals after curve fitting will be of use in judging the fit procedure.

The correction of background activity

Besides the correct analysis of time-activity curves, another major problem is the presence of background activity. In a myocardial region the activity measured not only originates from the metabolic process in the heart tissue, but also from the blood. Whether the activity of lipid pools is considered to belong to the metabolic process or to the background is a matter of choice.

Correction for free radioiodide

This background correction method corrects for I-123 in blood and interstitial space [11]. Two regions are taken into consideration, the myocardial region of interest and a background region, often chosen in the area of the superior caval vein. From both regions time-activity curves are constructed (Figure 8). At the end of a registration, Na-I is injected resulting in a stepwise increase in both time-activity curves. Registration is continued for about 10 min. In Figure 8 the increase in radioactivity due to Na 123-I in the myocardial time-activity curve is indicated with **a** and in the background area with **b**. It is assumed that the ratio **a/b** represents the ratio of free I-123 in the myocardial region and background region. Background correction is accomplished by multiplying the background time-activity curve with this ratio and by subtracting this result from the

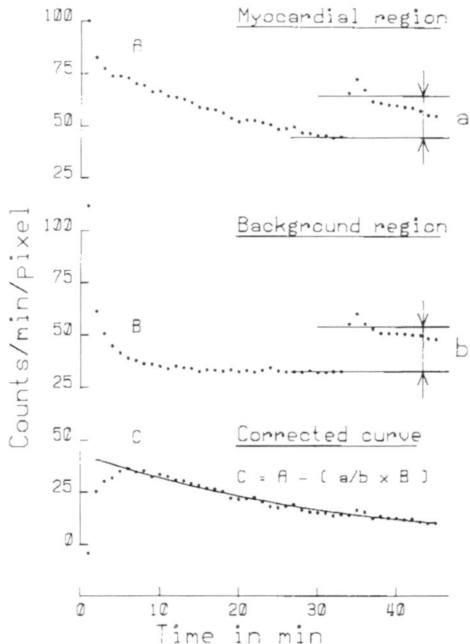

Figure 8. Background correction based on injection of NaI. Upper panel: time-activity curve from myocardial region (A); step in activity curve due to injection of NaI is indicated with a. Middle panel: time-activity curve from background region (B); increase in activity is indicated with b. Lower panel: corrected myocardial time-activity curve (C).

myocardial time-activity curve. The steps in a time-activity curve, **a** and **b**, are determined by subtracting the mean of the activities of the last two minutes before injection of Na-I from the mean of the activities at the second and third minute after the injection.

Some problems arise in applying this method and lead to inaccuracies in the corrected time-activity curve. As can be seen in Figure 8, noise impedes the exact determination of a step and thus also the determination of the ratio **a/b**. Because the activities of the myocardial region and background region converge to each other with time, small inaccuracies in the **a/b** ratio result in large deviations of the corrected curve. In some cases even negative count rates are found in the corrected curve. After injection of Na-I diffusion of this agent into tissues takes place. If this diffusion process is similar for in the myocardial region and the background region, the ratio **a/b** will not fulfill the assumption of this method. Because the process in the myocardial region depends on the clearance of iodide at least some inaccuracy will be the result. Of course this method does not correct for heptadecanoic acid stored in lipid pools.

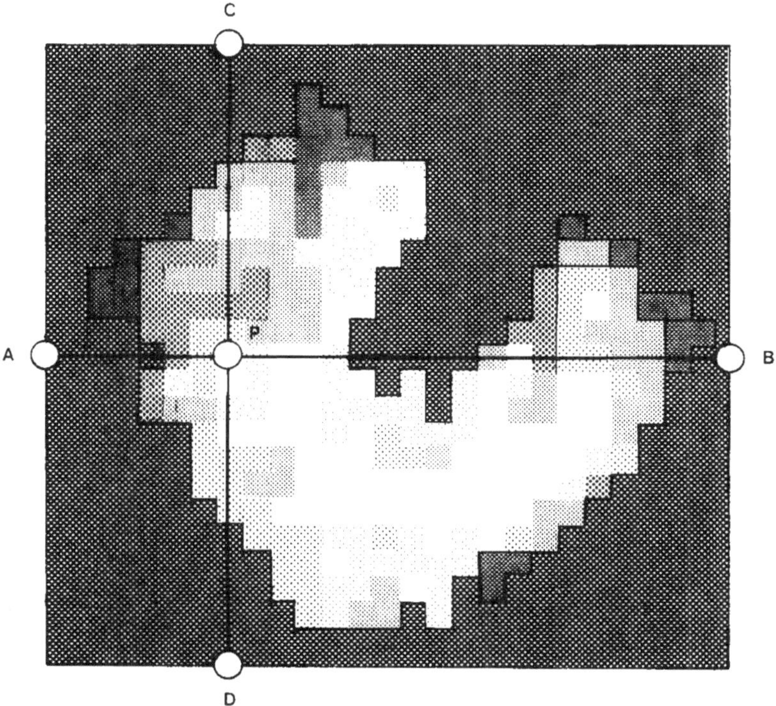

Figure 9. Interpolative background correction. Background of myocardial pixel P is calculated as the mean of two interdependent values derived from four pixels just outside the heart, A-D.

Interpolative background correction

This correction method proposed by Goris *et al.* [12] is based on the assumption that the background adjacent to the heart is not different from the background in the myocardial area. A rectangle is projected around the heart and the contribution of the background activity to every pixel in the area of the heart calculated based on the activities found on the rectangle. The method was modified by Watson *et al.* [13], who took also intense extracardiac activities into account. The procedure is shown in Figure 9. The procedure is based on interpolation of the background in the area around the heart. Besides this assumption problems arise if organs other than the heart overly the heart region.

Analysis of uncorrected time-activity curves

After some time the time-activity curve of a background area has an almost horizontal course (Figure 2). This corresponds very well with the model shown before. It is therefore reasonable to fit with a monoexponential plus a constant value. The background is represented by the constant value and the monoexponential is related to the metabolic process. Preliminary data indicate that this procedure is feasible. In a small group of patients with coronary artery disease, monoexponential curve fitting of uncorrected myocardial time-activity curves results in a high residual coefficient of variation values, indicating a bad fit. Also trends in the residuals confirm that monoexponential curve fitting is not the correct procedure. On the other hand, biexponential curve fitting led to interdependency of the parameters. Thus, the use of two parameters was not adequate and the use of four parameters too many. Curve fitting with a monoexponential plus constant, i.e. the use of three parameters, results in low residual coefficient of variation values, minimal trends in the residuals and a low interdependency of the parameters.

References

1. Most A S, Brachfeld N, Gorlin R, Wahren J (1969) Free fatty acid metabolism of the human heart at rest. J Clin Invest 48: 1177 - 1188
2. Poe N D, Robinson G D jr, MacDonald N S (1975) Myocardial extraction of labeled long-chain fatty acid analogs. Proc Soc Exp Biol Med 148: 215 - 218
3. van der Wall E E, den Hollander W, Heidendal G A K, Westera G, Majid P A, Roos J P (1981) Dynamic myocardial scintigraphy with I-123 labeled free fatty acids in patients with myocardial infarction. Eur J Nucl Med 6: 383 - 389
4. Visser F C, van Eenige M J, Westera G, den Hollander W, Duwel C M B, van der Wall E E, Heidendal G A K, Roos J P (1985) Metabolic fate of radioiodinated heptadecanoic acid in the normal canine heart. Circulation 72: 565 - 571
5. Visser F C, van Eenige M J, van der Wall E E, Westera G, van Engelen C J, van Lingen A, De Cock C C, den Hollander W, Heidendal G A K, Roos J P (1984) The elimination rate of I-123-heptadecanoic acid after intracoronary and intravenous administration. Eur J Nucl Med 11: 114 - 119
6. Rabinovitch M A, Kalff V, Allen R, Rosenthal A, Albers J, Das S K, Pitt B, Swappson D P, Maigner Th, Royers W L, Thrall J N, Beierwaltes W N (1985) 123-I-Hexadecanoic acid metabolic probe of cardiomyopathy. Eur J Nucl Med 10: 222 - 227
7. Dudczak R, Kletter K, Frischauf J, Losert U, Angelberger P, Schmoliner R (1984) The use of 123-I-labeled heptadecanoic acid (HDA) as metabolic tracer: Preliminary report. Eur J Nucl Med 9: 81 - 85
8. Machulla H J, Knust E J (1984) Recent developments in the field of 123-I-radiopharmaceuticals. Eur J Nucl Med 23: 111 - 118
9. Fridrich L, Pichler M, Gassner A, Vagner M, Mostbeck G, Eghbalian F (1985) Tracer elimination in J-123-heptadecanoic acid: half-life, component ratio and circumferential washout profiles in patients with cardiac disease. Eur Heart J 6(Suppl B): 61 - 70

10. Freundlieb C, Hoeck A, Vyska K, Feinendegen L E, Machulla H J, Stoecklin G (1980) Myocardial imaging and metabolic studies with (17-I-123)iodoheptadecanoic acid. J Nucl Med 21: 1043 - 1050
11. Hoeck A, Freundlieb C, Vyska K, Loesse B, Erbel R, Feinendegen L E (1983) Myocardial imaging and metabolic studies with (17-I-123)iodoheptadecanoic acid in patients with idiopathic congestive cardiomyopathy. J Nucl Med 24: 22 - 28
12. Goris M L, Daspit S G, McLaughlin P, Kriss J P (1976) Interpolative background subtraction. J Nucl Med 17: 744 - 747
13. Watson D D, Campbell N P, Read E K, Gibson R S, Teates C D, Beller G A (1981) Spatial and temporal quantitation of plane thallium myocardial imaging. J Nucl Med 22: 577 - 584

6. Experimental studies on myocardial metabolism of iodinated fatty acids: a proposal for a new curve analysis technique

M. COMET

Introduction

Currently, the most commonly used radioisotope for the study of cardiac muscle is thallium-201 (^{201}Tl). This tracer allows us to study coronary artery perfusion but provides no information of cardiac metabolism. Under aerobic conditions, most of the energy needed by the myocardium is provided by free fatty acid (FFA) degradation [1]. Evans and Gunton were the first, in 1965, who used, in dogs [2] and in men [3], a FFA labeled with iodine-131 to perform myocardial imaging studies. This work has been continued by Robinson and Poe: they demonstrated the need for labeling the FFA in ω position and proposed the use of 16-iodo-9-hexadecenoic acid [4-8]. The objective of using iodinated FFA is to determine by external means the amount of cellular uptake and the percentage distribution between storage and degradation. To reach this objective the observation of solely the scintigraphic image is of course insufficient. It is only possible to obtain quantitative information on metabolism if myocardial time-radioactivity curves are analysed.

After intravenous [IV] injection of ^{123}I labeled FFA, myocardial radioactivity reaches its maximal value within a few minutes, and decreases gradually afterwards (Figure 1). Until now, the curve analysis consisted only of measurements of the half-time period of the curve, which is arbitrarily fitted with a decreasing exponential [8-10]. In dogs, it has been demonstrated that following two successive injections of the iodinated FFA, results from measuring this half-time period are reproducible, provided the animal is in a steady state [11]. Compared to the values obtained in the basal state, perfusion of glucose associated with insulin and potassium [12] and lipid perfusion [12] leads to a significant increase of the half-time period of the curve. However, there is no significant change of this curve period under the influence of isoproterenol or propranolol [13], drugs which are known to have effects on FFA myocardial metabolism [14,15]. Similarly, other authors have not found abnormal half-time periods under ischemic conditions [16] or under a doxorubicin treatment [17] in animals. In men, it has been demonstrated that,

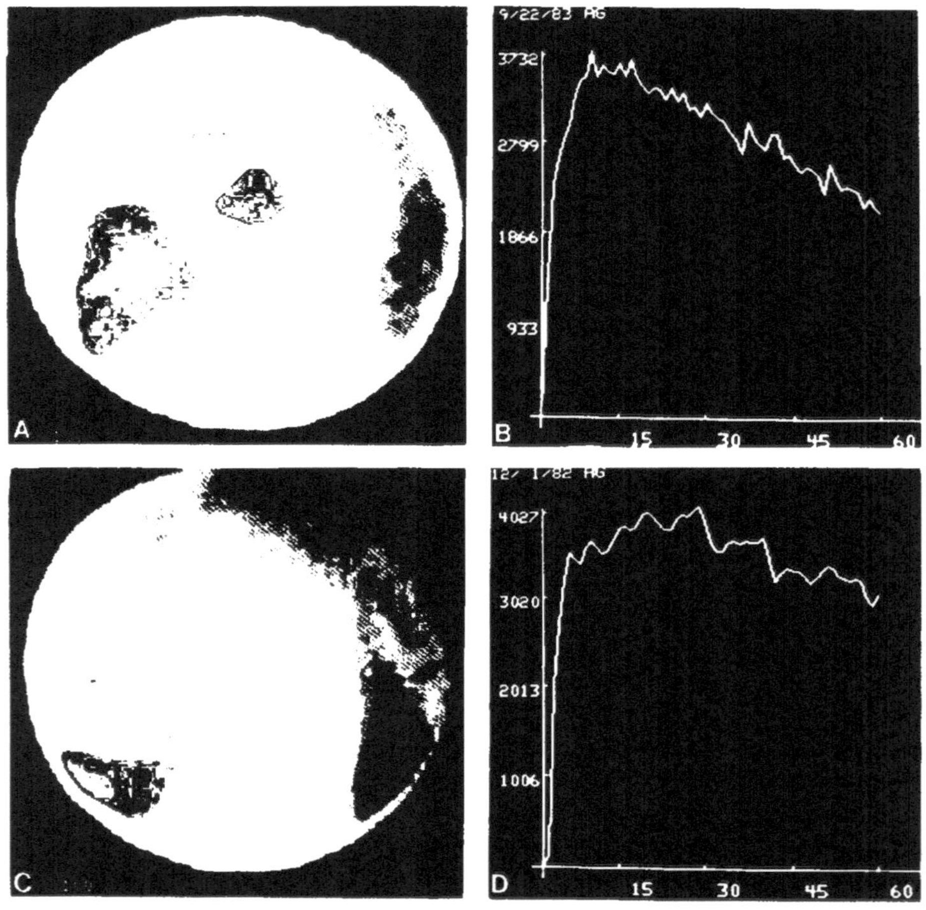

Figure 1. (A) Myocardial scintigraphy between 5 and 10 min after IV injection of 4 mCi of IHA in a normal patients. Myocardial and vascular regions of interest are outlined. (B) Myocardial time-activity curve during 60 min following injection. (C) Myocardial scintigraphy in a patient with cardiomyopathy. (D) Myocardial activity curve obtained from this patient with cardiomyopathy.

compared to the period measured in normally perfused areas, the half-time period measured in ischemic areas is longer [18] whereas the one measured in an infarcted zone is shorter [19]. In cardiomyopathies, this period is normal or increased [20,21]. Finally, it seems hazardous to link a given myocardial metabolic state to a value of the half-time period. The technique for analysis of the curve, besides its totally empirical character, does not take into account other important parts of the curve, i.e. the early ascending part and the late plateau phase, which appear to be very much modified in the case of, for example, a patient with cardiomyopathy.

Therefore it seems necessary, before appropriate clinical use of any iodinated FFA, to answer the following questions:

- Is uptake of the iodinated FFA similar to that of the physiological FFA?
- In the myocardial cell, is there a nonspecific deiodination process of the molecule? In other words, is the release of iodide from the cell only the result of mitochondrial degradation of the iodinated FFA?
- What is the intracellular fate of the iodinated FFA? Is it similar to that of the physiological FFA?

If there is no intracellular nonspecific deiodination and if the intracellular fate of the iodinated FFA is known, it is possible to construct a mathematical model. This model enables us to analyse the external detection curve and may provide us the desired information.

That is why the Grenoble group, after having developed a technique of labeling the FFA with ^{123}I, directed its research towards finding an answer to these questions.

Labeling technique

Robinson and Poe clearly demonstrated that the FFA molecule should be labeled in ω position with the radionuclide [5]. However, the labeling method proposed by the authors had the disavantage of having a yield of about 60% and needed therefore a purification step before injection. The labeling technique we proposed [22,23] and will discuss in this chapter has a 95% yield and therefore a purification step is not needed.

Choice of the molecule

It is necessary to select an iodinated FFA molecule of which the cadiac metabolism is very similar to that of the physiological FFA. Various molecules have been proposed: 16-iodo-9-hexadecenoic acid [4], 17-iodo-heptadecanoic acid [20], phenyl-iodo-pentadecanoic acid [24]. The latter has been used because it allows a fast urinary elimination of the metabolic degradation products of the FFA. However, it seems that the presence of a phenyl group obviously impairs the cellular metabolism of the FFA [25].

After IV injection of the labeled FFA, the course of the myocardial activity depends on the characteristics of the labeled molecule such as chain length [26], nature and position of the label in the molecule [5,27]. The evaluation of the relative importance of each of these factors is quite difficult to achieve from published studies because of the differences in the experimental procedures. Experimental protocols generally differ in the choice of the animal species (rats or mice) and in the time intervals after injection at which activity is measured. In order to choose a labeled molecule, we injected various FFA, which differed

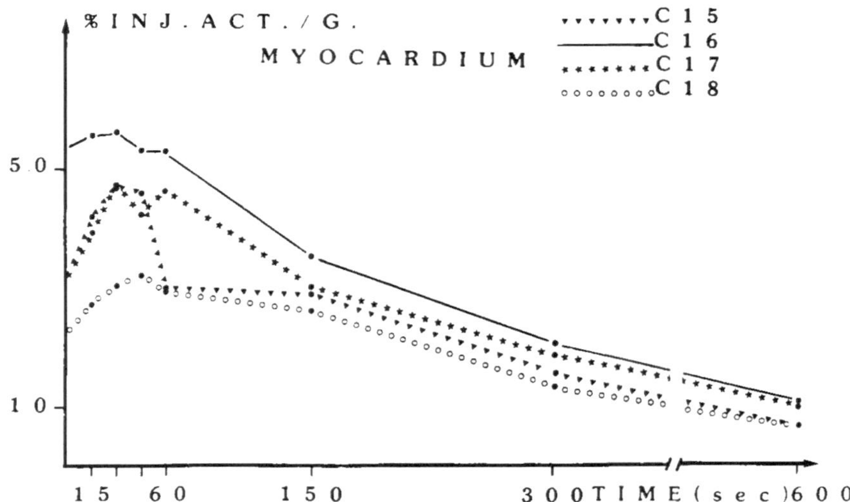

Figure 2. In mice, evolution of myocardial radioactivity after IV injection of ω-iodo-fatty acids of chain length C15, C16, C17, C18. Activity is expressed as percentage of injected dose per gram.

in chain length, saturation, nature and position of the radioactive label into mice [28-30]. Myocardial and blood activities were measured at very short time intervals after injection, especially during the first minute. FFA cellular uptake and metabolism appeared to be very rapid phenomena. Indeed, in mice, 300 seconds post injection, myocardial activity changes will indicate fatty acid metabolism only in a very indirect way. Iodinated FFA uptake is the highest for a chain length of 16 carbons. Maximal uptake increases when the chain length of saturated FFA varies from C8 to C16, and decreases with increasing chain length from C17 to C20 (Figure 2).

In blood the time-activity course is similar for all FFA. However there is an obvious hydrolysis of short chains, with iodide release. Robinson [4] reported similar results. Myocardial activity of the 16-carbon labeled FFA, whether saturated or with a double bond, has the same maximal value and a similar time course [29]. These results are consistent with those reported by others [5]. Concerning the influence of the composition of the FFA molecule, no difference appears in the time-activity course after injection between the cis and the trans form of the labeled FFA. The bromine labeled FFA has the same myocardial uptake as the iodine labeled FFA, but activity decreases faster. Such a difference in the time course of myocardial radioactivity could be due to the different membrane permeabilities of the two halogens [31]. In summary, among all the FFA studied, 16-iodohexadecanoic and 16-iodo-9-hexadecenoic acids showed the highest myocardial uptake. Since it is known that in man physiologically unsaturated FFA have a better myocardial extraction [32], it seems that 16-iodo-9-hexadecenoic acid, initially proposed by Poe [5], is well suited to allow external studies of myocardial metabolism in man.

Measurement of the myocardial extraction fraction of 16-iodo-9-hexadecenoic acid (IHA)

In order to confirm results obtained from mice, we measured in dogs the extraction fraction of IHA, ^{201}Tl, and ^{131}I-9-iodo-10-chloro-stearic acid, according to the Weich technique [33,34].

Technique

In a normal dog, which has been anesthetized, intubated and air-ventilated, three catheters are used: one in the left atrium, the second into the femoral artery and the last into the coronary sinus via the jugular vein. A solution of ^{131}I human serum albumin (HSA) with the FFA to be tested — from which an aliquot has been taken in order to determine activity ratio — is rapidly injected into the left auricle. Simultaneously, a blood sample is taken from the coronary sinus and the femoral artery with a syringe. The sampling of blood takes 4 seconds and a total of six samples are taken from each of the two catheters within 24 seconds. The volume of each sample varies between 2 to 5 ml. The activity of 1 ml of each sample is measured with a scintillation counter.

We consider the first pass completed when the sample activity decreases below 50% of the maximal activity. We do not take into account the samples that follow. The extraction fraction (EF) is calculated from the formula [33,34]:

$$EF = 1 - \frac{Ba}{Aa} \times \frac{Av}{Bv} \times 100\%$$

in which: $\dfrac{Ba}{Aa} = \dfrac{^{131}\text{I HSA activity}}{\text{Test molecule activity}}$

and $\dfrac{Av}{Bv} = \dfrac{\text{Sum of the activities of the test molecule}}{\text{sum of the activities of } ^{131}\text{I HSA}}$

The activities are measured from the aliquot of the injected solution. The activities of all samples from the coronary sinus taken during the first pass of the radioactive bolus are summed up.

Results

The extraction fractions were as follows:

^{201}Tl : 88.3% ± 2.5%
IHA : 64,3% ± 3.4%
^{131}I-9-iodo-10-chloro-stearic acid : 32% ± 5.6%.

The extraction fraction measured for ^{201}Tl is similar to that obtained by Weich [34]. Also, the results obtained with ^{131}I-9-iodo-10-chlorostearic acid and with IHA are identical with those obtained by Poe [5] who however used a different technique.

Study of the IHA myocardial distribution as a function of the local coronary flow

After IV injection of IHA, when maximal activity is reached, the problem is to know whether the local distribution always mirrors that of the local coronary flow. The study of IHA myocardial uptake has been performed 1) in dogs under normal conditions, 2) after acute myocardial infarction due to the occlusion of a coronary artery ligated 48 h before, and 3) during hyperemia secondary to clamping of a coronary artery for 20 s. When the heart is normally perfused, radioactivity is homogeneously distributed, both globally and regionally (subendocardium and subepicardium). However the discrete heterogeneity of the distribution reflects that of the local blood flow, measured with ^{99}Tc microspheres, since there is a significant correlation ($r>0.90$) for each dog between the coronary flow distribution and that of IHA [35].

In infarcted dogs, the ratio of the flow in the infarcted zone to that in the normally-perfused zone is, on average, 0.31 in the endocardium and 0.55 in the epicardium. With IHA, this ratio is, on average, 0.38 in the subendocardium and 0.50 in the subepicardium. In all dogs, the correlation between IHA distribution and that of ^{99m}Tc microspheres is highly significant.

In dogs with a post-ischemic hyperemia the ratio of the flow in the hyperemic zone to that of the of the normal zone is on average 2.54 in the endocardium and 3.39 in the epicardium. With IHA the activity ratio equals 1.05 in endocardium and 1.20 in epicardium. The absence of any significant increase of IHA uptake in the hyperemic zone could have several causes. The duration of the hyperemic reaction following a occlusion of 20 s is about 1 min [36]. Whereas microspheres represent the coronary flow distribution during hyperemia, it is very likely that IHA continues to be extracted for at least 2 min after the hyperemia is finished. As a next cause, cellular metabolic disturbances that are always found when ischemia lasts longer than 6 s [37] could explain the lack of any increase in uptake. In fact, in case of ischemia, FFA myocardial uptake is lower; this decrease could be due to metabolic impairments secondary to ischemia rather than a simple consequence of the flow reduction [38]. Similar results have been obtained in dogs under the same experimental conditions with arachidonic acid [39]. These findings confirm previous reports which state that the behaviour of IHA is different to that of ^{201}Tl during hyperemia [40,41]. In summary, IHA myocardial distribution cannot be considered as a true image of the coronary flow distribution as measured with microspheres. ^{201}Tl myocardial scintigraphy is not representative in all cases of the initial distribution of the iodinated FFA.

Intracellular and subcellular distribution of IHA

For iodinated FFA to be useful for the study of cardiac metabolism it is essential that myocardial iodide elimination results only from the complete oxidation of the FFA molecule [42,43]. Many authors [44,45] believe that a non-specific deiodination of the iodinated FFA occurs in the myocardial cell and they suggest therefore the use of iodophenylated FFA which do not undergo such a nonmetabolic process. To verify that nonspecific intracellular deiodination of IHA, if it exists, represents only a minor phenomenon leading to iodide production within the myocardial cells, we have analysed intracellular distribution of IHA administered as a bolus injection at the entrance of the coronary network of isolated rat hearts. This study has been performed with different glucose concentrations in the perfusion medium. Then, for a given time after injection, we have compared the intracellular distribution of the IHA to that of 1-^{14}C palmitic acid. As a result of this work, the following points seem to prove that FFA intramitochondrial oxidation is the most important phenomenon leading to a high intracellular iodide production.

(1) IHA is taken up by the myocardial cell, then enters the mitochondria where most of the radioacitivity is present in the organic phase. Activities found in the mitochondrial triglycerides and FFA are similar to those of 1-^{14}C oleate [46].

(2) A modification of glucose concentration in the perfusion medium induces changes in cellular activity distribution between aqueous and organic phases and also in subcellular activity distribution. In the presence of glucose, triglycerides and polar lipids show a significantly higher level of activity. In the presence of an exogenous substrate, the isolated heart is able to esterify a larger amount of IHA as shown by triglyceride accumulation in the cytoplasm.

(3) The presence of an exogenous substrate (glucose) in the perfusion medium modifies iodide elimination in the coronary effluents: elimination

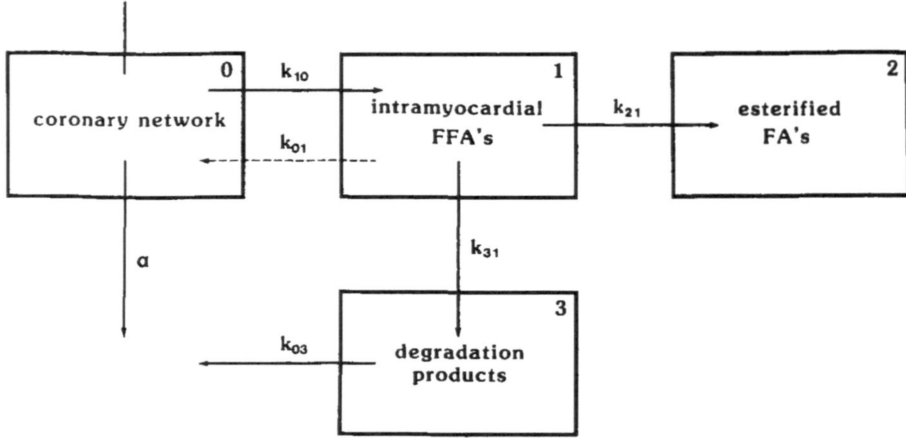

Figure 3. Compartmental model of the myocardial metabolism of an ω iodo fatty acid. FFA = free fatty acids (for explanation see text).

of iodide decreases in the presence of glucose which indicates a decrease of IHA oxydation. This decrease in iodide elimination is furthermore coupled to a slower total cardiac activity decrease. On the other hand, this time-activity curve in the eluate is quite similar to that obtained with iodophenyl-pentadecanoic acid [47] which is supposed not to undergo nonspecific deiodination.

(4) The very high activity found in the aqueous phase immediately after injection cannot be considered as an argument in favor of a nonspecific deiodination, because 90 s post injection of 1-^{14}C palmitate, activity distribution between aqueous and organic phases is similar to that measured in the same conditions for IHA.

From all these arguments it can be concluded that IHA extracted by the myocardial cell enters the mitochondria where it is oxidized with subsequent iodide release in cytoplasm and in the blood. Even if we cannot exclude the possibility of a nonspecific partial deiodination, the production of iodide due to a complete IHA oxidation is a phenomenon of sufficiently major importance to determine the configuration of the myocardial time activity curve.

Mathematical model of IHA cellular metabolism

We used a four-compartment model (Figure 3) [48]. Compartment 0 corresponds to free intravascular IHA, compartment 1 to free intramyocardial IHA, compartment 2 to esterified IHA and finally compartment 3 to free iodide resulting from mitochondrial degradation of IHA. We suppose the absence of back diffusion of the intramyocardial IHA into the vascular space and the absence of hydrolysis of the esterified forms of IHA during the time of measurement. The rate constants that characterize this model have the following physiological significances: k_{10} represents IHA uptake by the myocardial cells, k_{21} esterification of IHA, k_{31} mitochondrial degradation of IHA and finally k_{03} iodine output into the vascular space. At a given time t, q_1, q_2 and q_3 in the three myocardial compartments equal the following convolution products:

$$q_1(t) = k_{10} \cdot q_v(t) + e^{-(k_{21}+k_{31})t} \quad (1)$$

$$q_2(t) = k_{21} \cdot q_1(t) + \Gamma(t) \quad (2)$$

$$q_3(t) = k_{31} \cdot q_1(t) + e^{-k_{03}t} \quad (3)$$

with $q_v(t)$ = input function
$\Gamma(t)$ = step function

Theoretical myocardial activity $q_{mt} = q_1(t) + q_2(t) + q_3(t)$.

Mathematical model applied to a metabolic study on an isolated rat heart

The model was used for analysing time-activity course measured by external detection after an IHA bolus injection close to the coronary arteries of isolated Langendorff perfused rat hearts with various substrates (Figure 4) [49]. The measured cardiac activity $q_c(t)$ equals the sum of circulating IHA activity $q_v(t)$ and of myocardial activity $q_m(t)$. $q_v(t)$ was fitted with a decreasing exponential $q_v(t) = Ae^{\alpha t}$ where A is the maximum value of $q_c(t)$ curve. In order to know α, ^{131}I-HSA was injected into the coronary arteries of six Langendorff perfused isolated rat hearts. The decreasing part of the time-activity curve was considered as a decreasing exponential and the slope of the curve was calculated. The mean slope value thus obtained was 6.02 ± 1.25 min^{-1}. We searched for rate constants values k_{10}, k_{21}, k_{31} and k_{03} so that there is a fitting of $q_m(t)$ by $q_{mt}(t)$. The Gauss-Newton algorithm was used based on a least squares method. The iteration process was stopped when the sum of absolute values of relative variation of the four rate constants between two iterations was lower than 0.05. The convergence was verified by starting computation from other values of rate constants. Intracellular analysis allowed us to determine the myocardial radioactivity distribution between aqueous phase, organic phase and free fatty acids. The introduction into the equations (1), (2) and (3) of the rate constants values calculated with the model, allowed us to compute the expected values for $q_1(t)$, $q_1(t) + q_2(t)$ and $q_3(t)$ at time intervals corresponding with the intracellular measurements. These simulation studies demonstrated a very good correlation between time-activity curves of free IHA, esterified IHA and iodide obtained on one hand with the used model (Figure 5) and on the other hand with measurements of intracellular radioactivity.

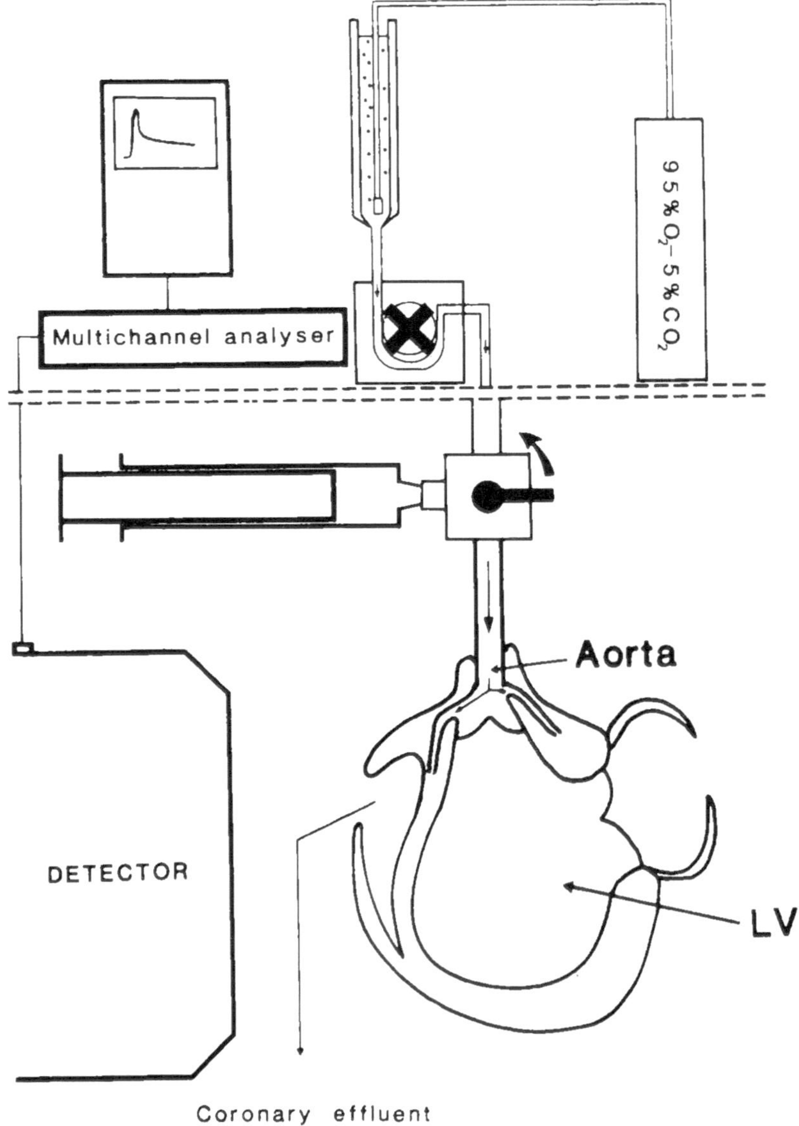

Figure 4. Experimental system for the measurement of the cardiac time-activity curve after injection of an iodinated fatty acid close to the coronary network of an isolated rat heart. LV = left ventricle.

Correlation coefficients between intracellularly measured activity results and those computed from the model were all higher than 0.85 which really indicates a good correlation. Results from our studies unequivocally demonstrate that the decreasing part of myocardial time-activity curve indicates in an indirect way modifications of myocardial metabolism because it is the sum of iodide

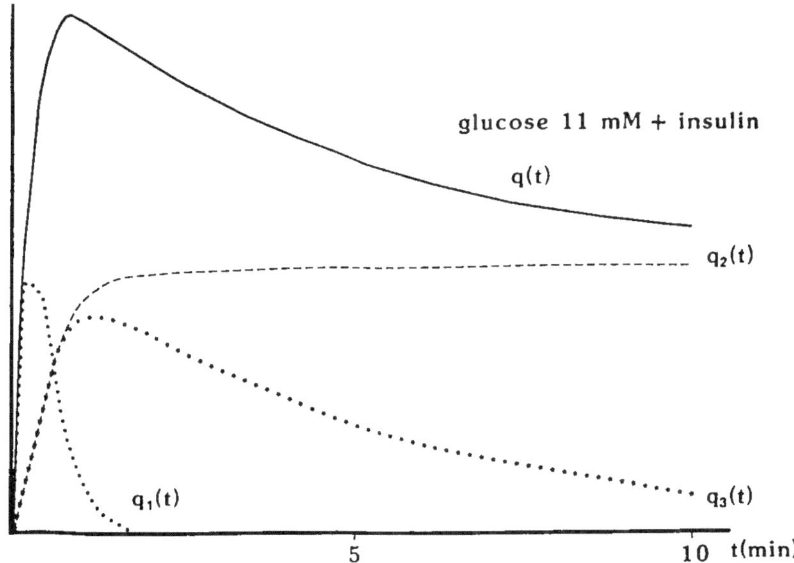

Figure 5a. Temporal evolution of the intracellular aqueous (q_3 (t)), organic (q_2 (t)), and FFA (q_1 (t)) fractions obtained after analysis with the model and the time-activity (q (t)) curve measured by external detection after injection of IHA at the entry of the coronary network of an isolated rat heart.

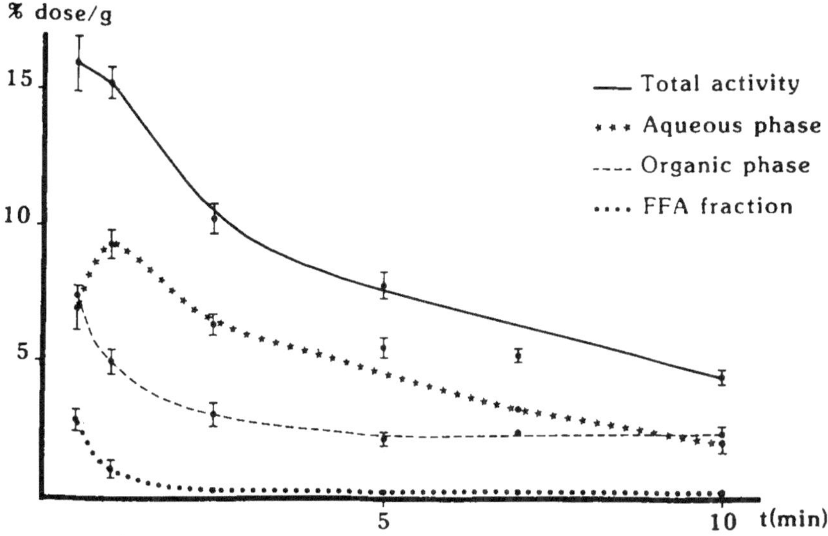

Figure 5b. Temporal evolution of the total radioactivity and of those of intracellular, aqueous, organic and FFA fraction after a bolus injection of IHA at the entry of the coronary network of an isolated rat heart.

and esterified IHA activities. Nevertheless, the shape of the decreasing part of the curve is essentially determined by iodide release. Curve analysis with this model has considerable advantages for the "slope" approach [50]. It takes into account the whole curve and in particular the initial part during which metabolic degradation and esterification occurs and it provides quantitative information of intracellular IHA metabolism. In conclusion, our model analysis of the cardiac time-activity curve after IHA injection appears to be the best adapted technique for studies on isolated rat hearts. This should allow us to recognise easily, by external detection, IHA cellular metabolic modifications induced by physiological or pharmacological interventions.

Mathematical model applied to *in vivo* studies

In vivo, three additional problems appear.

(a) There is a circulating activity due to a release of cellular degradation products of FFA into the plasma and also due to circulating IHA activity. The activity measured in the cardiac zone is the sum of myocardial activity and circulating activity. In order to substract circulating activity two techniques have been proposed.

The first one consists of the assessment of the amount of activity variations *a* and *b* at the level of a vascular zone and a cardiac zone respectively, following an IV injection of $Na^{123}I$ [9]. We can state that:

$$\frac{a}{b} = \frac{Ac1}{A1\text{-}Am}$$

in which

$$Am = A1 - \frac{a}{b} Ac2$$

where Ac1 is the circulating activity, Ac2 the activity in the vascular zone, A1 total cardiac activity and Am the myocardial activity after the injection of iodinated FFA.

We have proposed [11] a different method. Following the IV injection of IHA, we record the evolution of cardiac radioactivity over 30 to 60 min. Then we inject IV 370 MBq (10mCi) of ^{99m}Tc HSA. Activity is recorded for 10 min following injection. To substract circulating activity and to obtain myocardial time-activity evolution, we define two regions of interest (ROI): the first one (zone 1) includes the whole cardiac image and the other (zone 2) is outlined above the cardiac image at the level of the large vessels, without interfering with lung tissue. Time-activity curves are plotted at the level of these two zones after the IHA injection and the ^{99m}Tc HSA injection. After the IHA injection, activity in the cardiac region of interest A1 equals the sum of myocardial activity Am and circulating activity (Ac1)

$$A1 = Am + Ac1$$

Activity Ac2 in zone 2 has a constant ratio K with circulating activity in zone 1.

$$\frac{Ac2}{Ac1} = K$$

The value of K is measured after the ^{99m}Tc HSA injection: when circulating activity of ^{99m}Tc HSA is constant, we measure ^{99m}Tc HSA activity ratio between zones 1 and 2. Knowing K, we obtain the value for Am:

$$Am = A1 - \frac{Ac2}{K}$$

This technique has the advantage to allow, after the metabolic study, the assessment of myocardial function by the measuring the left ventricular ejection fraction. The choice of the extracardiac ROI is crucial: the ROI should be strictly centered on a vascular zone and should not interfere with the lungs. In fact, there is pulmonary extraction of iodinated FFA, since the ratio between ^{99m}Tc HSA and IHA activities is higher in a strictly vascular zone than in zones which include partially or exclusively pulmonary tissue. It has been demonstrated that 1.3% of the ^{14}C-palmitate injected into mice is found in the lungs 1 min after IV injection, and that from this amount 42,6% is esterified in phosphatidylcholine [51]. The turnover is slow, since the biological half-life of pulmonary palmitate is 14 h in rats [52].

(b) In man it is hardly possible to carry on myocardial activity recording for more than 60 to 90 min. However, measurements for a longer period of time are necessary if we want to obtain a value for the rate constant indicating esterification. That is why we had to further simplify the model by removing the storage compartment.

(c) The input function poses the final problem. The fate of IHA in plasma after injection depends on the metabolic state of the patient and his hepatic function etc. In order to know the input function it seems necessary to measure the IHA evolution curve in plasma after IV injection. This requirement seriously aggravates the problem if the curve is greatly different from one patient to the other, and if, therefore, a mean value of this input function cannot be used.

Conclusion

Our knowledge of the IHA intracellular fate seems sufficient to elaborate a mathematical model. The problem is to know whether the necessarily simplified mathematical model that will be used for the analysis of curves obtained *in vivo* will be just as reliable as the one used for the analysis of curves obtained from isolated hearts. Whatever the outcome, the use of a model, both for iodinated FFA and ^{11}C-labeled FFA [53], seems the only way to obtain quantitative information on cardiac FFA metabolism by externally employed imaging techniques.

References

1. Oliver M F (1976) The influence of myocardial metabolism on ischemic damage. Circulation 53(Suppl I): 168 - 170
2. Evans J R, Gunton R W, Baker R G, Beanlands D S, Spears J C (1965) Use of radioiodinated fatty acid for photoscans of the heart. Circ Res 16: 1 - 10
3. Gunton R W, Evans J R, Baker R G, Spears J C, Beanlands D S (1965) Demonstration of myocardial infarction by photoscans of the heart in man. Am J Cardiol 16: 482 - 487
4. Robinson G D, Lee A W (1975) Radioiodinated fatty acids for heart imaging. Iodine monochloride addition compared with iodide replacement labeling. J Nucl Med 16: 17 - 21
5. Poe N D, Robinson G D, MacDonald N S (1975) Myocardial extraction of labeled long chain fatty acid analogs. Proc Soc Exp Biol Med 148: 215 - 218
6. Poe N D, Robinson G D, Graham L S, MacDonald N S (1976) Experimental basis for myocardial imaging with ^{123}I labeled hexadecenoic acid. J Nucl Med 17: 1077 - 1082
7. Robinson G D (1977) Synthesis of ^{123}I-16-iodo-9-hexadecenoic acid and derivatives for use as myocardial perfusion imaging agents. Int J Appl Radiat Isot 28: 149 - 156
8. Poe N D, Robinson G D, Zielinski F W, Cabeen W R, Smith J W, Gomes A S (1977) Myocardial imaging with ^{123}I hexadecenoic acid. Radiology 124: 419 - 424
9. Freundlieb C H, Höck A, Vyska K, Feinendegen L E, Machulla H J, Stöcklin G (1980) Myocardial imaging and metabolic studies with (17-^{123}-I) Iodoheptadecanoic acid. J Nucl Med 21: 1043 - 1050
10. van der Wall E E, Westera G, den Hollander W, Visser F C (1981) External detection of regional myocardial metabolism with radioiodinated hexadecenoic acid in the dog heart. Eur J Nucl Med 6: 147 - 151
11. Comet M, Wolf J E, Pilichowski P, Dubois F, Busquet G, Mathieu J P, Pernin C, Riche F, Vidal M (1983) Scintigraphie myocardique après injection IV d'acide ^{123}I-hexadecene 9 oique. Etude de la reproductibilité des résultats chez le chien. J Biophys Med Nucl 7: 139 - 145
12. Comet M, Pilichowski P, Wolf J E, Busquet G, Dubois F, Mathieu J P, Pernin C, Riche F, Vidal M (1983) Scintigraphie myocardique après injection IV d'acide 16 ^{123}I hexadecene-9 oique. Etude de l'influence des concentrations plasmatiques des acides gras et du glucose. J Biophys Med Nucl 7: 151 - 157
13. Comet M, Wolf J E, Pilichowski P, Busquet G, Dubois F, Mathieu J P, Pernin C, Riche F, Vidal M (1983) Scintigraphie myocardique après injection intraveineuse d'acide 16^{123}I hexadécène 9 oique, étude de l'influence de l'isoprotérénol, du propranolol, du dipyridamole et de l'isoptine. J Biophys Med Nucl 7: 185 - 190
14. Takenaka F, Takeo S (1976) Effects of isoproterenol on myocardial lipid metabolism in rat hearts perfused with and without exogenous substrates. J Mol Cell Cardiol 8: 925 - 940

15. Opie L H, Thomas M (1976) Propranolol and experimental myocardial infarction. Postgrad Med J 52(Suppl 4): 124 - 133
16. Okada R D, Elmaleh D, Werre G S, Strauss H W (1983) Myocardial kinetics of ^{123}I-labeled-16-hexadecenoic acid. Eur J Nucl Med 8: 211 - 217
17. Styles C B, Noujaim A A, Jugdutt B I, Sykes T R, Bain G O, Shnitka T K, Hooper H R (1983) Effects of doxorubicin on (ω-I-131) heptadecanoic acid myocardial scintigraphy and echocardiography in dogs. J Nucl Med 24: 1012 - 1018
18. van der Wall E E, Heidendal G A K, den Hollander W, Westera G, Roos J P (1981) Metabolic myocardial imaging with ^{123}I-labeled heptadecanoic acid in patients with angina pectoris. Eur J Nucl Med 6: 391 - 396
19. van der Wall E E, den Hollander W, Heidendal G A K, Westera G, Majid P A, Roos J P. Dynamics myocardial scintigraphy with ^{123}I-labeled free fatty acids in patients with myocardial infarction. Eur J Nucl Med 6: 383 - 389
20. Höck A, Freundlieb C, Vyska K, Lösse B, Erbel R, Feinendegen L E (1983) Myocardial imaging and metabolic studies with (17-^{123}I) iodoheptadecanoic acid in patients with idiopathic congestive cardiomyopathy. J Nucl Med 24: 22 -28
21. Rabinovitch M A, Kalff V, Allen R, Rosenthal A, Albers J, Das S K, Pitt B, Swanson D P, Mangner T, Rogers, W L, Thrall J H, Beierwaltes W H (1985) ω^{123}I-hexadecenoic acid metabolic probe of cardiomyopathy. Eur J Nucl Med 10: 222 - 227
22. Mathieu J P, Riche F, Coornaert S, Bardy A, Busquet G, Godart J, Comet M, Vidal M (1982) Marquage d'acides gras en position ω par les isotopes de l'iode. J Biophys Med Nucl 6: 233 - 237
23. Riche F, Mathieu J P, Comet M, Coornaert S, Conti M L, Vidal M (1982) Synthesis of 16-iodo-9 hexadecenoic acid labeled with iodine 123. Radiochem Radioanal Lettter 53: 225 - 230
24. Machulla H J, Marsmann M, Dutschka K (1980) Biochemical concept and synthesis of a radioiodinated phenylfatty acid for in vivo metabolic studies of the myocardium. Eur J Nucl Med 5: 71 - 73
25. Schmitz B, Reske S N, Machulla H J, Egge H, Winkler C (1984) Cardiac metabolism of ω-(p-iodo-phenyl)-pentadecanoic acid: a gas liquid chromatographic-mass spectrometric analysis. J Lipid Res 25: 1102 - 1108
26. Otto C A, Brown L E, Wieland D H, Beierwaltes W H (1981) Radioiodinated fatty acids for myocardial imaging. Effect of chain length. J Nucl Med 22; 613 - 618
27. Machulla H J, Stöcklin G, Kupfernagel Ch, Freunlieb Ch, Höck A, Vyska K, Feinendegen L E. Comparative evaluation of fatty acids labeled with C11, C1-34m, Br-77, and I-123 for metabolic studies of the myocardium. Concise communication. J Nucl Med 19: 298 - 302
28. Riche F, Mathieu J P, Comet M, Vidal M, Pernin C, Marti-Batlle D, Busquet G, Bardy A (1983) Influence de la longueur de chaîne et du nombre pair ou impair d'atomes de carbone sur le comportement biologique des acides gras iodés. J Biophys Med Nucl 7: 97 - 106
29. Riche F, Mathieu J P, Busquet G, Vidal M, Godart J, Comet M, Pernin C, Benabed A, Bardy A (1983) Etude biologique d'acide gras en C16 marqués par un atome radioactif. J Biophys Med Nucl 7: 87 - 95
30. Keriel C, Bontemps L, Demaison L, Mathieu J P, Marti-Batlle D, Pernin C, Riche F, Vidal M, Godart J, Cuchet P, Comet M (1985) Influence on the myocardial and blood activity course on the characteristics of the labeled fatty acid injected IV into mice. Eur Heart J 6(Suppl B): 13 - 19
31. Kloster G, Stöcklin G (1982) Determination of the rate limiting step in halo-fatty acid turnover in the heart. In: Egerman H (ed) Radioaktive Isotope in Klinik und Forschung, 15 Badgasteiner Int Symp 15: 235 - 241
32. Harris P, Chlouverakis C, Gloster J, Howel-Jones T (1962) Arteriovenous differences in the composition of plasma free fatty acids in various regions of the body. Clin Sci 22: 113 - 118

33. Weich H F, Strauss H W, D'Agostino R, Pitt B (1977) Determination of extraction fraction by a double tracer method. J Nucl Med 18: 226 - 230
34. Weich H F, Strauss H W, Pitt B (1977) The extraction of thallium-201 by the myocardium. Circulation 56: 188 - 191
35. Riche F, Busquet G, Pilichowski P, Wolf J E, Mathieu J P, Vidal M, Vincens M, Godart J, Comet M, Pernin C (1981) Etude de la fixation myocardique de l'acide 16 I (131) hexadecene 9 oique en fonction du débit sanguin local chez le chien. J Biophys Med Nucl 5: 153 - 158
36. Fedor J M, MacIntosh D M, Rembert J C, Greenfield J C Jr (1978) Coronary and transmural myocardial blood flow responses in awake domestic pigs. Am J Physiol 235: H435 - H444
37. Olsson R A, Gregg D E (1965) Metabolic responses during myocardial reactive hyperemia in the unanesthetized dog. Am J Physiol 208: 231 - 236
38. Weiss E S, Hoffman E J, Phelps M E, Welch M J, Henry P D, Ter Pogossian M M, Sobel B E (1976) External detection and visualization of myocardial ischemia with 11C-substrates in vitro and in vivo. Circ Res 39: 24 - 32
39. Berger H, Addabbo M, Wolk S, Thakur M, Zacharis H, Caride V, Gottschalk A, Zaret B (1979) Myocardial arachidonic acid uptake and distribution in acute infarction and reactive hyperemia: relation to thallium 201. Circulation 60(Suppl II): II-269
40. Strauss H W, Harrison K, Langan J K, Lebowitz E, Pitt B (1975) Thallium 201 for myocardial imaging. Relation of thallium 201 to regional myocardial perfusion. Circulation 51: 641 - 645
41. Doyon B, Pilichowski P, Mathieu J P, Rossignol B, Comet M, Lacroix M, Pernin C (1980) Etude de la fixation myocardique du ^{201}Tl en fonction du débit sanguin local chez le chien. J Biophys Med Nucl 4: 95 - 101
42. Bontemps L, Demaison L, Keriel C, Pernin C, Mathieu J P, Marti-Batlle D, Vidal M, Fagret D, Comet M, Cuchet P (1985) Kinetics of 16^{123}I iodohexadecenoic acid metabolism in the rat myocardium. Influence of glucose concentration in the perfusate and comparison with 1-^{14}C palmitate. Eur Heart J 6(Suppl B): 91 - 96
43. Cuchet P, Demaison L, Bontemps L, Keriel C, Mathieu J P, Pernin C, Marti-Batlle D, Riche F Vidal M, Comet M (1985) Do iodinated fatty acids undergo a nonspecific deiodination in the myocardium? Eur J Nucl Med 1: 505 - 510
44. Goodman M M, Kirsch G, Knapp F F Jr (1984) Synthesis and evaluation of radioiodinated terminal p-iodophenyl-substituted α-and β-methyl branched fatty acids. J Med Chem 27: 390 - 397
45. Otto C A, Brown L E, Scott A M (1984) Radioiodinated branched chain fatty acids: substrates for beta oxidation? Concise communication. J Nucl Med 25: 75 - 80
46. Gloster J, Achillea M, Harris P (1978) Subcellular distribution of 1^{14}C palmitate and 1^{14}C oleate incorporated into lipids in the perfused rat heart: a comparison under isothermal and hypothermic conditions. J Mol Cell Cardiol 10; 439 - 448
47. Reske S N, Machulla H J, Sauer W, Hulsmann G, Schienle A, Breull W, Winkler C (1982) Flussdeterminierte myocardiale Aufnahme von (p ^{123}I-phenyl) pentadecansäure. Nucl Compact 13: 295 - 299
48. Dubois F, Depresseux J C, Demaison L, Mathieu J P, Bontemps L, Keriel C, Vidal M, Cuchet P, Comet M (1984) Mathematical model of iodinated fatty acid metabolism in the myocardium. J Mol Cell Cardiol 16(Suppl 2): 73
49. Dubois F, Bontemps L, Keriel C, Demaison L, Marti-Batlle D, Mathieu J P, Pernin C, Coornaert S, Comet M, Cuchet P (1984) Modèle mathématique du métabolisme myocardique des acides gras iodés du coeur isolé de rat. J Biophys Med Nucl 8: 204 - 205
50. Sherratt HSA, Gatley S J, Degrado T R, Ng C K, Holden J E (1983) Effects of 2(5(4-chlorophenyl)pentyl) oxidase-2-carboxylate on fatty acid and glucose metabolism in perfused rat hearts determined using iodine 125-I-16-iodo-hexadecanoate. Biochem Biophys Res Commun 117: 653 - 657
51. Darrah H K, Hedley-Whyte J (1973) Rapid incorporation of palmitate into lung. Site and metabolic fate. J Appl Physiol 34: 205 - 213

52. Tierney D F, Clements J A, Trahan H J (1967) Rates of replacement of lecithins and alveolar instability in rat lungs. Am J Physiol 213: 671 - 676
53. Schelbert H R, Phelps M E (1984) Positron computed tomography for the in vivo assessment of regional myocardial function. J Mol Cell Cardiol 16: 683 - 693

7. Radioiodinated free fatty acids: a clue to myocardial metabolism?

F.C. VISSER and G. WESTERA

Introduction

Metabolism is the basic process of the heart. Complex biochemical reactions are needed to build and maintain the cellular structures and to perform its ultimate task for myocardial contraction. Because physiological conditions of the heart vary widely with the demands of the body, the metabolic processes have to be extremely flexible to respond accordingly. Also the different fuels, which are transported to the heart by the blood, vary in concentration, needing a fine tuned mechanism of combined stubstrate utilization.

On the other hand, biochemical derangements inside the cardiac cell, e.g. in cardiomyopathy, can lead to malfunction of the contractile properties.

These considerations emphasize the importance of studying cardiac metabolism in patients and preferably in a noninvasive way. Because oxidation of longchain free fatty acids (FFA) contributes for 60-70% to the energy required for contraction, they form an excellent starting point for studying cardiac metabolism. The ideal fatty acids to use are those labeled with a radioisotope of the elements carbon, hydrogen and oxygen. Of these, C-11 is the only one feasable for biological studies. As decribed elsewhere in this book (Chapter 10), C-11-palmitic acid is successfully employed to investigate the heart metabolism under normal and pathological conditions.

High costs for production of this isotope and for the tomographs to detect the annihilation radiation limit the use of positron emitters in routine clinical practice. Therefore fatty acids labeled with gamma-emitting isotopes have been investigated to see if they could imitate the metabolic behaviour of the natural fatty acids under the different pathophysiological conditions.

In 1975 Poe [1] proposed to use fatty acids labeled with I-123 in the omega position because the terminal iodine had a similar size as a methyl group, therefore not interfering with biological properties such as uptake.

Since then numerous radioiodinated fatty acids have been developed and used in animal and patient studies. At this moment the most commonly used fatty acids are radioiodinated heptadecanoic acid, hexadecenoic acid and phenylpentadecanoic acid. Sofar clinical studies are promising: under ischemic conditions the elimination rate of the radioactivity was diminished as demonstrated by van der Wall in patients with exercise induced angina pectoris and in patients with unstable angina [2,3]. The same observation was made by Reske showing impaired iodo-phenyl pentadecanoic acid metabolism during exercise in patients with coronary artery disease [4]. Also at rest after intracoronary and intravenous administered heptadecanoic and phenylpentadecanoic acid the uptake and elimination pattern were clearly different from normal in patients with coronary artery disease [4-10]. In the acute stage of myocardial infarction in some patients a rapid washout of the radioactivity was observed, therefore discriminating the ischemic from necrotic myocardium [11]. The slow elimination rate of radioactivity in coronary artery disease may return to normal after several therapeutic interventions: after coronary dilatation [12], after bypass surgery [7] and cardiac rehabilitation [13]. In patients with cardiomyopathy a heterogeneous accumulation pattern and a wide scatter of elimination rates were found [14]. Simultaneous administration of glucose, insuline and heptadecanoic acid slowed the observed elimination rate of the radioactivity [15]. Thus the radioiodinated free fatty acids appear to be promising in studying cardiac metabolism in patients with various manifestations of clinical heart disease.

It must be pointed out that animal experimental work did not confirm these findings. Okada [16] demonstrated in his dog model that there was no difference in elimination rate between normal and ischemic canine myoardium. Schoen reported the absence of a relation between the myocardial oxygen consumption and the elimination rate [17], the former being an index of cardiac work.

This leads us to the most intriguing question in the application of omega-radioiodinated free fatty acids: what is actually measured in the time-activity curve, detected by the gamma camera? When looking at the time-activity curve four different components can be seen (Figure 1). The first part in which the activity rises and reaches its peak is obviously related to appearence of the fatty acid in the coronary bed and uptake in the myocardial cells. The rapid decline thereafter is related to tracer washout from the coronary bed and interstitial spaces. The third, slower washout of the radioactivity is related with the oxidation of the fatty acid and subsequent liberation of the radiolabel. The fourth almost flat part of the curve is related to turnover from the fatty acids incorporated into the various lipids.

It must be pointed out that most of these interpretations are derived from experiments with C-11 or C-14 palmitic acid, meaning that they are not necessarely transferable to radioiodinated fatty acids. Although comparable with C-11 palmitate, substantial differences are present.

The most obvious one (apart form its hetero-character) is the position of the radiolabel. In palmitic acid the radiolabel is in the alpha position, whereas the radioiodine is bound to the last carbon atom of the fatty acid chain. Secondly,

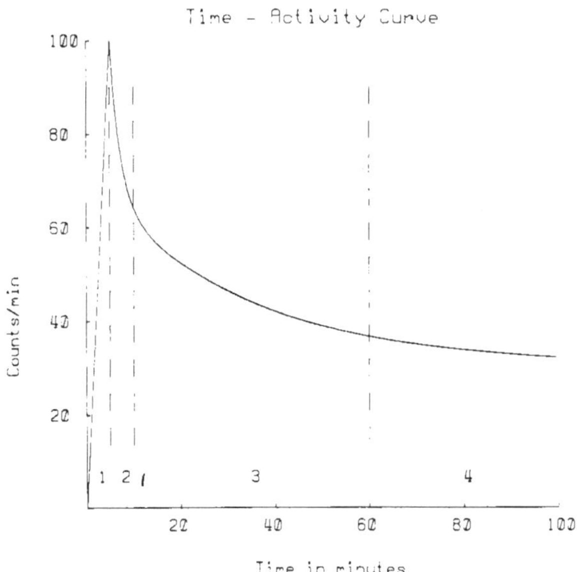

Figure 1. A schematic representation of the time-activity curve in counts per minute after radiolabeled fatty acid administration. The ordinate represents the counts per minute, the abscissa time in minutes. Phase 1 represents the arrival of the fatty acid in the heart; phase 2 washout of the fatty acid from the coronary bed after uptake; phase 3 is related to oxidation of fatty acids and liberation of the radiolabel into the systemic circulation; phase 4 the disappearance of radioactivity from radiolabeled lipids.

the C-11 element after oxidation has occurred, is incorporated in CO_2. Radioiodine is either liberated as free iodide in the case of heptadecanoic and hexadecenoic acid or as iodobenzoic acid in the case of phenylpentadecanoic acid. C-11-O_2 is rapidly cleared from the myocardial cells whereas free radioiodide being a polar ion may have difficulties to pass the several membranes before entering the systemic circulation.

The most important phases to consider in patient studies are phase 3 and 4. Phase 1 and 2, uptake and release from the coronary bed occur more or less simultaneously, especially after intravenous administration of the fatty acid. In phase 3 the oxidation and subsequent release of the radiolabel takes place. Therefore this part of the time-activity curve might be an index of the amount and rate of fatty acid oxidation. Using palmitic acid the relation has clearly been demonstrated. Increasing heart rate and cardiac work increased the slope of elimination of the radioactivity. Furthermore a relation with myocardial oxygen consumption was established.

In radioiodinated fatty acids data of the relation between the elimination rate and cardiac work are conflicting. As stated previously no relation was found with myocardial oxygen consumption in experiments by Schoen [17]. However in our dog experiments the elimination rate increased with higher blood pressure. With a mean blood pressure of 66 mmHg the half-time value of the elimination rate was 22 min, decreasing to 14 min in dogs with a mean blood pressure of 92 mmHg. Therefore the main object of our recent work has been to establish the relation of the externally observed elimination rate with fatty acid metabolism. Or more specifically, can we actually measure fatty acid metabolism parameters using radioiodinated free fatty acids?

Before going into details, the term metabolism has to be defined further because the term is used for the whole process of transfer of the fatty acid into the myocardial cell to washout of endproducts of cardiac combustion. Three main components can be discerned: 1) uptake of fatty acids into the myocyte, 2) distribution into the various pools, 3) the oxidative pathways and clearance of oxidation products. As is known from natural analogues, fatty acids are taken up by either passive and/or active transport. Thereafter a part is stored as lipids, mainly triglycerides and phospholipids. A major part is transported via the carnitine shuttle to the mitochondria where oxidation occurs to produce energy-rich phosphate bonds. So the important questions are: is uptake similar to the natural fatty acids? Is the biochemical distribution pattern comparable and is the oxidation phase detectable using the time-activity curve?

Uptake

The topic uptake is discussed elsewhere in this book. In short, differences in uptake exist between the various radioiodinated fatty acids. This is more pronounced during ischemia. When comparing extractions, iodo-heptadecanoic acid is preferentially taken up. The extraction fraction of C-11 palmitate is reported to be 70-80% in normal flow conditions whereas the measured extraction of iodo-heptadecanoic acid is 40-50% [18]. Although somewhat less, the uptake is proportional to flow like with the natural fatty acids.

Relation of the time-activity curve with beta-oxidation

Schematically, the kinetics of the fatty acids can be presented in a simplified compartment model (Figure 2). The radioiodinated fatty acids are transported into the mitochondria (k_3). Inside the mitochondria they are oxidized by beta-oxidation pathways (k_5), leaving the halide ions or iodobenzoic acid behind as final catabolites (x^-) which eventually leave the cell (k_9). For clinical evaluation it is essential to know the rate of the different steps and especially which one is rate determining. In general the slowest step is responsable for the observed time-activity curve, unless two have about the same speed. It would be highly desirable for the clinical setting that the oxidation rate (k_5) is the slowest one, because then the elimination rate could be related to fatty acid oxidation, as suggested by Otto [19].

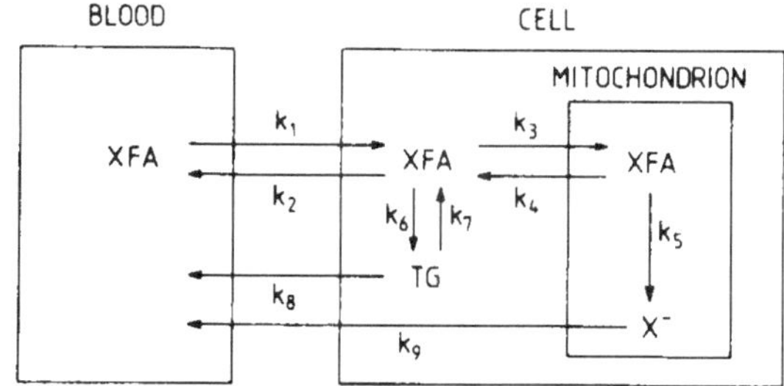

Figure 2. Simplified compartment model for the turnover of radiolabeled fatty acids in heart muscle. X=halogen; FA=fatty acids; TG=triglycerides.
(from Kloster e.a. (3) with permission)

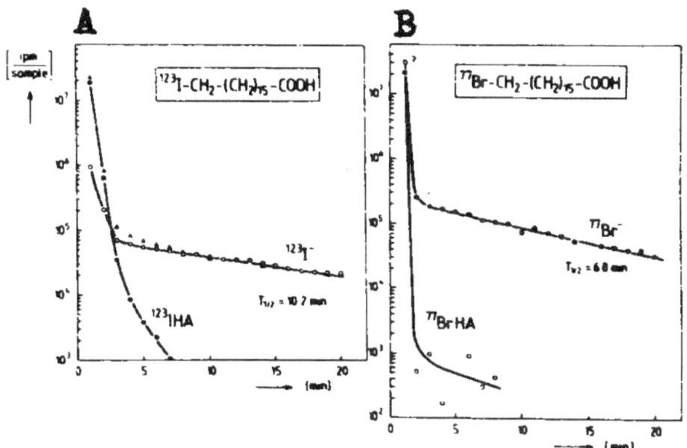

Figure 3. Typical kinetics of elimination of free iodide (A) and bromide (B) from isolated perfused Guinea-pig hearts after bolus injection of IHA and BHA respectively (no carrier added). Also shown the washout of the halofatty acid from the extracellular space. HA = heptadecanoic acid. (from Kloster e.a. (3) with permission)

Kloster and Stoecklin [20] investigated the perfusate of isolated Guinea-pig hearts after bolus injection of halo-fatty acids and after perfusing the heart during 40 min with radioactive halide ions alone. As seen from Figure 3, after fatty acid administration, the halide ions are the only catabolites to be eliminated from the heart. The half-time values of halide catabolites corresponded well with the half-time values of the radioactivity after equilibration of the heart with halide ions alone (Table 1).

Table 1. Elimination half-times (in minutes) of radioactivity after halo-fatty acid and halide administration to myocardium of Guinea-pigs

Tracer injected	Half-time value	Tracer injected	Half-time value
17-I-123-IHA	9.8 ± 0.3	I-123	10.3 ± 0.5
17-Br-77-BHA	5.1 ± 1.6	Br-77	6.5 ± 0.3
17-F-18-FHA	16.7 ± 2.0	F-18	13.2 ± 0.6

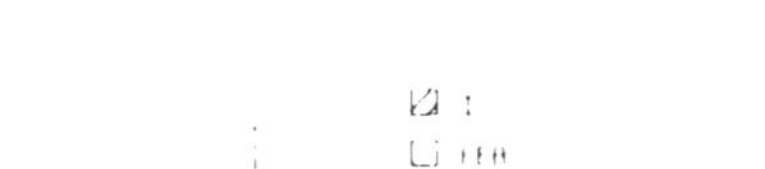

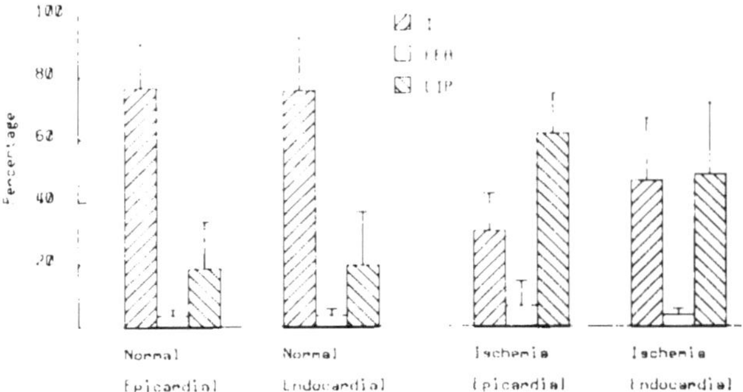

Figure 4. Proportion of free radioiodide (I), radioiodinated free fatty acids (FFA) and radioiodinated lipids (LIP) in normal and ischemic subepi- and subendocardium. The proportion was determined 5 min after injection of I-HDA.

These data suggest that the rate determining step is related to transport of ions from inside the mitochondria to the vascular space (k_9). Nonetheless, only the perfusate was measured and not the intracellular metabolites. We therefore undertook an experiment in which the intracellular metabolites were measured in canine myocardium [21]. Ten open-chest dogs were studied. In four of them, 5 min after I-131-heptadecanoic acid (I-HDA) administration, the heart action was arrested, the whole heart cut-out and immediately stored in iced water to stop further cardiac metabolism. Of pieces normal myocardium the composition of injected I-HDA, free iodide and radiolabeled lipids were determined (Figure 4). As can be seen, 5 min after I-HDA injection the major part appears to be free iodide: 76%. Only 5% of the radioactivity is present as I-HDA, whereas the remainder 19% are lipids. Thus after uptake, a part of I-HDA is stored as lipids and the major part is immediately oxidized, leaving the free iodide behind. To get a better insight into the dynamic kinetics, in the same dog model seven serial myocardial tissue samples were taken from the myocardium within a time period of 30 min (Figure 5). In the biopsies the radioactivity increased during the first 5 min due to uptake of recirculating I-HDA in blood (Figure 6). Thereafter the radioactivity decreased. This curve was paralleled by the decrease of free radioiodide, having a half-time value of 25 min. Because the phospolipids, triglycerides and cholesterolesters remained constant, the elimination rate as observed during a scintigraphic study is related to washout of free radioiodide [18]. Thus there appears to be no relation with the oxidation rate of radioiodinated free fatty acids.

Influence of ischemia

From studies with natural fatty acids under ischemic condition is known that

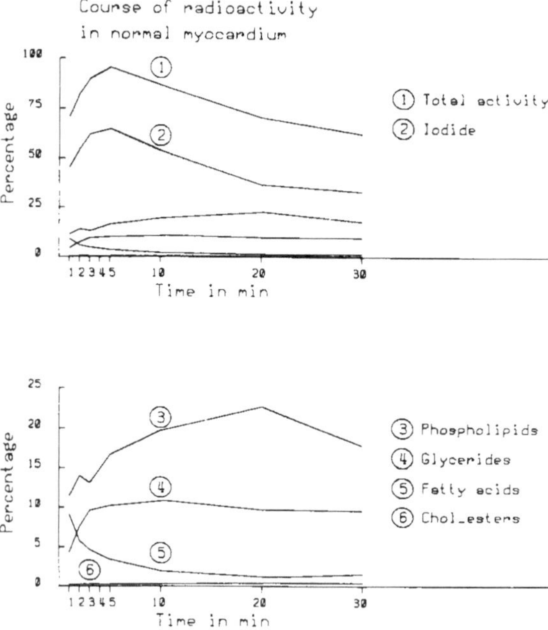

Figure 5. Course of radioactivity, normalized to peak count rate (100%) and distribution over I-HDA, free radioiodide and various lipids with incorporated I-HDA (mono-, di-, triglycerides, phospholipids and cholesterolesters).

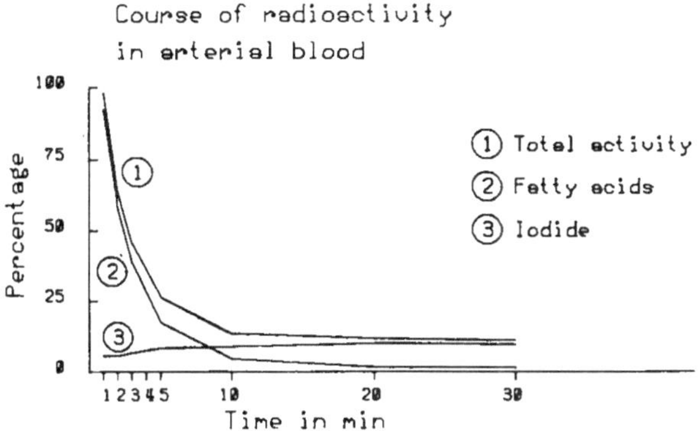

Figure 6. Course of radioactivity in arterial blood after I-HDA injection. Data were normalized to peak value of activity found in the first minute. The distribution over I-HDA and free radioiodide is given.

uptake of FFA is decreased. This is not only due to decreased flow and subsequent decreased supply of FFA but also due to a reduction of extraction. Inside the cell metabolic breakdown is diminished and a proportionally larger fraction of FFA is diverted into the lipid pool. To test if the altered kinetics are also applicable to radioiodinated free fatty acids the same dog experiment was

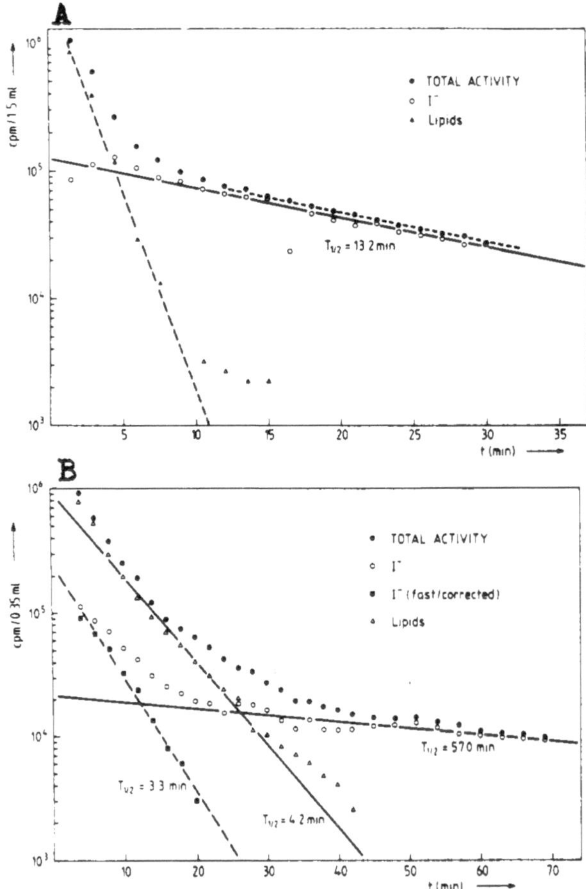

Figure 7. (A) Time course of radioactivity in perfusate after bolus injection of IHA in normoxic perfused rabbit heart and chemical form of radioactivity in different fraction as determined by chromatographic analysis. (B) Time course of radioactivity in perfusate after bolus injection of IHA in globally ischemic perfused rabbit heart and chemical form of radioactivity in different fractions as determined by chromatographic analysis (half-times for iodide elimination derived by curve stripping). (from Kloster e.a. (22), with permission)

used as described above. In six dogs a part of the myocardium was made ischemic by ligation of the left anterior descending artery. Figure 4 shows the results: uptake of I-HDA in the ischemic part was 33% of normal myocardium. Thirty-nine percent was free radioiodide, 6% was FFA and 55% were lipids. This indicates that I-HDA behaves with respect to uptake and distribution under ischemia like the natural fatty acids. Kloster [22] studied the washout pattern of catabolites during normal perfusion and ischemia. In the experiments with isolated Guinea-pig hearts the washout of control hearts had a half-time of 14.3 min. When the hearts were made globally ischemic, the behaviour of I-HDA changed dramatically: 1) washout of lipids was more prolonged; the half-time of lipid washout was 4.0 min compared to 0.7 min in normoxic animals; 2) the elimination of iodide ions became biphasic with a fast component of 3.8 min and a second slow one of 60.5 min (Figure 7).

Analysis of these experimental results indicates that during ischemia the time-activity curve shows a different kinetic behaviour compared to non-ischemic myocardium. This is in agreement with patient studies in which ischemia causes a decrease in the rate of elimination of radioactivity. Because no direct relation is present with the oxidation rate, it is tempting to speculate on the underlying mechanism. Two factors are possibly responsible: chronic ischemia causes shrinking and loss of mitochondria. It is expected that this will result in a slower iodide transport inside the cell. Secondly, capillary blood flow and venous return of the coronary circulation might be delayed in the affected areas of obstructive coronary artery disease, influencing the intra-extracellular concentration gradient of free iodide. The combined effects can result in slowing down the elimination of radioactivity. In acute ischemia and infarction mitochondria swell and mitochondrial and cellular membranes show increased porosity. This can lead to increased washout (and thus to an increase of the observed elimination rate) of metabolites of fatty acids.

Biochemical distribution pattern

Under influence of several interventions the ratio between fatty acids to be oxidized and to be stored in lipids can vary. It is known from *in vitro* experiments that addition of glucose and insuline results in decreased fatty acid oxidation and increased esterification to glycerides which are then more slowly utilized. The same observation was made using C-11-palmitate and glucose/insuline infusion. Dudczak [15] studied the kinetics of I-HDA in patients and found reduced uptake during glucose/insuline infusion and an abolishment of the biexponential elimination curve, present in control studies. In our dog experiments the distribution pattern was also investigated during glucose infusion. In Figure 8A the results obtained from a control dog are shown and in Figure 8B from a dog during glucose administration. It can be recognized that during glucose infusion a larger amount of I-HDA is stored as lipids. In contrast to Dudczak's findings [15] however, the elimination rate of free iodide remained unaltered.

The same observation of distribution patterns was made by Bontemps [23] in isolated rat heart during glucose in which the aqueous phase (free iodide and water soluble metabolites) decreased and the organic phase (lipids) increased.

The influence of ischemia has been discussed. Figure 4 shows that during ischemia a larger amount of fatty acids is stored in the lipids and less I-HDA is oxidized, resulting in diminished free iodide.

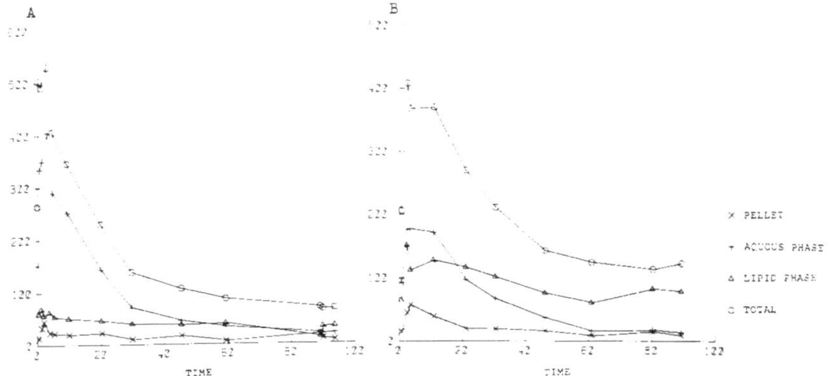

Figure 8. Time-activity curve in myocardium after injection of radioiodinated free fatty acids in control dog (A) and during glucose infusion (B). The distribution over the aqueous phase (free iodide) and organic phase (lipids) is given. Half-time values of the aqueous phase in A and B were 12 and 14 min respectively.

Conclusions

It can be concluded from our experimental data that uptake, distribution and elimination of radioiodinated free fatty acids are comparable with natural fatty acids and therefore provide evidence for the feasibility of using the fatty acids as indicators of myocardial metabolism.

However, detailed analysis of fatty acid kinetics in patients in the same way as in the experimental conditions can be difficult. First of all, after intravenous injection in man, other organs such as liver and muscles metabolize the fatty acid giving rise to high background activity from circulating free iodide. Background correction can be difficult and may result in improper analysis of the time-activity curve (van Eenige, Chapter 5). Furthermore, because a time-activity curve is obtained from patients using one specific view of the gamma camera, there will be overlapping of anatomical structures and lack of depth resolution. Also overlap between normal and ischemic myocardium may be present averaging the half-time values of normal and abnormal tissue. Finally, a diseased part of the myocardium may be missed in the one projection used during scintigraphy of the patient.

Although these difficulties are present, data of uptake and distribution patterns and of half-time values in patients with known cardiac disease justify the use and further clinical investigation of radioiodinated free fatty acids.

Acknowledgement

We are indepted to Prof. Dr G Stoecklin who allowed us to use some of his results in detail for this contribution.

References

1. Poe N D, Robinson jr G D, MacDonald N S (1975) Myocardial extraction of labeled long-chain fatty acid analogs. Proc Soc Exp Biol Med 148: 215 - 218
2. van der Wall E E, Heidendal G A K, den Hollander W, Westera G, Roos J P (1981) Metabolic myocardial imaging with I-123 labeled heptadecanoic acid in patients with angina pectoris. Eur J Nucl Med 6: 391 - 396
3. van der Wall E E, den Hollander W, Heidendal G A K, Westera G, Roos J P (1983) Myocardial scintigraphy with I-123 labeled heptadecanoic acid in patients with unstable angina pectoris. Postgrad Med J 59(Suppl 3): 38 - 40
4. Reske S N, Leddar R, Nitsch J, Kluenenberg H, Winkler C (1985) Impaired cardiac I-123-phenyl fatty acid turnover in CAD after repeated submaximal exercise. Circulation 72 (Suppl 3): 358
5. Visser F C, van Eenige M J, van der Wall E E, Westera G, van Engelen C J, van Lingen A, de Cock C C, den Hollander W, Heidendal G A K, Roos J P (1985) The elimination rate of I-123-heptadecanoic acid after intracoronary and intravenous administration. Eur J Nucl Med 11: 114 - 119
6. Dudczak R, Schmoliner R, Pichler M, Frischauf H, Moesslacher H (1981) Myocardial imaging with I-123-heptadecanoic acid assessment of regional myocardial fatty acid metabolism. In: Schmidt H A E, Roesler H (eds) Proceedings of the 19th International Annual Meeting of the European Society of Nuclear Medicine, Bern, 1, p 173
7. Freundlieb C, Hoeck A, Vyska K, Erbel R, Feinendegen L E (1982) Fatty acid uptake and turnover rate in the ischemic heart before and after bypass surgery. In: Raynaud C (ed) Nucl Med Biol Proc third World Congr Nucl Med Biol Paris, II, Pergamon Press pp 1392 - 1395
8. Aurich D, Reske S N, Biersack H J *et al.* (1982) Biplanar sequential scintigraphy of the myocardium by means of 123-I-heptadecanoic acid. In: Raynaud C (ed) Proc third World Congr Nucl Med Biol Paris, II, Pergamon Press pp 1389 - 1391
9. Dudczak R, Schmoliner R, Kletter K, Frischauf H, Angelberger P (1983) Clinical evaluation of I-123-labeled p-phenylpentadecanoic acid (p-IPPA) for myocardial scintigraphy. J Nucl Med All Sci 27: 267 - 279
10. Reske S N (1985) I-123-phentylpentadecanoic acid as a tracer of cardiac free fatty acid metabolism. Experimental and clinical results. Eur Heart J 6(Suppl B): 39 - 47
11. van der Wall E E, den Hollander W, Heidendal G A K, Westera G, Majid P A, Roos J P (1981) Dynamic myocardial scintigraphy with I-123 labeled free fatty acids in patients with myocardial infarction. Eur J Nucl Med 6: 383 - 389
12. Vyska K, Freundlieb C, Hoeck A, Feinendegen L E, Machulla H J, Stoecklin G (1980) Myocardial imaging and measurement of myocardial fatty acid metabolism using omega-I-123-heptadecanoic acid. Adv Clin Cardiol 1: 422 - 436
13. Hoeck A, Freundlieb C, Vyska K *et al.* (1982) The influence of rehabilitation training on fatty acid metabolism in patients with myocardial infarciton. In: Faivre G, Bertrand A, Cherrier F, Amor M, Neimann J L (eds) Noninvasive methods in ischemic heart disease. Nancy: Specia pp 300 - 300
14. Hoeck A, Freundlieb C, Vyska K, Loesse B, Erbel R, Feinendegen L E (1983) Myocardial imaging and metabolic studies with 17-I-123 iodoheptadecanoic acid in patients with idiopathic congestive cardiomyopathy. J Nucl Med 24: 22 - 28
15. Dudczak R, Kletter K, Frischauf H, Losert U, Angelberger P, Schmoliner R (1984) The use of I-123-labeled heptadecanoic acid (HDA) as metabolic tracer: preliminary report. Eur J Nucl Med 9: 81 - 85
16. Okada R D, Elamaleh D, Werre G S, Strauss H W (1983) Myocardial kinetics of I-123-labeled-16-hexadecanoic acid. Eur J Nucl Med 8: 211 - 217
17. Schoen H R, Senekowitsch R, Berg D, Schneidereith M, Moellenstaedt S, Kriegel H,

Pabst H W, Bloemer H (1984) Kinetics of I-123-heptadecanoic acid in normal myocardium. In: Amersham (ed) Eur Nucl Med Congr, Helsinki. Heidelberg: Brausdruck, p 58
18. Visser F C, van Eenige M J, Westera G *et al.* (1985) Metabolic fate of radioiodinated heptadecanoic acid in the normal canine heart. Circulation 72: 565 - 571
19. Otto C A, Brown L E, Wieland D M, Beierwaltes W H (1981) Radioiodinated fatty acids for myocardial imaging: effects of chain length. J Nucl Med 22: 613 - 618
20. Kloster G, Stoecklin G (1982) Determination of the rate-determining step in halofatty acid-turnover in the heart. Radioaktive Isotope in Klinik und Forschung, Vol 15. Verlag H Egermann: Wien, pp 235 - 241
21. Visser F C, van Eenige M J, Westera G, den Hollander W, Roos J P (1985) Kinetics of radioiodinated heptadecanoic acid and metabolites in the normal and ischaemic canine heart. Eur Heart J 6 (Suppl B): 97 - 101
22. Kloster G, Stoecklin G, Smith E F, Schroer K (1984) Omega-halofatty acids: A probe for mitochondrial membrane integrity. In vitro investigations in normal and ischaemic myocardium. Eur J Nucl Med 9: 305 - 311
23. Bontemps L, Demaison L, Keriel C, Pernin C, Mattieu J P, Marti-Batlle D, Vidal M, Fagret D, Comet M, Cuchet P (1985) Kinetics of 16-I-123-iodohexadecenoic acid metabolism in the rat myocardium, influence of glucose concentration in the perfuse and comparison with I-14-C palmitate. Eur Heart J 6 (Suppl B): 91 - 96

8. Cardiac metabolism of I-123 phenyl-pentadecanoic acid

S.N. RESKE

Introduction

Probably the first tracer experiment for investigation of a metabolic reaction sequence was published in 1905 by Knoop [1]. He fed dogs and rabbits with odd- and even-numbered free fatty acids (FFA), which were substituted or labeled at the terminal C-atom with a phenyl-residue. It was found that odd-numbered FFA were excreted with urine as benzoic acid and even-numbered as phenyl-acetic acid. It was concluded from these experiments that FFA are degraded by subsequent cleavage of C-2 fragments.

In 1980 Machulla [2], with Knoop's early experiments in mind, proposed para-I-123-phenyl fatty acids for noninvasive investigation of cardiac FFA-metabolism, thus avoiding problems encountered with *in vivo* deiodination of aliphathic radioiodinated FFA [3,4].

The final catabolites of iodinated phenylpentadecanoic acid (I-PPA), the most widely used compound of this type of radioiodinated fatty acids, are finally excreted with urine as I-benzoic acid, I-hippuric acid and probably also I-benzoic glucuronide (Figure 1) [5]. The application of radiolabeled FFA for investigating cardiac energy metabolism is especially meaningful since

(1) FFA are the main fuel for energy production of the heart muscle at rest;
(2) regional FFA-uptake is very closely linked to that of regional myocardial blood flow (rMBF) over a wide range of normal and reduced flow rates;
(3) degradation of FFA in β-oxidation is most sensitive to oxygen deprivation, and
(4) local derangements of cardiac FFA metabolism are known to occur in certain cardiomyopathies.

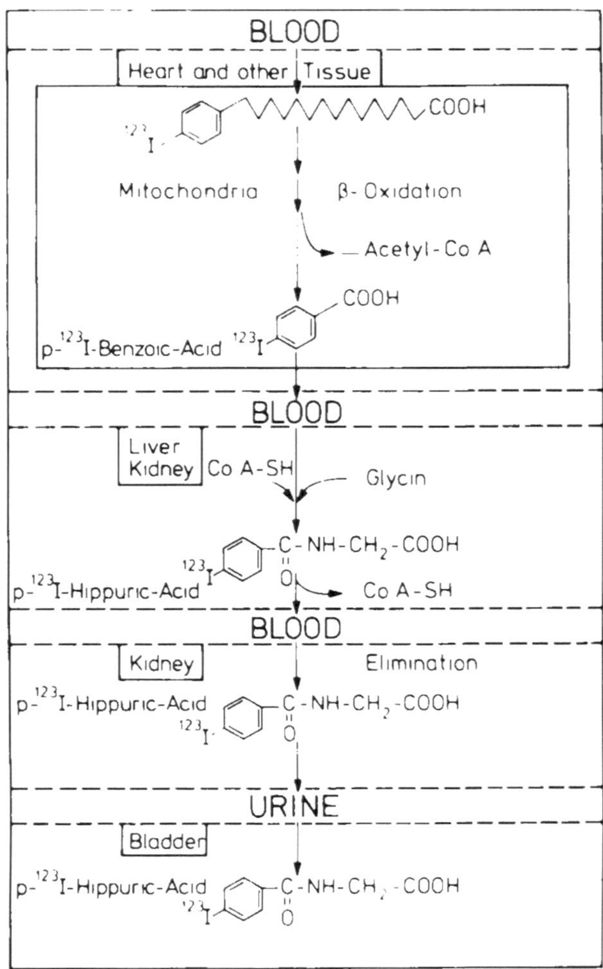

Figure 1. Scheme of the metabolic fate of I-PPA, i.e. β-oxidation, conjugation, elimination and finally excretion in the urine

Cardiac metabolism of iodinated phenyl-pentadecanoic acid (I-PPA) ascertained in animal experiments

The following article will review some of the major results of animal experimental as well as of clinical studies of cardiac I-PPA metabolism and will give a framework for future investigations in this field.

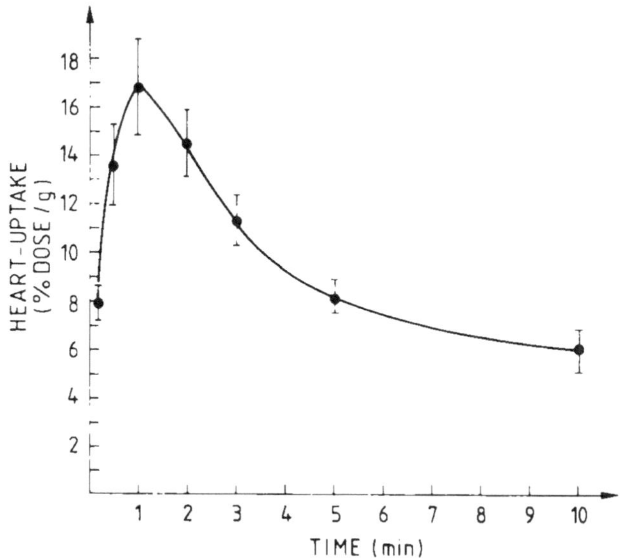

Figure 2. Kinetics of heart uptake of I-PPA in non-fasted mice.

Animal experimental studies

Pharmacokinetics

Uptake and turnover of I-PPA has been studied in murine experiments [6,7]. After intravenous (i.v.) tracer application a rapid cardiac uptake of about 4-5% of the injected dose was achieved within 2-3 min. Maximal cardiac uptake was followed by a two-component tracer clearance. Half-times of about 2-3 min and 20-30 min were determined for the rapid first and late second component respectively. Two-component cardiac tracer clearance was observed in both fasted and fed animals, the latter however showed a somewhat delayed cardiac tracer clearance (Figure 2) [8].

Intracellular lipid distribution was studied after lipid extraction according to a modified Folch method [9,10] and subsequent thin-layer-chromatography (TLC) of the lipophilic and hydrophilic metabolites. Labeled hydrophilic metabolite concentration rapidly increased during the first 2-3 min after tracer application. Thereafter a quick washout of these metabolites from the heart was found, indicating a rapid oxidation of a substantial fraction of I-PPA [11]. These findings were substantiated in a recent gas-chromatographic mass-spectrometric study, in which I-benzoic acid, I-phenylpropionic acid and I-phenylpropenoic acid were identified as major catabolites of I-PPA [12]. Comparable cardiac clearance slopes of ^{51}Cr-EDTA, which was injected simultaneously with I-PPA in a set of experiments [7] (which is cleared exclusively from the extracellular space) and that of hydrophilic I-PPA-metabolites (which are

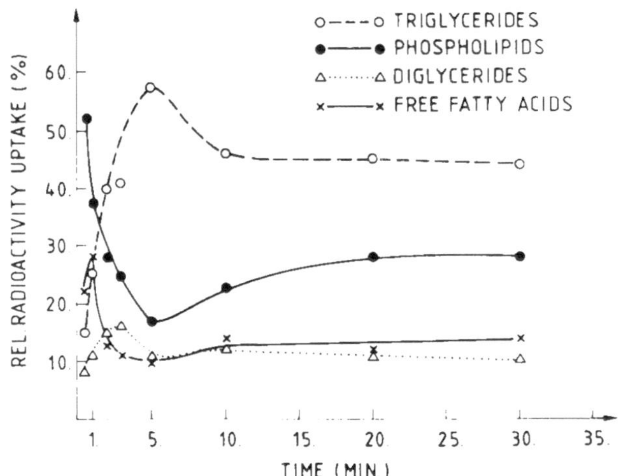

Figure 3. Kinetics of uptake of I-PPA in cardiac lipids.

cleared from the mitochondrial compartment) argue against major transport barriers during the washout of I-PPA oxidation products from mitochondria to blood vessels.

The major cardiac lipid fractions, i.e. FFA, phospholipids (PL), diglycerides (DG) and triglycerides (TG) are rapidly labeled after i.v. injection of I-PPA (Figure 3). In normoxic heart muscle, where metabolic fate of FFA is primary related to oxidation [13], relatively low equilibrium concentrations of I-PPA — recovered in FFA and DG-fraction — were encountered (Figure 3). A moderate uptake of I-PPA in labeled PL (20-30% of lipid-bound radioactivity) was found. I-PPA-uptake into PL probably reflects incorporation into structural membrane lipids, characterized by a rather slow metabolic rate. The initial rapid radioactivity clearance from labeled PL might reflect incorporation of I-PPA into phosphatidic acid, a common precursor molecule of PL- and TG-synthesis [14]. Correspondingly, a rapid and high uptake of I-PPA into TG fraction was observed. About 50-60% of labeled lipids were recovered as labeled TG in fasted compared to about 80-90% in fed animals [15], demonstrating the influence of nutritional state on cardiac I-PPA metabolism.

Interestingly, the high cardiac metabolic rate of FFA seemed to be associated with a relatively high TG-labeling pattern. In contrast, tissues with a comparatively low FFA-oxidation rate, like lung or spleen tissue, had significantly lower uptake of I-PPA into TG-fraction [7,11]. These findings question the conventional view of TG-fraction as a "lipid-storage pool" but might rather indicate a physiological role of cardiac TG-pool as a "buffer compartment" for intracellular FFA. The physiological role of such a buffer compartment might involve the regulation of cytosolic FFA-concentration at low values in order to prevent the detrimental effects of a high concentration of intracellular FFA. Such a metabolic buffer would be especially advantageous

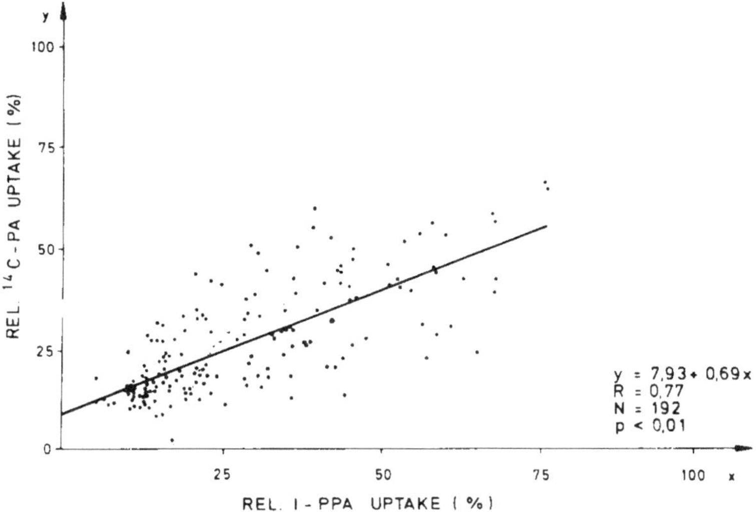

Figure 4. Correlation of I-PPA and C-14 palmitic acid uptake in cardiac lipids. Kinetics of I-PPA uptake in the respective lipid fractions.

for short-term regulation of cytosolic FFA-concentration in states of rapidly varying amounts of FFA supply and demand.

Comparison with C-14 palmitic acid

Myocardial metabolism of I-PPA was investigated together with a "standard" FFA i.e. 1-^{14}C-palmitic acid (CP), in a dual tracer experiment in order to compare both tracers in an identical metabolic environment [6]. Cardiac uptake and intracellular lipid distribution of both tracers were determined as described previously [6]. Uptake and turnover of both global radioactivity incorporated into heart muscle tissue as well as in extracted hydrophilic and lipophilic metabolites were significantly correlated (Figure 4) [6].

Highest uptake of CP and I-PPA was found in TG-fraction, an intermediate amount in PL-fraction (somewhat higher values for CP than for I-PPA after the initial equilibration period) and a significant amount in DG- and FFA-fraction (Figure 5). Uptake and kinetics of both tracers in the main cardiac lipid fractions were significantly correlated ($r=0.5$ - 0.9, $p<0.05$ - 0.001, $N=142$). It was concluded from these findings, first, that I-PPA is metabolized in heart muscle tissue very similar to CP and second, that cardiac turnover of both tracers is significantly related.

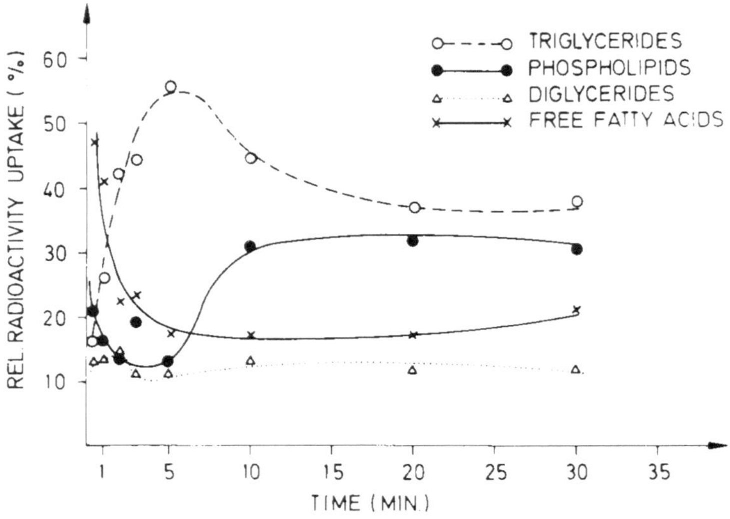

Figure 5. Kinetics of C-14 palmitic acid uptake in cardiac lipids.

Metabolic interventions

In a series of experiments, cardiac metabolism was investigated in the isolated perfused Langendorff rat heart both at rest as well as after isoproterenol (2μg) mediated stimulation or lactate-induced suppression (2 and 20 μmol) of cardiac lipid metabolism [16].

In a first set of experiments, metabolites produced by I-PPA during perfusion of rat heart with Krebs-Henseleit buffer were characterized by gas chromatography-mass spectometry (GC-MS) [12]. This study yielded the following results: 1) heart triglycerides contained 73% of I-PPA and only small amounts of unesterified I-PPA were found in myocardium; this finding correlated well with radioactivity uptake measurements in these fractions, which were determined simultaneously; 2) three catabolites could be identified and characterized in the effluents ω(p-iodo-phenyl-) propionic acid, ω(p--iodophenyl-)propenoic and p-iodo-benzoic acid. These short-chain catabolites were only detected in the perfusion medium which indicated that they were not unriched but rapidly eliminated from heart muscle tissue [12]. These findings conclusively show that I-PPA is degraded in heart muscle to short-chain catabolites (mainly I-benzoic acid) which are rapidly released from this tissue.

In a second set of experiments, CP and I-PPA were simultaneously applied to isolated Langendorff-perfused rat hearts during isoproterenol-mediated stimulation or lactate-induced suppression (2.0 and 20.0 μmol lactate in the perfusion medium) of cardiac lipid metabolism [16]. $^{14}CO_2$ and hydrophilic

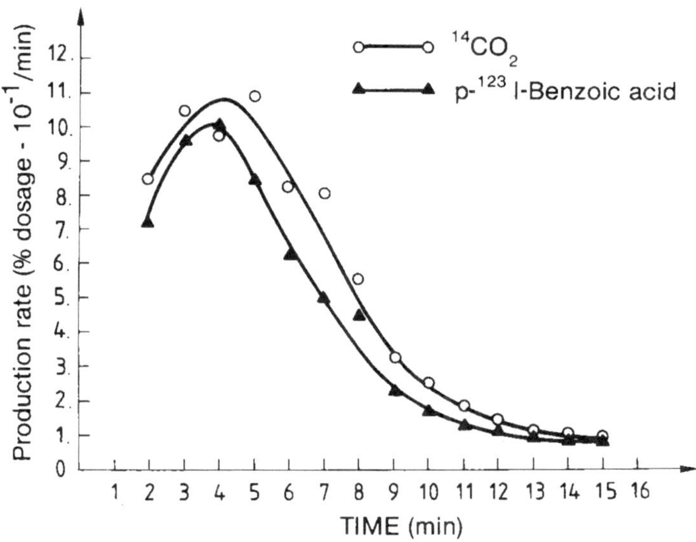

Figure 6. CO_2 and I-benzoic acid production after simultaneous ^{14}C palmitic acid and I-PPA application to isolated perfused Langendorff rat hearts.

metabolites of I-PPA were measured in the effluent. In addition, the time-course of precordial radioactivity clearance and the I-PPA uptake in cardiac lipid fractions — extracted after the 20 min perfusion period — were determined.

$^{14}CO_2$-production was correlated at the basal state as well as after a suppressed and stimulated lipolysis with the production of hydrophilic catabolites (Figure 6) ($r=0.87$, $p<0.005$, $N=35$). The slope of $^{14}CO_2$-washout from the heart and that of hydrophilic catabolites was also significantly correlated during the metabolic intervention ($r=0.92$, $p<0.05$, $N=30$), indicating identical directional changes of the rate of cardiac oxidation of both FFA.

The slope of the externally recorded release of radioactivity from heart muscle showed significant changes during enhanced or suppressed lipolysis: isoproterenol caused a 63% reduction of elimination half-time, i.e. increased radioactivity turnover, whereas lactate slowed down radioactivity release considerably (42% and 200% increased elimination half-times).

Isoproterenol treatment did not change relative I-PPA-uptake into cardiac lipids. Administration of lactate shifted the uptake of I-PPA into TG-fraction.

Based on these studies the following conclusions can be made:

1) Cardiac I-PPA metabolism is correlated to that of CP in different metabolic states;
2) These changes can be assessed by recording precordial tracer clearance;
3) These changes reflect the rate of overall FFA-oxidation and intermediary storage in tissue lipid esters.

Uptake and rMBF

Robinson and Poe [17] as well as Okada *et al.* [18] found a very close correlation of regional myocardial blood flow (rMBF) and regional uptake of I-heptadecanoic acid in normal and ischemic myocardium. Also initial I-PPA uptake is mainly governed by rMBF in both normally perfused and acutely ischemic myocardium [19]. During pacing-induced (195 bpm) stimulation of rMBF, however, only a moderate increase of regional I-PPA uptake disproportionate to rMBF-increase was observed in the canine heart [20]. At rMBF values exceeding 150-170 ml/min × 100 g a threshold value of regional I-PPA uptake was found, indicating a limited capacity of FFA-utilization in this experimental model. The exact relation of rMBF and regional I-PPA uptake during more physiological conditions and the modulating influence of alternate substrate supply on regional I-PPA uptake remain to be established.

Uptake in reperfused myocardium

In a limited number of canine experiments, regional I-PPA uptake was studied after a temporary (30 min) occlusion of the LAD and subsequent reperfusion [21]. Whereas all control dogs with permanent occlusion showed a concordant reduction of rMBF and regional I-PPA uptake, reperfusion restored both regional rMBF to about 120% of control values and regional I-PPA uptake to about 100% of the pre-occlusion values. Thus a sustained regional cardiac metabolic function, as assessed by means of the uptake of I-PPA, was found in potentially salvable myocardium after a short-term occlusion of a coronary artery. Evaluation of regional I-PPA uptake after a reversible occlusion of a coronary artery may thus provide a new diagnostic technique for short-term therapy control after coronary thrombolysis. The relation of local cardiac I-PPA uptake in jeopardized myocardium after prolonged acute ischemic events will currently be investigated.

SPECT-imaging of acute myocardial ischemia

The utility of myocardial imaging and assessment of regional myocardial metabolism of I-PPA by means of single photon emission tomography (SPECT) has been recently shown by our group [22] and others [23]. High quality cross-sectional images of dog hearts with clear delineation of left ventricular walls can be obtained. Normal myocardium shows a uniform left ventricular radioactivity uptake as well as a homogeneous radioactivity clearance. Myocardial infarcts are visualized as areas of deficient radioactivity accumulation (Figure 7). Regional elimination expressed in half-times of I-PPA, as determined by SPECT measurements, were significantly prolonged in

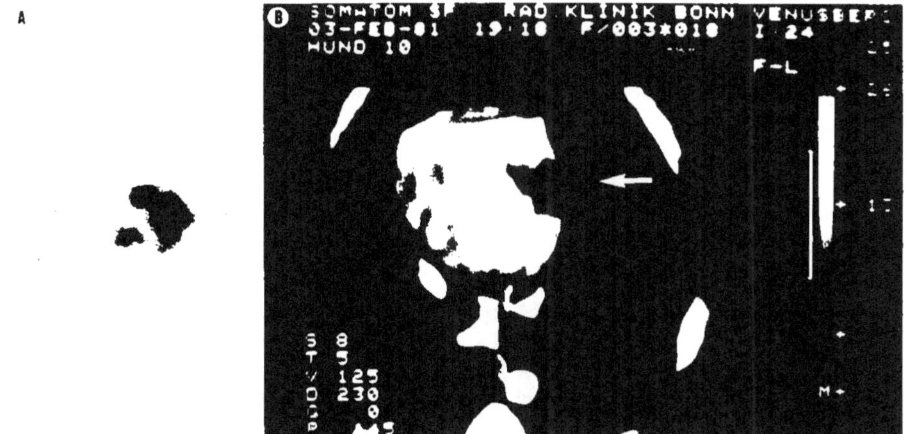

Figure 7. Detection of acute ischemia with SPECT. Two hours after ligation of the LAD a clearly defined I-PPA uptake defect is seen in the anterolateral wall of a dog heart (midventricular level, tranversal slice(A)). For comparison the cardiotransmission CT, recorded during contrast infusion, is shown (B). The acute ischemic myocarium is clearly delineated as hypodense area in the anterolateral wall of the left ventricular myocardium. L = left, A = anterior; R = right; P = posterior.

reperfused myocardium after a reversible occlusion of the supplying coronary artery [23]. I-PPA clearance was – 5.2% in reperfused myocardium compared to + 30.4% in nonischemic control segments [23]. Permanent occlusion of a coronary artery resulted in a slow gradual increase of radioactivity into the corresponding segment of – 9.4% during a 40 min imaging period, compared to + 15% radioactivity decrease in unaffected control segments [23]. These data suggest a great potential of noninvasive imaging of regional FFA metabolism by means of I-PPA and SPECT in acute ischemia and after therapeutic interventions aimed to restore rMBF and cardiac metabolic function.

Clinical studies

Turnover after intracoronary tracer application

Myocardial turnover of I-PPA has been assessed by measuring precordial radioactivity clearance and coronary venous blood sampling after intracoronary (i.c.) tracer injection in a limited number of patients with coronary artery disease [24]. Patients with valvular heart disease and normal coronary arteries served as controls. After i.c. I-PPA injection 45-53% of the applied tracer was extracted during a single passage of I-PPA through the coronary vascular bed. Patients with a significant (<50%) luminal obstruction of the respective cor-

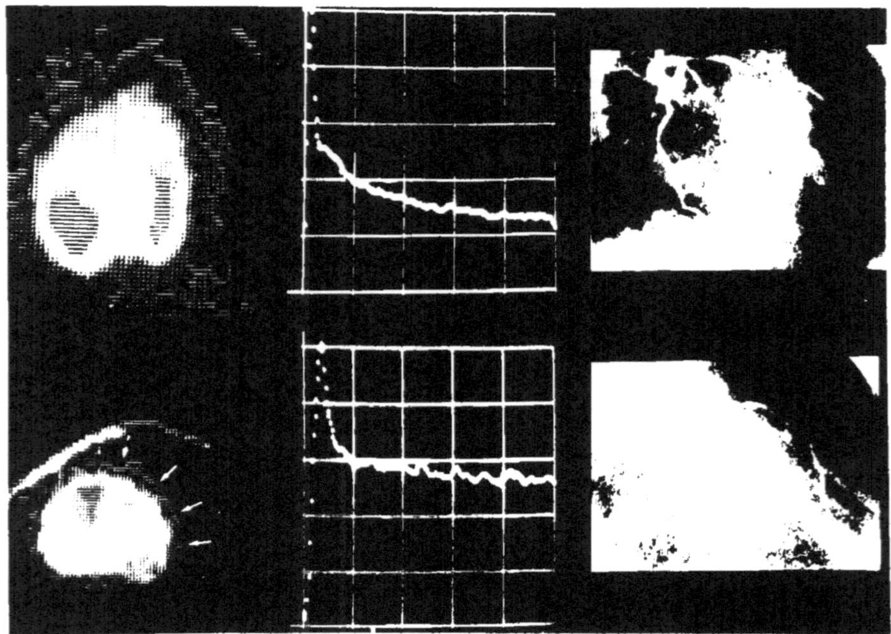

Figure 8. I-PPA uptake and turnover after intracoronary (left mainstem) injection. The control patient (upper row) shows homogeneous uptake in the anterolateral and septal walls (45 LAO projection and multicomponent tracer clearance. In contrast, a patient with a subtotal proximal LAD-stenosis shows reduced uptake in the anterolateral wall (arrows) and monocomponent tracer clearance following the first vascular spike. The patient with CAD in the lower row was recorded in anterior projection.

onary artery showed a normal to reduced (34-61%) extraction fraction, depending probably on the degree and number of stenoses in the respective vessels.

Myocardial tracer uptake was significantly reduced in the territory of stenosed vessels compared to normally supplied segments (Figure 8). Three-component cardiac I-PPA tracer clearance was found in normal myocardium. Cardiac tracer kinetics were very similar to that of ^{11}C-palmitic acid studied by means of positron emission tomography (PET) [25].

In segments, supplied by stenosed vessels, tracer clearance was significantly delayed as compared to normally perfused segments of control patients [24], indicating a compromised cardiac FFA-oxidation due to CAD. Since all patients in this small series suffered from advanced CAD with high grade (>90%) stenoses in the respective vessels, at least in these cases regional metabolic derangements could be detected already at rest. The relation of regional I-PPA uptake and clearance and the grade of luminal vessel obstruction, the number and probably also chronology of coronary stenoses need a further detailed evaluation.

In coronary sinus blood increasing amounts of hydrophilic catabolites of

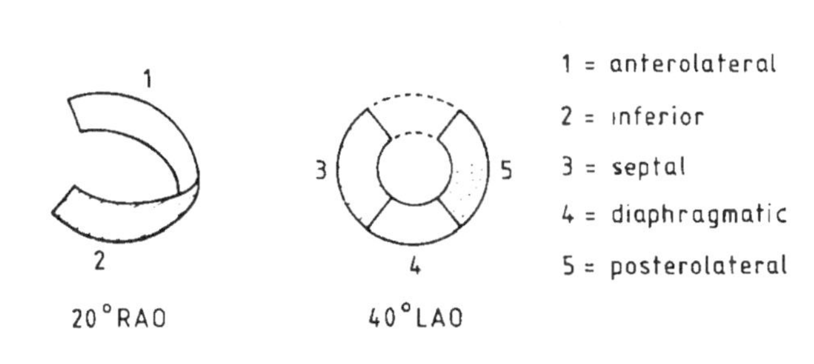

Figure 9. Scheme of cardiac segments visualized by the bilateral collimator.

I-PPA were found [24] indicating oxidation of I-PPA to short-chain catabolites (mainly I-benzoic acid) also in humans. It was concluded from these studies that I-PPA is metabolized by the heart muscle in patients and that in advanced CAD the rate of cardiac oxidation of I-PPA may be delayed already at rest. These studies encouraged us to investigate regional I-PPA metabolism of the heart in a greater number of patients with CAD by means of a more non-invasive approach, i.e. peripheral tracer injection and conventional imaging techniques.

Resting I-PPA turnover in control patients

Cardiac turnover of I-PPA was studied in control patients with a probability of CAD $< 3\%$, as assessed by clinical history, age, sex, risk factors, clinical findings and noninvasive stress tests. Myocardium was imaged after i.v. tracer injection by means of a bilateral collimator, visualizing the heart simultaneously in 20° RAO and 40° LAO projection (Figure 9). In a first series of examinations, sequential scintigraphy was performed for 90 min.

Segmental cardiac uptake was visually evaluated and catagorized according to the criteria: normal, markedly decreased or deficient. In addition, after background correction according to the Goris-procedure [26], segmental radioactivity turnover was determined. The slope of the segmental cardiac time-activity curves was fitted with two exponential functions or, when appropriate, with a monoexponential function.

Immediately after i.v. injection of I-PPA the blood pool is visualized due to albumin binding of the tracer. I-PPA is rapidly cleared from peripheral blood ($T\frac{1}{2}$=1-2 min) and accumulated in the normal myocardium and liver. The normal left ventricular myocardium is visualized with homogeneous tracer uptake, at a maximum about 8-12 min after tracer injection. Thereafter a gradual decrease of the tracer from the heart muscle is observed. Essentially only left ventricular myocardium is visualized due to its greater muscle mass

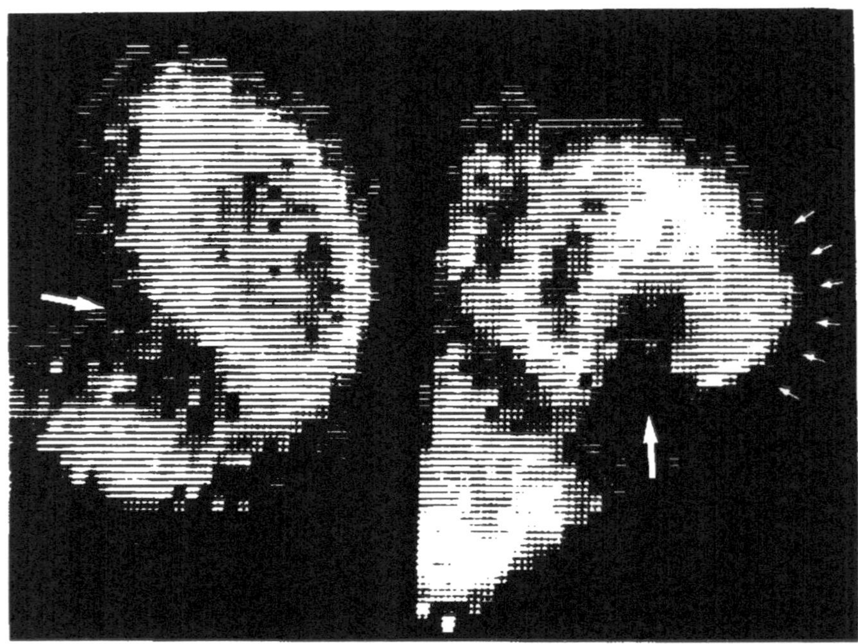

Figure 10. I-PPA uptake 10 min after tracer injection in a patient with CAD and a history of an inferior wall infarction. Note deficient uptake in the inferior segment and reduced uptake in the posterolateral wall due to high grade LCX-stenosis.

and rMBF. The right ventricle is normally only faintly to be seen but right ventricular uptake may be markedly increased and even exceed that of the left ventricle in chronic volume and/or pressure overload.

Regional time-activity curves show a quite homogeneous two-component tracer clearance from normal myocardium. Regional time-activity curves, recorded only for 40-60 min can be rather accurately fitted with a monoexponential function (T½~ 50 min) [27]. This relatively long elimination half-time results from the dissection of the late slow component of the cardiac clearance curve. From this observation it has been erroneously concluded that the metabolism of I-PPA is slowed compared to "naturally" occurring FFA due to the terminal I-phenyl residue [28]. If cardiac tracer clearance is correctly analyzed, i.e. for 90 min, and curve peeling of the late slow component is accurately performed, half-times of about 50-60 min (late slow component) and 10-12 min (first rapid component) are found [29]. The "compartment ratio" [30] of these components (i.e. the fraction of the intercept of the first component over the sum of both intercepts) is 0.45-0.55. This kinetic behaviour is very similar to that described for ^{11}C-palmitic acid in humans [31].

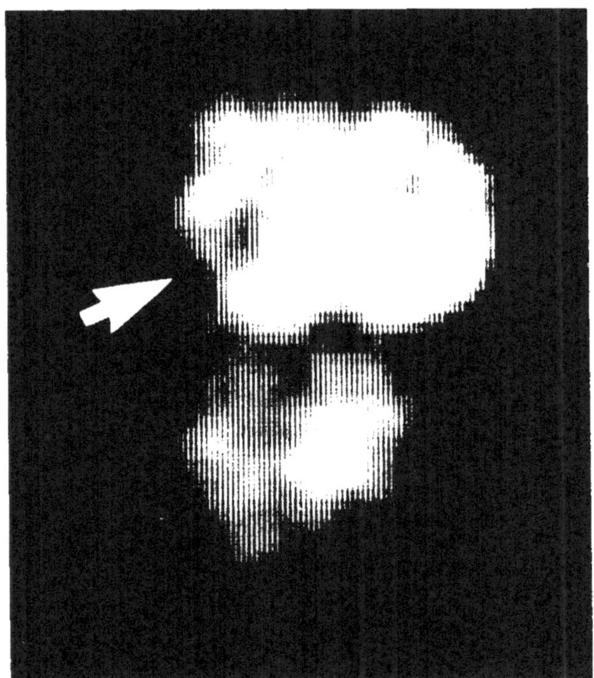

Figure 11. Myocardial scan of a 3-month old infant with a large interventricular septal defect and a myocardial scar in the enlarged right ventricle assessed by ventriculography. Note localized reduced tracer uptake in the inferolateral wall of the enlarged and hypertrophied right ventricle. (500 μCi I-PPA i.v., 45 LAO view 10 min post injection)

Metabolic patterns in CAD

Detection of myocardial infarction

In a series of 23 patients with CAD, proven by coronary angiography, 17 patients had a history (3 months to 12 years) of a transmural myocardial infarction. Eleven patients had an anterior wall infarction and six patients a posterior or posterolateral wall infarction. In 90% these infarcts were detected as areas of a highly reduced or deficient tracer uptake (Figure 10) irrespective of the location of the lesion. These data indicate a significant potential of this imaging modality for infarct detection, localization and conceivably quantitation especially in conjunction with SPECT [22]. Occasionally even a right heart infarction may be detected (Figure 11).

Detection of CAD

A moderately reduced regional I-PPA uptake is indicative of a significantly stenosed coronary artery. In our first series, detection of significantly stenosed

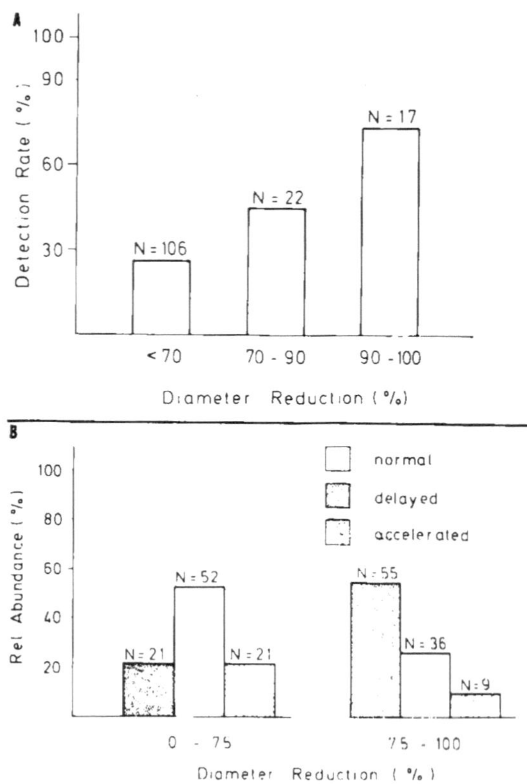

Figure 12. (A) Reduced regional I-PPA uptake in patients with CAD in dependence on diameter reduction of coronary arteries. Infarcted regions were excluded from this analysis. (B) Regional turnover in CAD. Note increased number of pathological findings in advanced disease.

coronary arteries in other than the infarct-related vessels is depicted in Figure 12. With increasing diameter reduction detection rate increases from about 30% (0-70% stenosed vessels) to about 50-75% (70-99% stenoses). Similar to results of Tl-201 stress scintigraphy [32,33], in multivessel disease only the most stenosed vessel(s) are detected by a regionally reduced I-PPA uptake. An interesting effect of cardiac collaterals was observed: noncollateralized, more than 75% stenosed vessels, had a reduced uptake in about 60% compared with 30% in collateralized vessels. The undisturbed I-PPA supply at rest in the stenosed and collateralized arteries may indicate a protective effect of cardiac collaterals in a subset of patients with CAD.

Thus the relation of regional cardiac I-PPA uptake and extent of coronary artery disease is obviously complex and dependent on several variables: regional uptake is dependent on substrate supply (i.e. blood concentration of the tracer and rMBF), integrity of an oxidative tissue metabolism, the amount (and number?) of coronary artery stenoses as well as collateralization and extent of concomitant stenoses in the other vessels. A clearly reduced tracer uptake in the distribution of moderately stenosed vessels, where a flow-restriction is not expected at rest, may indicate a "biochemical defect" on the basis of repetitive ischemic events [34,35]. Intriguing problems are the relation of these uptake patterns to patient prognosis and the reversibility of oxidative FFA-tissue metabolism after adequate therapy. Also the effects of acute and chronic pharmacological interventions remain to be clarified.

Cardiac radioactivity clearance is homogeneous in the heart after i.v. injection of I-PPA. I-PPA elimination half-times of 11.2 ± 1.41 min and 75.8 ± 31.6 min ($x \pm SD$, $N=40$) for the first and second component of cardiac tracer clearance were observed. Based on these normal values about 55% of segments supplied by < 75% stenosed coronary arteries had a normal I-PPA turnover; whereas another 22% of < 75% stenosed vessel showed either an enhanced or delayed turnover. Cardiac segments dependent on highly obstructed vessels (75-99%) had only in 36% a normal I-PPA turnover; in 55% a significantly delayed or accelerated (9%) I-PPA turnover was found (Figure 7).

Delayed cardiac I-PPA turnover may be interpreted as metabolic sequelae of reduced oxygen delivery and consequently reduced FFA-oxidation [13,36]. Biochemically the metabolic fate of I-FFA might be shifted from predominant primary oxidation to turnover in cardiac lipid-esters.

Markedly accelerated turnover of I-PPA in the territory of some highly stenosed coronary arteries was found in a subset of patients. The interpretation of these findings is unclear as yet, since cardiac lipid turnover is expected to be rather slow in these segments. Interestingly, however, marked ultrastructural changes of cardiac tissue (increased amount of functionally incompletely decoupled mitochondria) have been observed in heart muscle specimens of patients with severe CAD [37,38]. Thus accelerated cardiac lipid turnover might be related to certain ultrastructural and/or functional disturbances of the heart muscle in advanced CAD. In addition, incomplete I-FFA oxidation [39] or increased lipid washout, documented in acutely ischemic myocardium [36], has to be taken into consideration. Further studies are needed to elucidate this very interesting metabolic pattern, since increased cardiac turnover of I-PPA has been observed in our laboratory exclusively in severe CAD, suggesting a doubtful prognosis of patients who manifest this special metabolic pattern.

Metabolism after maximal exercise

During acute ischemia cardiac FFA-metabolism is markedly changed [13] (Figure 12). Concomitant with a reduction of MBF, FFA utilization i.e. FFA-uptake, is reduced and there is a metabolic shift from primary oxidation of cytosolic CoA activated FFA to intermediary storage in tissue lipid-esters. As a consequence, global cardiac FFA-turnover is significantly delayed.

We thus compared cardiac I-PPA-turnover, assessed by externally recording

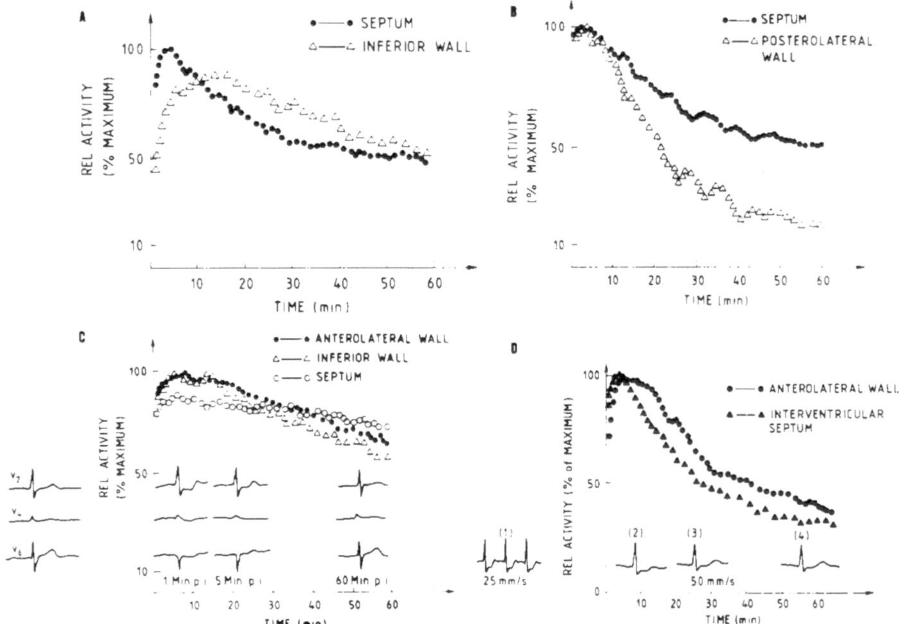

Figure 13. Pathological turnover patterns of I-PPA metabolism in CAD after symptom-limited bicycle stress. (A) Regional delayed turnover in inferior wall; (B) regional enhanced turnover in the posterolateral wall; (C) global persistent delayed turnover in all cardiac segments in three vessel disease; (D) regional reversible delayed turnover in the anterolateral wall. All segments with a pathological turnover were supplied by significantly stenosed coronary arteries.

the precordial radioactivity clearance of normal patients (< 3% probability of CAD) to that of patients with CAD assessed by coronary angiography. Patients were studied after symptom-limited supine bicycle exercise. Myocardial turnover of I-PPA was evaluated as described above. Background-corrected cardiac time-activity curves of normal patients and normally perfused segments of patients with CAD were characterized by a rapid tracer accumulation and a subsequent biexponential tracer clearance. The half-times of the rapid first and slow late component were 6.3 ± 1.3 minutes and 83.7 ± 40.1 minutes respectively ($x \pm SD$, N=42). These values were significantly shorter than those obtained from normal perfused segments at rest. All segments in the distribution of significantly obstructed coronary arteries (> 75%) showed different clearance patterns; concomitant with clinical and electrophysiological signs of ischemia several different patterns of altered FFA-turnover were found (Figure 13):

(1) Regional delayed clearance;
(2) Regional accelerated clearance;
(3) Global, i.e. in all cardiac segments, delayed clearance; and
(4) Regional reversible delayed clearance.

Reversible delayed cardiac tracer clearance was reverted towards normal with relief of chest pain and normalization of the ECG. These findings suggest that acute ischemia-related alterations of cardiac FFA-metabolism can be detected by means of myocardial scintigraphy with I-PPA and may be used for detection and localization of jeopardized myocardium. The prognostic implications of the different metabolic patterns are currently investigated.

Cardiac metabolism after submaximal exercise

The main substrates of cardiac energy metabolism, i.e. FFA, glucose and lactate, are, at least to a certain degree, interchangeable [13]. When supplied to the heart simultaneously, lactate appears to be the preferred substrate. These metabolic properties pose significant problems when patients are stressed at maximum and arterial lactate concentrations are significantly elevated. Indeed arterial lactate concentrations may rise as high as 7 times the baseline values during maximal exercise. In this situation the rate of cardiac FFA-oxidation is on one hand stimulated by increased demand but on the other hand subjected to the inhibiting influence of high lactate utilization. Thus the effect on the rate of cardiac FFA-oxidation depends on the balance of suppressive and enhancing stimuli. Indeed we observed after extensive exercise in healthy volunteers only a very small rapid turnover fraction of I-PPA whereas the slow turnover fraction of cardiac I-PPA turnover dramatically increased. Thus the optimal work load, where FFA-oxidation is yet stimulated and the arterial lactate level is not that high to suppress cardiac FFA-oxidation, is hardly to predict in patients in a clinical setting. We tried to avoid this dilemma by stressing patients repeatedly at only submaximal levels [40]: exercise was repeated in order to maximize initial flow mediated cardiac I-PPA uptake after the first stress. After imaging the heart in three views, submaximal exercise was repeated at the same work load in order to increase differences of regional I-PPA turnover.

Cardiac tracer uptake and turnover were analyzed by the circumferential profile method in early and delayed background-corrected scans. In a series of 15 patients with CAD studied as yet, only two patients developed angina and one patient ECG-changes indicative of ischemia during this stress regimen. In contrast, a reduced tracer uptake was found in about 75% of regions supplied by $>$ 50% stenosed vessels. In normally supplied segments I-PPA uptake was reduced in the late scans compared to the early scans by $38 \pm 16\%$ ($x \pm$ SD, N=52). Twelve of 15 patients of this series had a regional delay in cardiac I-PPA turnover, which was defined as a reduction of late uptake less than the mean minus two standard deviations of normal control segments (Figure 14). In about 50% of patients with CAD a net increase of I-PPA uptake in at least one segment was found. In contrast, control patients with a low probability of CAD ($<$ 3%) studied after repeated submaximal exercise, had a general homogeneous reduction of cardiac tracer uptake in late compared to the early scans of about 40-50%. It was concluded from this study that nonhomogeneous cardiac I-PPA turnover is found in patients with CAD already after submaximal exercise. Exercise-induced impairment of cardiac I-PPA turnover is an

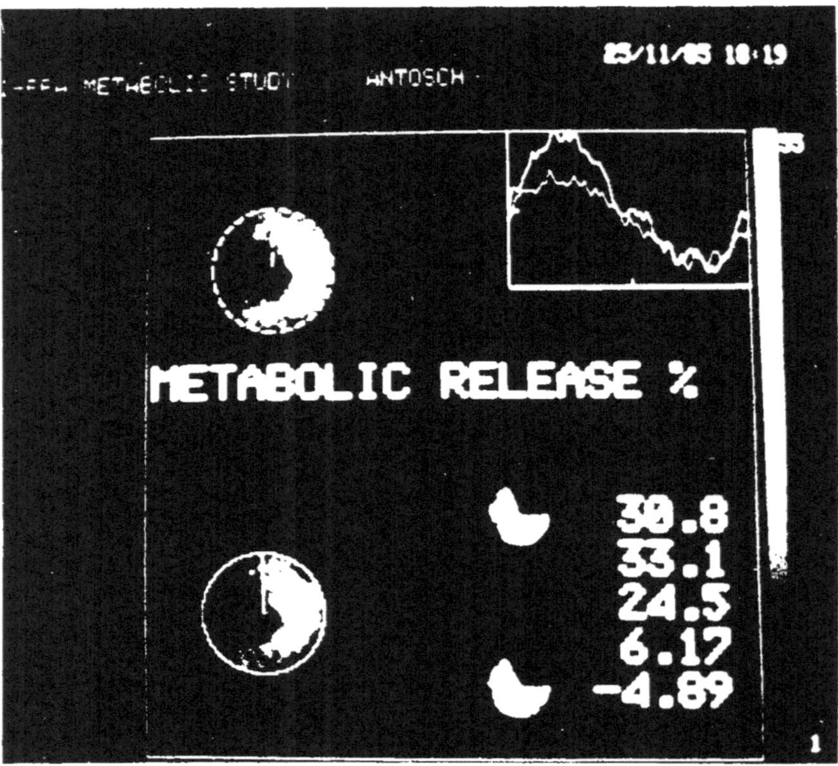

Figure 14. Inhomogeneous metabolism of I-PPA after repeated submaximal bicycle stress in a patient with CAD and a history of an anteroseptal myocardial infarct (45 LAO projection). The upper row depicts the early background corrected scan and the circumferential profiles (early profile in white, late profile in gray). The lower row shows the late scan and the segmental metabolic release after the second stress test about 25 min post injection. Note highly reduced cardiac metabolic function in the peri-infarcted area. Segmental metabolic function is depicted clockwise from the valve plane, starting from the high posterolateral wall.

early event, developing probably before overt clinical or electrophysiological signs of ischemia are detected. These findings provide additional support that oxidative cardiac FFA metabolism is indeed most sensitive to oxygen deprivation.

References

1. Knoop F (1905) Der Abbau aromatischer Fettsäuren im Tierkörper. Beitr Chem Physiol Pathol (Braunschweig) 6: 150 - 153
2. Machulla H J, Marsmann M, Dutschka K (1980) Biochemical synthesis of a radioiodinated phenyl fatty acid for in vivo metabolic studies of the myocardium. Eur J Nucl Med 5: 171 - 173

3. Freundlieb C, Höck A, Vyska K, Feinendegen L E, Machulla H J, Stöcklin G (1980) Myocardial imaging and metabolic studies with 17(I-123 Iodo)heptadecanoic acid. J Nucl Med 21: 1043 - 1050
4. Visser F C, van Eenige M J, Westera G, den Hollander G, Duwel C M B, van der Wall E E, Heidendal G A K, Roos J P (1985) Metabolic fate of radioiodinated heptadecanoic acid in the normal canine heart Circulation 72: 565 - 571
5. Tubis M, Blahd W H, Endow J S, Ronwalay S S (1964) The metabolism of ortho-I-131 Iodobenzoic acid. Its use as a possible liver function test. J Nucl Med 5: 532 - 541
6. Reske S N, Sauer W, Machulla H J, Winkler C (1984) 15(123-I-iodophenyl-)pentadecanoic acid as tracer of lipid metabolism. Comparison with 1-14C-palmitic acid in murine tissues. J Nucl Med 25: 1335 - 1342
7. Reske S N, Sauer W, Machulla H J, Knust J, Winkler C (1985) Metabolism of 15(p-I-123 Phenyl-)Pentadecanoic acid in heart muscle and non-cardiac tissues Eur J Nucl Med 10: 228 - 234
8. Reske S N, unpublished observation
9. Egge H, Murawski U, Müller J, Zilliken F (1970) Mikrolipid-Analysen aus Serum mit dem Eppendorff-System 3000. Z Klin Chem Klin Biochem 8: 488 - 491
10. Reske S N, Fuchs R, Machulla H J, Winkler C (1982) Radio-chromatographic microanalysis of myocardial lipids prelabeled with radioiodinated fatty acids. Radiochem Radioanal Lett 55: 257 - 264
11. Reske S N (1983) Jod-123-Phenyl-Pentadecansäure — Ein neuer Tracer zur Untersuchung des myokardialen Metabolismus freier Fettsäuren. Nuklearmedizin 1: 25 - 46
12. Schmitz B, Reske S N, Machulla H J, Egge H, Winkler C (1984) Cardiac metabolism of ω(p-iodo-phenyl-)pentadecanoic acid: a gas chromatographic mass spectrometric analysis. J Lipid Res 25: 1102 - 1108
13. Neely J R, Morgan H E (1974) Relationship between carbohydrate and lipid metabolism and the energy balance of heart muscle. Annu Rev Physiol 34: 413 - 458
14. van Golde L M G, van den Bergh S G (1977) In: Snyder F (ed) Lipid Metabolism in Mammals, Vol 1. New York: Plenum Press, pp 35 - 116
15. Reske S N, Machulla H J, Winkler C (1982) Metabolism of 15(p-123-I-phenyl-)pentadecanoic acid in hearts of rats. J Nucl Med 23: P 10
16. Reske S N (1985) I-123 Phenylpentadecanoic acid as tracer of cardiac free fatty acid metabolism. Experimental and clinical results. Eur Heart J 6(Suppl B): 39 - 47
17. Poe N D, Robinson G D, Graham L S, Mac Donald N S (1976) Experimental basis for myocardial imaging with 123-I-labeled hexadecanoic acid J Nucl Med 17: 1077 - 1082
18. Okada R, Elmaleh P, Werre G S, Strauss H W (1983) Myocardial kinetics of I-123-labeled hexadecanoic acid. Eur J Nucl Med 8: 215 - 217
19. Reske S N, Schön S, Knust E J *et al.* (1984) Relation of myocardial blood flow and initial cardiac uptake of 15(p-123-I-phenyl-)pentadecanoic acid in the canine heart. Nuklearmedizin 2: 83 - 85
20. Reske S N, Schön S, Eichelkraut W, Hahn N, Machulla H J (1983) Flow-dependence of uptake of I-123 phenylpentadecanoic acid in the canine heart J Nucl Med 24,: P 12
21. Schön S, Reske S N, Schmitt H, Machulla H J, Knopp R, Winkler C (1984) Sustained I-131 phenylpentadecanoic acid uptake in salvaged myocardium. J Nucl Med 25: P 80
22. Reske S N, Biersack H J, Lackner K, Machulla H J, Knopp R, Hahn N, Winkler C (1982) Assessment of regional myocardial uptake and metabolism of ω-(p-123-I-phenyl-)pentadecanoic acid with serial single-photon emission tomography. Nucl Med 21: 249 - 253
23. Rellas G S, Corbe H J R, Kulkarni P, Morgan C, Devous M D, Bieja U, Bush L, Parkey R W, Willerson J T, Lewis S E (1983) I-123 Phenylpentadecanoic acid: detection of acute myocardial infarction and injuring in dogs using an iodinated fatty acid and single photon emission tomography. Am J Cardiol 52: 1326 - 1332

24. Reske S N, Koischwitz D, Reichmann K, Machulla H J, Simon H, Winkler C (1984) Cardiac metabolism of I-123 phenylpentadecanoic acid after intracoronary tracer application. Eur J Radiol 4: 144 - 149
25. Goldstein R A, Klein M S, Welch M J, Sobel B E (1980) External assessment of myocardial metabolism with C-11-palmitate in vivo. J Nucl Med 21: 342 - 348
26. Goris M L, Daspit S G, McLaughlin P, Kriss J P (1976) Interpolative background correction. J Nucl Med 17: 744 - 747
27. Reske S N, Simon H, Machulla H J, Biersack H J, Knopp R, Winkler C (1983) Myocardial turnover of p-(123-I-phenyl-)pentadecanoic acid in patients with CAD. J Nucl Med 23: P34
28. van der Wall E E, Heidendal G A K, den Hollander W, Westera G, Roos J P (1981) Metabolic myocardial imaging with I-123 labeled heptadecanoic acid in patients with angina pectoris. Eur J Nucl Med 6: 391 - 396
29. Reske S N (1985) ^{123}I-phenylpentadecanoic acid as a tracer of cardiac metabolism. Experimental and clinical results Eur Heart J 6 (Suppl B): 39 - 47
30. Dudzcak R, Kletter K, Frischauf H, Dosert U, Angelberger P, Schmoliner R (1984) The use of I-123 labeled heptadecanoic acid (HDA) as metabolic tracer: preliminary report. Eur J Nucl Med 9: 81 - 85
31. Schelbert H R, Phelps M E, Shine K I (1983) Imaging metabolism and biochemistry — a new look at the heart Am Heart J 105: 522 - 526
32. Rigo P, Becker L C, Griffith L *et al.* (1979) Influence of coronary collateral vessels on the results of Tl-201 myocardial stress imaging. Am J Cardiol 44: 452 - 458
33. Gibson R S, Tayler G J, Watson D D *et al.* (1981) Predicting the extent and location of coronary artery disease during the early postinfarction period by quantitative thallium-201 scintigraphy. Am J Cardiol 47: 1010 - 1019
34. Braunwald E, Kloner R A (1982) The stunned myocardium: prolonged, postischemic ventricular dysfunction. Circulation 66: 1146 - 1149
35. Geft I L, Fischbein M C, Ninomiya K *et al.* (1982) Intermettent brief periods of ischaemia have a cumulative effect and may cause myocardial necrosis. Circulation 66: 1150 - 1153
36. Henze E, Grossmann R G, Huang S C *et al.* (1982) Myocardial uptake and clearance of C-11 palmitic acid in man: effects of substrate availability and cardiac work. J Nucl Med 23: P12 - P3
37. Flameng W, Suy R, Schwarz F *et al.* (1981) Ultrastructural correlates of left ventricular contraction abnormalities in patients with chronic ischaemic heart disease: Determinants of reversible segmental asynergy postrevascularization surgery. Am Heart J 102: 846 - 857
38. Schaper W (1983) Pathophysiologie der Koronarinsuffizienz. In: Köhler E, Noack E, Schrey A (eds) Mononitrat. München: Wolf u. Sohn, pp 66 - 77
39. Moore K H, Radloff J F, Hull F E, Sweely C C (1980) Incomplete fatty acid oxidation by ischaemic heart: β-hydroxy fatty acid production. Am J Physiol 239(8): H257 - H265
40. Reske S N, Ledda R, Nitsch J, Klunenberg H, Winkler C (1985) Impaired cardiac I-123 Phenyl fatty acid turnover in CAD after repeated submaximal exercise. Circulation 72 (Suppl III): 358

9. The development of radioiodinated 3-methyl-branched fatty acids for evaluation of myocardial disease by single photon techniques

F.F. KNAPP Jr, M.M. GOODMAN, K.R. AMBROSE, P. SOM, A.B. BRILL, K. YAMAMOTO, K. KUBOTA, Y. YONEKURA, R. DUDCZAK, P. ANGELBERGER and R. SCHMOLINER

Introduction

The measurement of regional myocardial "release-rates" after intravenous administration of iodine-123-labeled fatty acids such as 17-iodoheptadecanoic acid (HDA) [1-6] and 15-(p-iodophenyl)pentadecanoic acid (IPP) [7-13] has been well documented. These agents have proven useful to probe regional aspects of fatty acid metabolism in ischemic heart disease. Studies with (^{123}I)HDA have als shown an unusual and unexpected relation between uptake and release rates in cardiomyopathies [14]. These agents were designed to exhibit extraction similar to natural fatty acids and enter the β-oxidation catabolic chain. Since free radioiodide and short-chain metabolites are released rapidly, the measurement of regional "release-rates" is presumed to reflect the metabolic activity of the myocardial tissue. The structures of these agents and structurally-modified fatty acids discussed in this chapter are shown in Figure 1.

Over two decades ago it was reported that the energy requirements of the normal heart in the basal state are usually met by catabolism of free fatty acids [15,16] with little contribution by oxidation of glucose and lactate. The regional distribution of radioiodinated oleic acid in the myocardium was studied in dogs and humans [17,18] in an effort to develop a diagnostic agent which could be used to evaluate ischemic heart disease by identification of perfusion defects. The preliminary studies in humans with documented myocardial infarction, however, showed decreased fatty acid uptake on images in only about 39% of the cases. It was thus concluded that radioiodinated fatty acids were not practical diagnostic agents for detection, location and estimation of size of myocardial infarcts [18]. Because of these findings, no further investigations in this area were reported for over a decade. In the 1970 decade a renewed interest in the fatty acid research was stimulated. The need for an improved flow related tracer was realized [19-21] and investigators suggested the attachment of ^{123}I to a fatty acid for this purpose [22]. The regional distribution of 16-(^{123}I)iodohexa-decenoic acid was compared to ^{43}K in series of dogs with acute myocardial infarction to evaluate the possibility of using the fatty acid as a marker of

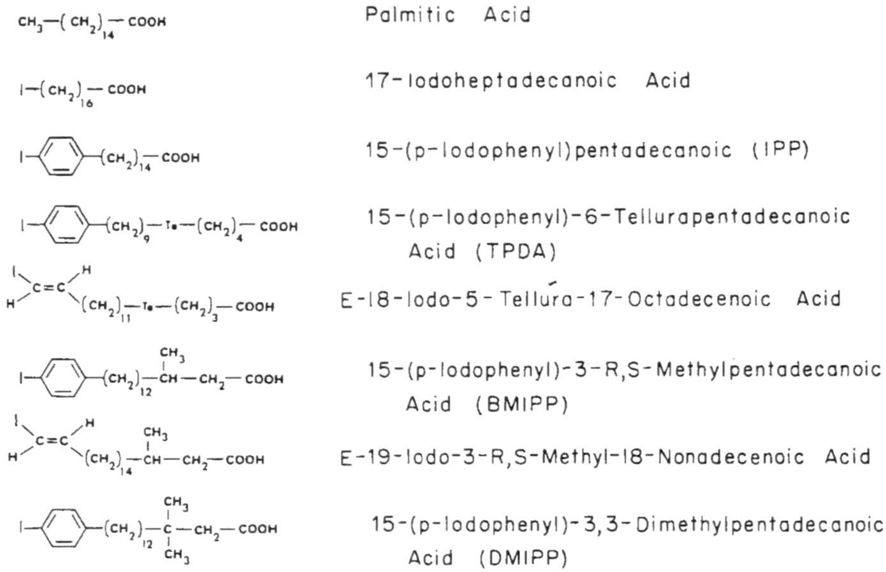

$CH_3{-}(CH_2)_{14}{-}COOH$	Palmitic Acid
$I{-}(CH_2)_{16}{-}COOH$	17-Iodoheptadecanoic Acid
$I{-}C_6H_4{-}(CH_2)_{14}{-}COOH$	15-(p-Iodophenyl)pentadecanoic (IPP)
$I{-}C_6H_4{-}(CH_2)_9{-}Te{-}(CH_2)_4{-}COOH$	15-(p-Iodophenyl)-6-Tellurapentadecanoic Acid (TPDA)
$I(H)C{=}C(H){-}(CH_2)_{11}{-}Te{-}(CH_2)_3{-}COOH$	E-18-Iodo-5-Tellura-17-Octadecenoic Acid
$I{-}C_6H_4{-}(CH_2)_{12}{-}CH(CH_3){-}CH_2{-}COOH$	15-(p-Iodophenyl)-3-R,S-Methylpentadecanoic Acid (BMIPP)
$I(H)C{=}C(H){-}(CH_2)_{14}{-}CH(CH_3){-}CH_2{-}COOH$	E-19-Iodo-3-R,S-Methyl-18-Nonadecenoic Acid
$I{-}C_6H_4{-}(CH_2)_{12}{-}C(CH_3)_2{-}CH_2{-}COOH$	15-(p-Iodophenyl)-3,3-Dimethylpentadecanoic Acid (DMIPP)

Figure 1. Structures of radiolabeled fatty acids which have been developed for myocardial imaging.

regional perfusion [19-21]. These reports led to the synthesis of the 16-carbon unsaturated fatty acid agent 16-(^{123}I)iodo-9-hexadecanoic acid [22]. Myocardial images with this new agent were compared to ^{43}K and (^{11}C)stearic acid and (^{11}C)palmitic acid. Within the first 5-10 min after intravenous injection the blood clearance, myocardial uptake and kinetics were found to be similar for these three fatty acids. The myocardial clearance of 16-(^{123}I)hexadecanoic acid was found to be relatively rapid with clearance of more than 66% of the radioactivity within 2-20 minutes after injection. Although this rapid clearance pattern posed a significant problem for routine clinical imaging, investigators suggested that the rate of clearance of the radiolabel from the heart could be related to fatty acid utilization and should be quantified [19,20]. More recently, several fatty acid analogues labeled with radionuclides such as ^{11}C and ^{123}I have been studied extensively for myocardial imaging as well as for noninvasive measurement of regional fatty acid metabolism [1,23-27]. Following intravenous injection, natural fatty acids such as palmitic acid accumulate rapidly in the myocardium, and the uptake and clearance kinetics are felt to be a measure of "metabolism" as discussed earlier (*vide ante*). This rapid clearance of such agents may limit their use for many routine clinical studies of cardiac metabolism and function.

The design of structurally-modified fatty acids that show normal extraction but are not readily catabolized through the oxidation chain has also been explored. These agents would be used in a different manner to evaluate myocardial energy metabolism since they would not be catabolized with the subsequent measurement of the release of catabolites. A variety of tellurium-123m (^{123m}Te) and I-123-labeled tellurium fatty acids have been designed for this purpose [27-33] and show the unique property of rapid, high extraction with essentially irreversible retention by the myocardium. These agents thus offered for the first time an opportunity to evaluate the uptake phase of fatty acid "metabolism". In essence, they behave like a "molecular microsphere" but can be administered intravenously. This noninvasive use offered an attractive alternative to the invasive intracoronary administration of radiolabeled microspheres, for example, to accurately measure coronary perfusion. A canine model was developed to evaluate the salvage of threatened myocardium following occlusion of a coronary artery. Since the structurally-modified 15-(p-iodophenyl)-6-tellura-pentadecanoic acid (TPDA) shows no redistribution and its initial distribution is "frozen", the administration of a second injection of TPDA after release of a coronary artery ligature allows an accurate evaluation of the degree of viable tissue [34]. A second application only recently demonstrated, for the use of structurally-modified agents is the discordance between the myocardial distribution of a perfusion marker such as thallium-201, and radioiodinated fatty acids such as 1-(^{14}C)-3-methylheptadecanoic acid in hypertensive rats [35-37]. Such a difference was not anticipated and could suggest that iodine-123 fatty acids that show slow washout could thus be used in conjunction with single-photon computerized tomography (SPECT) to identify regions of impaired fatty acid metabolism that cannot be detected with a flow-tracer such as ^{201}Tl. The goals of this chapter are to briefly review our efforts over the last few years to develop a radioiodinated fatty acid which could be used to evaluate regional myocardial uptake, and to discuss in detail our current studies with radioiodinated 3-methyl-branched fatty acids and their use as research tools to study regional fatty acid uptake in hypertensive rats by autoradiography. Also described are a series of patient studies with 15-(p-[^{123}I]iodophenyl)-3-R, S-methylpentadecanoic acid and a comparison of the properties of this agent and the straight-chain analogue 15-(p-iodophenyl)pentadecanoic acid.

The design and synthesis of radioiodinated 3-methyl-branched fatty acids

To overcome the technical problems associated with significant myocardial clearance of the radiolabel resulting from rapid myocardial metabolism, we sought to introduce unique structural features into the fatty acid molecule which would not decrease uptake from the plasma, but which would interfere with subsequent catabolism within the myocyte. Such a goal represented both a conceptual and synthetic challenge, because drastic structural modifications could lead to a molecule that would no longer resemble a fatty acid and thus would not be efficiently extracted by the myocardium. Our early studies involved the use of fatty acids containing stable, nonradioactivity tellurium

(Te) to interfere with β-oxidation to "trap" the fatty acid in the myocardium with iodine-123 attached as either an iodoalkyl, iodophenyl or iodovinyl group. A model agent, 15-(p-iodophenyl)-6-tellurapentadecanoic acid (TPDA), was prepared via introduction of radioiodide by decomposition of a triazene intermediate [38] and shows the expected high heart uptake and prolonged retention in rats [39]. We have also developed and evaluated a variety of telluraoctadecenoic acid analogues in which the radioiodide is stabilized as a vinyliodide [30,31]. The position of the Te heteroatom is found to be an important factor and 18-iodo-5-tellura-18-octadecenoic acid shows high myocardial uptake, high heart: blood ratios and prolonged retention as observed with TPDA [32].

Because of the special care required for the preparation and handling, and the potential toxicity of the Te fatty acids, we have recently investigated the use of methyl-branching in the 2- and 3-positions of the alkanoic acid chain to inhibit β-oxidation and prolong myocardial retention. Since 15-(p[^{123}I]iodophenyl)-pentadecanoic acid (IPP) has been used in large number of institutions and has been shown to be a safe agent in which radioiodide is stabilized and shows little *in vivo* deiodination (*vide ante*), we chose to prepare the 3-methyl analogue in which the only structural change would be the presence of the methyl group in position-3. Our initial synthetic strategy for the preparation of 14-(p-iodophenyl)-2-(R,S)methyltetradecanoic acid, which was the precursor for preparation of 15-(p-iodophenyl)-3-(R,S)methylpentadecanoic acid (BMIPP), involved the use of substituted oxazolines as the substrates for carbon-carbon bond formation [40]. In this agent the configuration at the β-carbon is racemic and the BMIPP consists of a racemic mixture of the 3R-and 3S-methyl isomers. The effect of methyl-branching at the 2- and 3-positions on myocardial retention in rats was assessed by a comparison of the distribution of the methyl-branched agents with the myocardial uptake of the corresponding straight chain analogues, 14-(p-[^{125}I]iodophenyl)tetradecanoic acid and 15-(p-[^{125}I]-iodophenyl)pentadecanoic acid. The increased myocardial uptake and retention of radioactivity following injection of (^{125}I) BMIPP in comparison to the 14-carbon fatty acids and the unbranched analogue, (^{125}I) IPP, suggested that methyl-branching at position-3 could be an effective means of inhibiting myocardial metabolism of radioiodinated terminal iodophenyl fatty acids. Our new methyl-branched fatty acid, 15-(p-iodophenyl)-3-R,S-methylpentadecanoic acid (BMIPP) showed much longer myocardial retention in rats than the straight chain IPP analogue [39-41]. This agent did not show, however, the irreversible retention demonstrated with Te fatty acids. A similar agent, 14-(iodophenyl)-3-R,S-methyltetradecanoic acid, showed less absolute heart uptake than BMIPP and the same washout properties [42,43]. The goals of this chapter are to briefly review the development of 3-methyl-branched fatty acids. Further investigation of the effects of methyl-branching have recently led to the development of a 3,3-dimethyl analogue of BMIPP.

The synthetic strategy developed earlier for the synthesis of BMIPP [40] has now been applied for the preparation of the new dimethyl analogue, DMIPP. Dimethylglutaric anhydride was used for introduction of the geminal dimethyl group. Iodination was accomplished by thallation in trifluoroacetic acid with thallium(III)trifluoroacetate followed by reflux with potassium iodide. Under these conditions [45] the para-iodoproduct is formed with greater than 95% regioselectivity. This new agent exhibits high myocardial uptake, high heart to blood ratios and prolonged retention as described in the following section.

One undesirable property accompanying the pronounced myocardial uptake of the terminal iodophenyl fatty acids is the high blood radioactivity levels which result in only modest heart to blood ratios. Special procedures are thus required to differentiate between the radioactivity in the cardiac muscle and that pooled within the cardiac chambers. In order to overcome the significant *in vivo* deiodination we observed in studies with iodoalkyl [38], iodoalkyl tellurium [39], and iodoalkyl methyl-branched long-chain fatty acids [40], we chose to stabilize radioiodide within the alkyl chain of the methyl-branched fatty acid as either a para-iodophenyl or (E)-iodovinyl group. Our recent studies with a model iodovinyl fatty acid, 18-(^{125}I)iodo-17-octadecenoic acid [46] shows initial high heart uptake (1 h, 1.90-2.28% dose/g) with high heart to blood ratios (7.3-7.8:1).

A variety of synthetic methods are available for the regiospecific introduction of radioiodide into the para position of terminal phenyl ring [30] and into the trans (E) position of iodovinyl long-chain fatty acids. The selection of the most attractive method is based upon a number of factors such as radiochemical yield, adaption to a microscale for the preparation of high specific activity radioiodinated products, rapid reaction times and ease of purification. In addition, the regiospecificity of the desired radioiodinated isomer for the simple isolation of the product by methods is within the scope of most clinical facilities. Further, the methods used to fabricate either the iodophenyl or iodovinyl moiety on the carboxylic acid should be compatible with the carboxylic acid functional groups present within the alkyl chain (-COOH, -$COOCH_3$). It is also important that the substrate used in the iodination step be readily accessible and a generally stable substance that can be stored for long periods of time. Since the ^{123}I-labeled fatty acids are not usually commercially available, all of these factors must be evaluated when planning the synthesis for a clinical facility.

To evaluate the effects of β-methyl-branching in a model agent in which radiodide has been stabilized as a terminal trans vinyl iodide, (E)-9-(^{123}I)iodo-3-(R,S)-methyl-18-nonadecanoic acid was prepared and studied in rats in comparison with the corresponding straight-chain analogue, 19-(^{125}I)iodo-18-nonadecanoic acid [41]. These studies were an extension of our earlier investigations in the iodophenyl series demonstrating that methyl-branching led to high myocardial uptake and good retention [31]. The synthesis of this new methyl-branched fatty acid involved a 15-step sequence of reactions climaxing with formation of the iodovinyl methyl-branched agent by iododestannylation

(Table 1) of methyl-(E)-19-(tri-n-butylstannyl)-3-(R,S)methyl-18-nonadecenoate. Methyl-branching was introduced at an early stage of the sequence using 3-methyl glutaric anhydride. This new agent shows high myocardial uptake, good heart: blood (H/B) ratios and significantly greater myocardial retention in fasted rats than the corresponding straight-chain analogue, 19-(^{125}I)iodo-18-nonadecenoic acid. Excellent myocardial images have been obtained after administration to rats and confirmed the slow myocardial washout over a 60 min period [41]. These data suggest that this agent may also be a good agent like BMIPP for evaluation of heart disease involving aberrations in fatty acid uptake imaging techniques such as single photon emission computerized tomography where redistribution or washout should be minimized. The use of radioiodinated BMIPP in salt-sensitive hypertensive rats to demonstrate regional differences in distribution by autoradiographic techniques is described later.

A compilation of methods that may be used for the preparation of para-iodophenyl substituted long-chain fatty acids is summarized in Table 2. Radioiodinated 15-(iodophenyl)pentadecanoic acid [7] has been prepared by electrophilic iodination of 15-phenylpentadecanoic acid (PPA). The distribution of radioactivity obtained using this iodination technique is 70% of the desired para-isomer and 30% of the ortho-isomer. Thus, isolation of para-isomer is only possible by a high pressure liquid chromotographic (HPLC) separation of the mixture of isomers. Because the separation of the para-isomer from the ortho isomer by HPLC is not always efficient as well as the limited availability of HPLC systems at clinical institutions, a rapid method involving radioiodide exchange from unlabeled IPP has more recently been developed. After an exchange period of 30 min at 170°C, it has been reported that 95% of the radioiodide was incorporated into the para-position of PPA (1 mg - p-IPP). This appears to be a very attractive method, however, yields may be

Table 1. Iodination methods for the preparation of radioiodinated (E)-(iodovinyl)-substituted fatty acids.

Method	Advantage	Disadvantage
Iodostannylation	High yield; rapid; regiospecific; high specific activity; stable substrates	
Iodide Boron displacement	High yield; regiospecific; rapid	Unstable substrates, substrates are difficult to prepare, moderate specific activity
Iododethallation	High specific activity; regiospecific; rapid; iodide as source of ^{123}I	Substrates are difficult to prepare, fresh preparation from toxic reagents
Iododemercuration	Regiospecific; stable substrates	Substrates difficult to prepare, moderate specific activity

dramatically reduced at microscale preparations with sources of iodine-123 containing impurities.

Iododemetallation reactions provide elegant methods for the introduction of radioiodide into the para-position of iodophenyl long-chain fatty acids. The iodide displacement of the p-(bis-(trifluoroacetoxy)thallium)phenyl-substrates has been the most thoroughly investigated procedure [31,40,41]. Thallation of the phenyl ring of mono-substituted phenylalkyl-substrates with the bulky thallium(III)trifluoroacetate gives primarily the para disubstituted isomer due to steric factors. The aryl thallium intermediate rapidly collapses to the p-(iodophenyl)-substituted fatty acid at 100°C in the presence of iodide. Although radioiodinated p-iodophenylalkyl fatty acids may be prepared in excellent radiochemical yield and high specific activity, the widespread clinical use of this method may be limited due to several disadvantages. This method requires the fresh preparation of the (bis(trifluoroacetoxy)thallium(III))phenyl intermediate from highly corrosive and toxic reagents. In addition the formation of the phenyl thallium intermediate may take several hours for completion prior to addition of radioiodide due to chelating effect of the carboxylic acid moiety. Three alternative iododemetallation methods which are probably more attractive approaches are iododestannylation, iododemercuration and boronic acid displacement. Tin, mercury and boron substituents rapidly are quantitatively displaced by the iodide anion in the presence of oxidizing agents such as peroxide and N-chlorosuccinimide. Tin, mercury, and boron substrates are stable reagents and may be fabricated in radiopharmaceutical kits. The major disadvantage to these alternative methods is that preparation of the organometallic substrates will required considerable chemical synthesis to direct the metal substituents to the para-position of the terminal phenyl substituted substrates.

Table 2. Iodination methods for the preparation of radioiodination para-(iodophenyl)-substituted fatty acids.

Method	Advantage	Disadvantage
Electrophilic iodination	Rapid; high specific activity	Postional isomers (ortho, para), requires HPLC separation
Iodide exchange	Rapid, high yield; high specific activity; regiospecific	High temperature; yields not reproducible at microscale
Iododemetallation Dethallation	High yield; regiospecific	Requires fresh preparation thallium substrate; long reaction times
Demercuration, Boronic acid displacement, Destannylation	Regiospecific; rapid; stable substrate; high yield	Substrates are difficult to prepare
Triazene decomposition	Regiospecific; rapid; stable substrates; high specific activity	Moderate yields

Another attractive approach we have investigated is the HI decomposition of triazene intermediates [41]. There are several advantages of this triazene decomposition reaction. In the presence of HI the phenyltriazenes undergo decomposition to yield exclusively the p-iodophenyl products. Secondly, the substrates are stable and the reaction can be readily adapted to the microscale, which is important in the development of radiopharmaceutical kits for high specific activity the regiospecific radioiodinated products. An additional advantage is, the reaction is rapid, proceeds within 45 min at room temperature and can be performed in clinics without the use of elaborate laboratory equipment. The major drawback of this method in comparison with those described above is that presently radiochemical yields are only modest (30-50%).

Another strategy we have investigated to stabilize radioiodide on fatty acids to overcome the problem of in vivo deiodination involves attachment of radioiodide to the sp^2 hybridized carbon of a vinyl moiety [41,46]. Methods have been developed similar to iododemetallation reaction in which iodide has been substituted on a phenyl ring. There are several advantages of fabricating an iodovinyl moiety on a carboxylic acid using the destannylation [41] reaction in contrast to alternative halodemetallation reactions (Table 2), such as those using boron or aluminum reagents. Unlike the reaction of either catecholborane [46] or diisobutyl aluminum hydride with acetylenic esters, the carbomethoxy group of terminal acetylenic ester substrate is inert to reduction with trialkyltin hydrides. Secondly, in the presence of I^+ the (E)-trialkyltin adducts rapidly undergo destannylation to yield exclusively the (E)-iodovinyl products. Finally, this method can be adapted to a "no carrier added" scale for preparation of high specific activity radioiodinated products.

In vivo properties of 3-methyl-substituted 15-(p-iodophenyl)pentadecanoic acid analogues

Detailed studies of the relative tissue distribution, myocardial uptake and retention of 15-(p-iodophenyl)-3-(R,S)-methylpentadecanoic acid (BMIPP) in fasted rats have demonstrated that this new agent shows the expected more prolonged retention in the myocardium in comparison to the straight chain IPP analogue. The myocardial washout half-times in fasted rats were found to be 5-10 minutes for IPP and 30-45 min for BMIPP [40]. In contrast, the new (^{125}I)DMIPP 3,3-dimethyl-substituted agent shows high myocardial uptake and prolonged retention in the hearts of fasted rats with a washout half-time of 6-7 h (Figure 2). Similar prolonged heart retention was observed in fed rats, although the blood levels remained higher resulting in lower heart to blood ratios. While BMIPP shows slow washout with approximately 40% loss of the initial high myocardial uptake in rats after 60 minutes [41], DMIPP exhibits prolonged retention with only~ 24% loss after even 4 h. In addition, within 15 minutes after injection, the mean heart to blood ratios are greater than 10:1 for

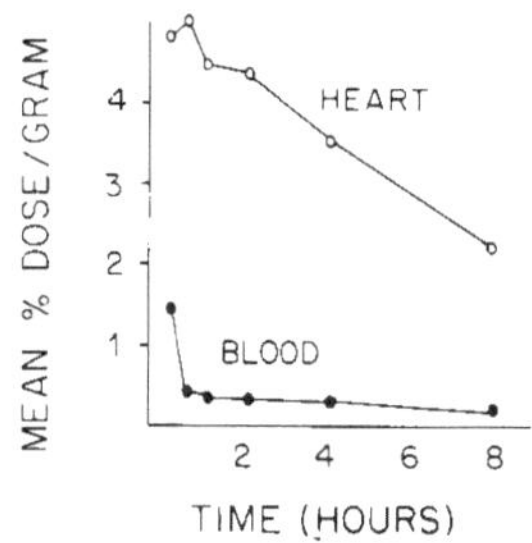

Figure 2. Comparison of the heart and blood levels of radioactivity following the administration of 15-(p-[^{123}I]iodophenyl)-3,3-dimethylpentadecanoic acid (DMIPP) to fasted female Fischer rats.

DMIPP, in contrast to a 3-4:1 ratio for BMIPP. Thus, introduction of dimethyl-branching into the IPP molecule not only results in substantial increase in the myocardial retention (Figure 3), but also results in a dramatic increase in the blood clearance resulting in much higher heart to blood ratios. Although an understanding of the consequences of this structural change on the molecular fate of DMIPP is not yet clear, (^{123}I)DMIPP may exhibit attractive properties for use as a "molecular microsphere" described earlier [34]. Iodine-123 DMIPP is the first example of a structurally-modified fatty acid that does not contain the Te heteroatom which exhibits the unique property of essentially irreversible myocardial retention over the first couple of hours after intravenous administration to unfasted rats. The higher heart-blood ratios and significantly increased myocardial retention observed with (^{125}I)DMIPP in comparison to the monomethyl (BMIPP) and unbranched (IPP) analogues are illustrated in Figure 3. These differences were further evaluated and confirmed in a triple-label experiment in which a (^{123}I)DMIPP/(^{131}I)DMIPP/(^{125}I)IPP mixture was administered to the same fasted rats. As expected from the large body of information available on the myocardial uptake of structurally-modified fatty acids, the initial uptake or "extraction" phase reflects regional perfusion and is very similar for these three agents. Within 10-15 min following injection, however, differences in retention are clearly evident in fasted animals.

Our earlier studies clearly demonstrated the higher myocardial uptake and longer retention observed with BMIPP in comparison with the IPP straight chain analogue [41]. The synthesis, radioiodination and myocardial uptake and retention of a similar 14-carbon agent, 14-(p-iodophenyl)-3-R,S-methyltetradecanoic acid (BMIPT), have also been reported [43]. Comparison of the relative myocardial uptake of (^{125}I)BMIPP and (^{131}I)BMIPT in dual label studies in rats and dogs have demonstrated that the 15-carbon BMIPP shows considerably greater uptake than the 14-carbon analogue although washout kinetics are similar (Strauss, Elmaleh *et al,* personal communication). Thus, total chain length is evidently a very important structured feature affecting

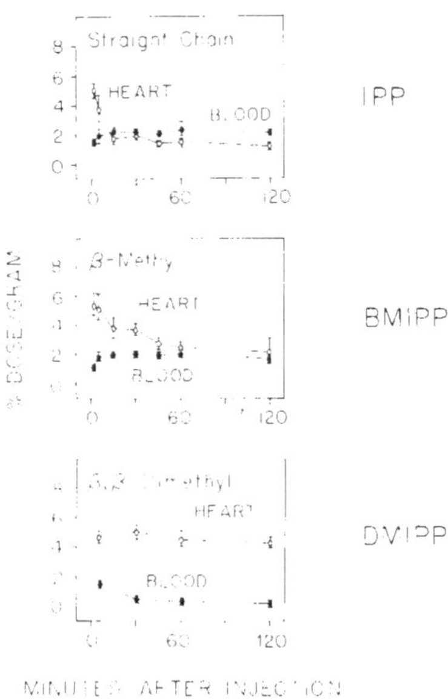

Figure 3. Comparison of the heart and blood levels of radioactivity in separate groups of unfasted female Fischer rats following intravenous administration of (^{125}I)IPP, (^{125}I)BMIPP or (^{125}I)DMIPP.

myocardial uptake of these modified agents. The introduction of the additional methylene group in BMIPP may appear subtle, but has dramatic effects on subsequent biological properties. Thus, the effects of structural changes cannot be predicted and a careful, systematic evaluation of many analogues is required to optimize the most attractive structural features.

In our most recent studies we have evaluated the effects of dimethyl-branching in the β-(3)-position of 15-(p-iodophenyl)pentadecanoic acid on the relative myocardial uptake and retention and heart to blood ratios after administration to rats. A number of early studies suggested that dimethyl-branching in the α- or β-positions would inhibit β-oxidation. In the rat, 2,2-dimethylstearic acid (Figure 4) was readily absorbed through the intestine when administered in olive oil [47] and 2,2-dimethyladipic acid was isolated from the urine. These studies were also performed with unlabeled and ^{14}C-labeled, 2,2-dimethylstearic acid in man [48]. Analysis of the thoracic lymph indicated the presence of both free 2,2-dimethylsuccinic acid, and incorporation into glycerides and phospholipids. These early studies thus demonstrated that although β-oxidation is inhibited by dimethyl-substitution in the α-position, activation still occurs with incorporation of the structurally-modified fatty acid into storage products (glycerides) and complex lipids. A similar dimethyl-branched fatty acid, 2,2-dimethylnonadecanoic acid, was also evaluated in rats and humans [49]. The analogous ω-oxidation products, 2,2-dimethyl glutaric acid and 2,2-dimethylpimetic acid, were isolated from the urine.

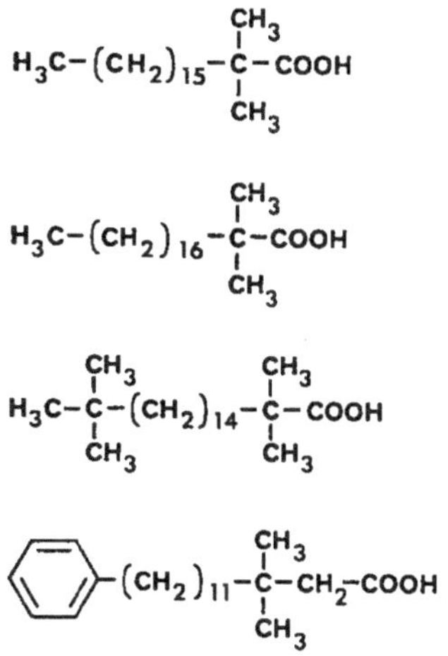

$H_3C-(CH_2)_{15}-C(CH_3)_2-COOH$ 2,2-Dimethylstearic Acid

$H_3C-(CH_2)_{16}-C(CH_3)_2-COOH$ 2,2-Dimethylnonadecanoic Acid

$H_3C-C(CH_3)_2-(CH_2)_{14}-C(CH_3)_2-COOH$ 2,2,17,17-Tetramethylstearic Acid

$C_6H_5-(CH_2)_{11}-C(CH_3)_2-CH_2-COOH$ 3,3-Dimethyl-14-phenylmyristic Acid

Figure 4. Structures of dimethyl-branched fatty acids used in early studies of the effects of alkyl-substitution on the incorporation into lipid pools *in vivo*.

Another dimethyl-substituted fatty acid, 3,3-dimethyl-14-phenylmyristic acid (e.g. 3,3-dimethyl-14-phenyltetradecanoic acid), has also been prepared and evaluated, and studies with this agent are pertinent to our experiments with DMIPP [50]. A phenyl ring was introduced into this fatty acid to inhibit ω-oxidation. This modified fatty acid bound well to albumin, indicating that these structural modifications do not interfere with binding and exhibited very slow clearance from the plasma. In addition, the fatty acid was not metabolized, supporting the proposition that dimethyl-branching in position-3 inhibits β-oxidation. More recently, studies by others with a model dimethyl-branched fatty acid, 14-(^{125}I)iodo-3,3-dimethyltetradecanoic acid, demonstrated that this agent showed very low heart uptake, high blood levels and significant *in vivo* deiodination [51,52]. These studies do not, however, provide any clear insight concerning the effects of dimethyl-branching on myocardial uptake since the agent had a shortchain length and iodide was attached as an iodoalkyl moiety, prone to facilitate deiodination.

The principal application using structurally-modified agents that show slow myocardial washout would include potential evaluation of regional differences in fatty acid uptake when the coronary arteries are normal and regional perfusion is not impaired. Structurally-modified fatty acids that show prolonged retention are also candidated for potential clinical evaluation of hypertensive heart disease as recently demonstrated in studies involving quantitative dual tracer autoradiography, a technique where the relative distribution of two agents is monitored [35-37]. The use of radioiodinated BMIPP and DMIPP for these types of stydies is described in a subsequent section of this chapter. As described earlier, there is also a need for diagnostic agents to evaluate ischemic "border zones" after reperfusion to determine the effectiveness of drug

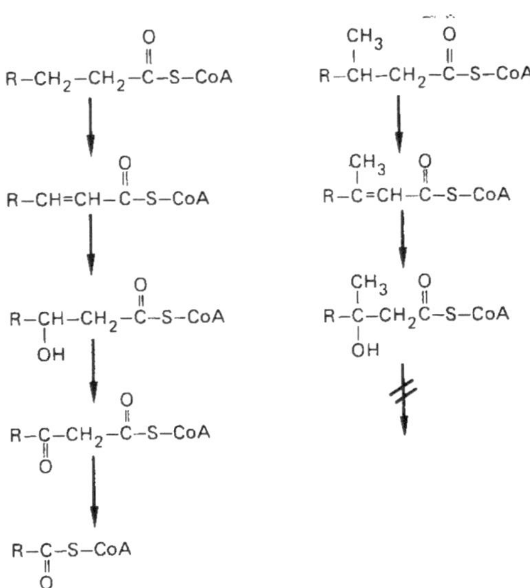

Figure 5. Sequential reactions involved in the normal β-oxidation of long-chain fatty acids.

treatment after an ischemic attack by revealing regional changes in myocardial blood flow.

The successful use of 17-(^{123}I)iodoheptadecanoic acid (HDA) involves evaluation of the differences in regional myocardial "release rates" [1-6]. The release rates are felt to reflect the release of free radioiodide which is formed by the β-oxidation of the injected agent. Although there is some controversy regarding the interpretation of differences in washout rates [53], increased "washout" rates have been correlated with increased catabolism of the HDA. Such an analysis may be much more complex since "washout" is now felt to only indirectly reflect catabolism since the diffusion of free radioiodide may be the rate-limiting factor rather than the rate of catabolism [54-56]. Many investigators have used the term metabolism synonymous with β-oxidation, although "metabolism" would include other events involving biochemical transformations, including activation to thioesters and incorporation into triglycerides and other lipid pools. Thus, a discussion of the use of structurally-modified fatty acids such as DMIPP to measure some aspects of metabolism is not necessarily related to catabolism resulting from β-oxidation.

Although the mechanism(s) responsible for the prolonged retention of DMIPP in comparison to BMIPP and IPP has not been delineated, the observation that all these agents show good initial uptake indicated that events subsequent to extraction are responsible for the increased retention of the β-methyl analogues. Catabolism by normal β-oxidation (Figure 5) in the usual manner is not possible with BMIPP (Figure 7). Although the possibility of α-hydroxylation followed by subsequent oxidation to the α-keto acid and then decarboxylation to yield a product with one less carbon has been discussed,

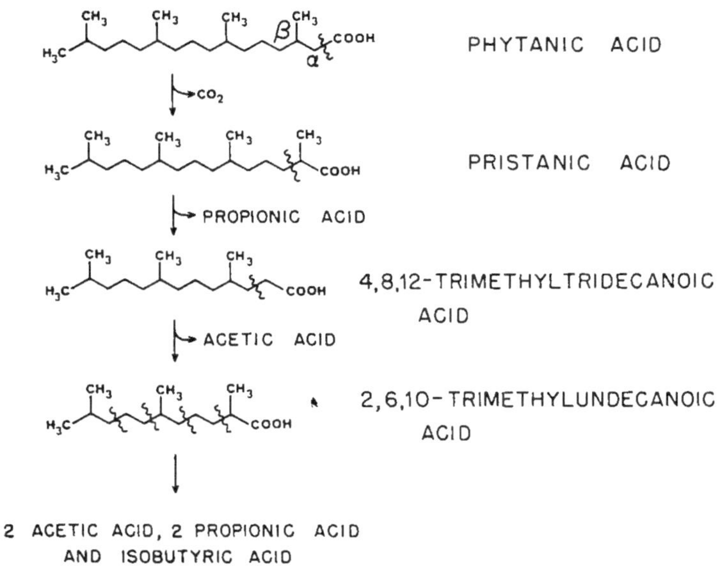

PHYTANIC ACID

CO_2

PRISTANIC ACID

PROPIONIC ACID

4,8,12-TRIMETHYLTRIDECANOIC ACID

ACETIC ACID

2,6,10-TRIMETHYLUNDECANOIC ACID

2 ACETIC ACID, 2 PROPIONIC ACID AND ISOBUTYRIC ACID

Figure 6. Normal catabolism of phytanic acid by initial α-hydroxylation.

there are several precedents for this process occurring. One example is the α-hydroxylation of lignoceric acid (n-tetracosonic acid) in brain tissue to give cerebronic acid (2-hydroxylignoceric acid) [57]. In brain, the α-hydroxy acids are important components of galactolipids, such as N-acyl-spingosine-β-galactoside (cerebrosides) and the corresponding cerebroside-3-o-sulfates. The α-hydroxy fatty acids are formed directly from the parent acids (not CoA-derivative) by a mixed-function oxidase [58]. More pertinent to the possible catabolism of BMIPP is the well established metabolism of phytanic acid [59-61] (3,7,11,15-tetramethylhexadecanoic acid) which proceeds with initial α-hydroxylation, oxidation and then decarboxylation, thus circumventing the inhibitory effect of β-methyl-branching interfering with the usual chain degradation by β-oxidation (Figure 6). In this manner, the original β-methyl group is transposed to the α-position of the decarboxylated product and subsequent chain degradation by β-oxidation can proceed. Accumulation of phytanic acid in the blood, liver, kidneys and other organs is presented in Refsum's diseases in individuals in whom the α-hydroxylase is absent, resulting in atypical retinitis pigmentosa, night blindness, nerve deafness, peripheral and cerebellar ataxia [62].

Metabolism of BMIPP in a similar manner could proceed as indicated in Figure 7. Even if the first step of the normal β-oxidative process could proceed by conversion of BMIPP (1) to (2) by the dehydrogenase and then subseqent regiospecific hydration to give (3), further oxidation by the alcohol dehydrogenase in the normal manner without carbon-carbon bond cleavage could not occur and thus (4) could not be formed. The alternative α-hydroxylation of (1)

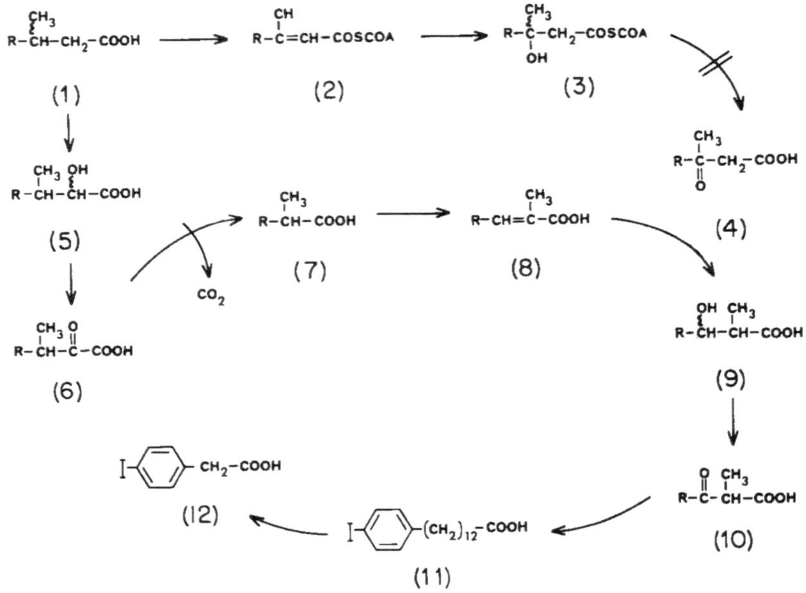

Figure 7. Possible catabolism of 15-(p-iodophenyl)-3-R,S-methylpentadecanoic acid (BMIPP) by either α- or β-oxidation. R = the remainder of the (p-iodophenyl)alkyl chain.

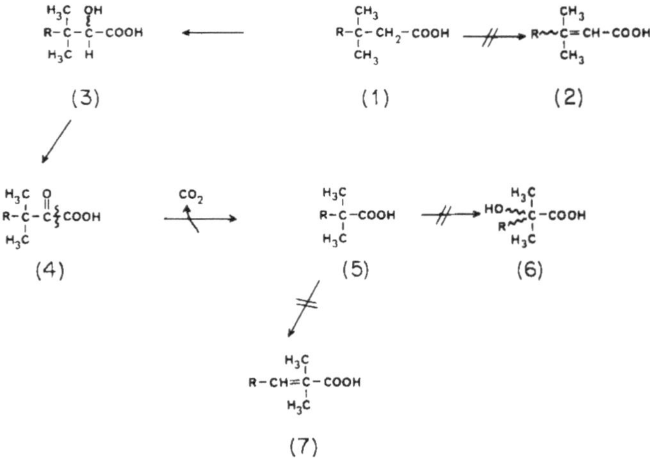

Figure 8. Potential catabolism of 15-(p-iodophenyl)-3,3-dimethylpentadecanoic acid (DMIPP) by α- or β-oxidation. R = remainder of the (p-iodo-phenyl)alkyl chain.

could give (5) which would be a substrate for subsequent oxidation to (6). Decarboxylation of (6) would then give the α-methyl acid (7), thus removing the impediment of the β-methyl group that was present in (1). Subsequent dehydrogenation to (8), hydration to (9) and oxidation would give (10), an activated α-methyl-β-keto acid. Cleavage of propionic acid from (10) would then yield 13-(p-iodophenyl)tridecanoic acid (11), a straight-chain analogue which could then be metabolized via the usual β-oxidative chain to give p-iodophenylacetic acid (12). Presumably, conjugation with glycine would then give an analogue of iodoaceturic acid. Thus, there are well established alternative routes of catabolism for β-methyl fatty acids such as BMIPP.

By an analysis of the established routes of α- and β-oxidation, the possible metabolism of DMIPP can be analyzed (Figure 8). Direct α,β-dehydrogenation of DMIPP (1) to (2) would not be possible without concomitant carbon-carbon bond cleavage. In a similar manner, α-hydroxylation of (1) to (3) could yield the α-hydroxy-β,β-dimethyl product (3) and dehydrogenation would yield the α-keto acid (4). Subsequent decarboxylation could give the α,α-dimethyl acid (5), but this would be a dead-end since neither α- nor β-hydroxylation of this product would be possible. Thus, dimethyl-substitution at the β-position would appear to inhibit catabolism by both α- and β-oxidative routes. Because of the complex spectrum of metabolites probably present in the body fluids (blood) and urine resulting from metabolism and excretion from various organ pools, an evaluation of the myocardial metabolism of BMIPP, DMIPP, etc., will probably only be possible with an adequate perfused heart system. Although such an analysis may explain why the dimethyl analogue DMIPP shows much longer myocardial retention than the monomethyl BMIPP and straight chain IPP analogues, the much higher heart to blood ratios observed with DMIPP are an unanticipated added bonus. These combined advantages of rapid, pronounced myocardial uptake, prolonged retention and high heart to blood ratios would suggest that the new 3,3-dimethyl-substituted DMIPP analogue is an excellent candidate to evaluate regional myocardial fatty acid uptake by SPECT.

Studies described in the next section were directed toward an assessment of the relative distribution of radioiodinated DMIPP, BMIPP and IPP within the intracellular organelles and also within the various fatty acid lipid pools of rat hearts. A correlation of these data with the retention of these agents observed in vivo may provide a clue regarding the relative metabolism and may also provide a clue to the mechanism(s) operative in the more prolonged retention of the DMIPP dimethyl analogue.

The effects of 3-methyl-branching on the distribution of radioiodinated 15-(p-iodophenyl)pentadecanoic acid analogues in subcellular fractions and lipid pools of rat myocardium

To gain insight to the metabolism of the 3-methyl-branched fatty acids, subcellular distribution studies and lipid analysis studies were performed using the BMIPP and DMIPP branched analogues and the IPP unbranched analogue. Fischer rats were injected intravenously with either (^{125}I)IPP, (^{125}I)BMIPP or

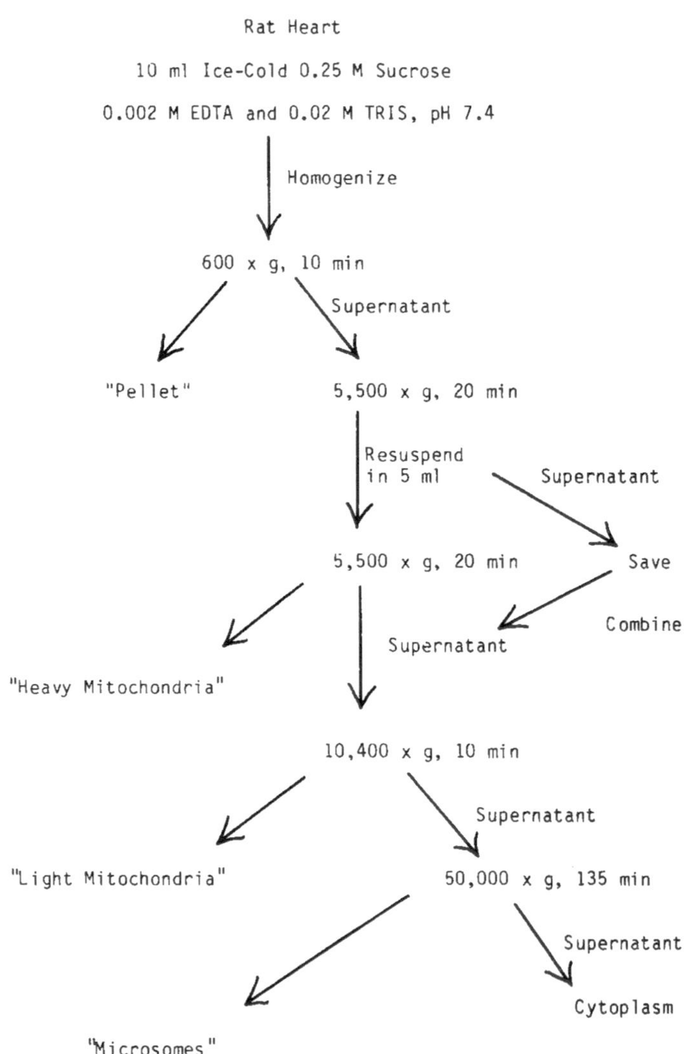

Figure 9. Summary of homogenization and differential centrifugation procedure for isolation of subcellular fractions.

(^{125}I)DMIPP complexed with 6% bovine serum albumin. For subcellular distribution studies, rat hearts were excised, immersed and sectioned in cold EDTA-Tris sucrose buffer to remove residual blood and then homogenized with the buffer using a ground glass homogenizer. The homogenate was then subjected to differential centrifugation (Figure 9) to obtain the crude pellet, mitochondrial, microsomal and cytoplasmic fractions. For extraction of lipids from either whole hearts or the isolated subcellular fractions, the tissue was

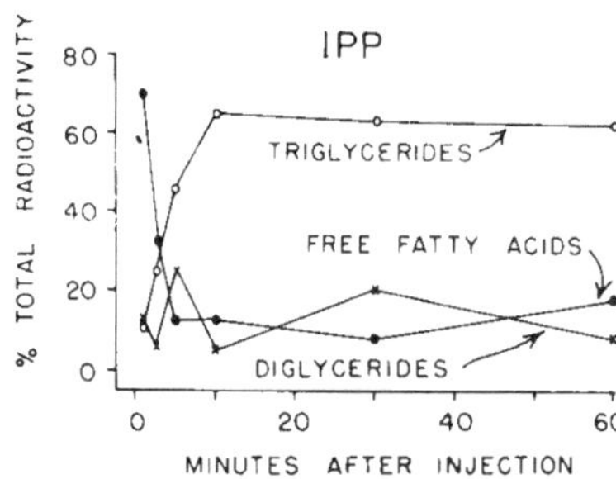

Figure 10. Distribution of radioactivity in lipid pools isolated by extraction of female Fischer rat hearts following intravenous administration of 15-([^{125}I]iodophenyl)pentadecanoic acid (IPP).

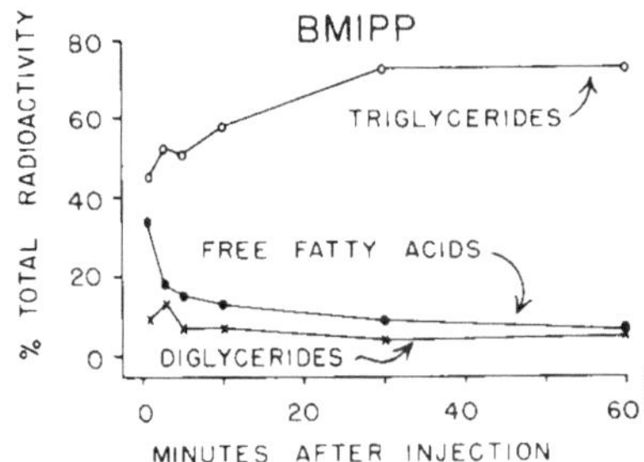

Figure 11. Distribution of radioactivity in lipid pools isolated by extraction of female Fischer rat hearts following intravenous administration of 15-([^{125}I]iodophenyl)-3-R,S-methylpentadecanoic acid (BMIPP).

homogenized in a 2:1 chloroform:methanol mixture using standard methods [63]. The extracted lipids were analyzed by thin-layer chromatography using a petroleum ether-ethyl ether-acetic acid (80:20:1) solvent system that adequately separates the various fatty acid pools; polar lipids (R_f origin), diglycerides (R_f=0.20), free fatty acids (R_f=0.50), and triglycerides (R_f=0.75). Sections of the plates were scrapped directly into vials and counted.

Initial studies involved an evaluation of the distribution of radioactivity in the lipid pools from whole hearts of fasted rats up to 1 h after administration of the radioiodinated fatty acid. Injection of the unbranched (^{125}I)IPP analogue results in initial high myocardial extraction followed by rapid washout of radioactivity. Lipid analysis demonstrated that the majority of the radioactivity was initally (1-3 min) present in the free fatty acid fraction. There is a rapid increase, however, of radioactivity associated with the triglyceride fraction and this increase is maximal at 10 min (Figure 10). Radioactivity in the diglyceride fraction is maximal at 5 min (20% total activity) and decreased slowly over the remainder of the assay period. With the BMIPP monomethyl-branched analogue, the majority of radioactivity at all assay times was found in the triglyceride fraction with radioactivity in the free fatty acid fraction significant

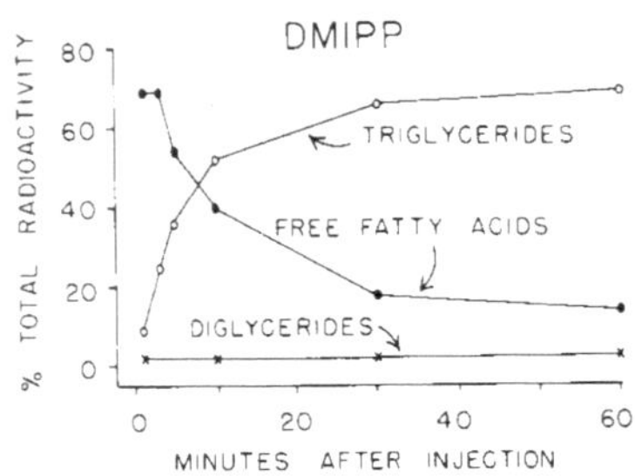

Figure 12. Distribution of radioactivity in lipid pools isolated by extraction of female Fischer rat hearts following intravenous administration of 15-(p-[^{125}I]oidophenyl)-3,3-dimethylpentadecanoic acid (DMIPP).

only at the earliest time periods (Figure 11). The radioactivity in the diglyceride fraction was maximal at 3-5 min (14% extracted activity), but fell similar to the activity in the free fatty acid fraction. With the DMIPP dimethyl-branched analogue, the free fatty acid fraction initally contained the majority of radioactivity. At later time periods the triglyceride fraction had the majority of the radioactivity (Figure 12). The rate of "conversion", however, was comparatively slower than with IPP. Similar studies with the three analogues were also conducted with unfasted rats demonstrating a faster incorporation into the triglyceride fraction with IPP and BMIPP and somewhat slower incorporation with DMIPP.

From the preliminary tissue distribution studies (Figure 3) 5 and 30 min time periods were chosen for examination of the lipid pools in the hearts of rats injected with the (^{125}I)IPP/(^{131}I)BMIPP/(^{123}I)DMIPP triple labeled mixture. This study was designed to eliminate the possible errors inherent in a comparison of the differences that may be detected in subcellular distribution and lipid pools between different groups of rats. In this manner, each measurement has essentially an internal control and differences observed with the three analogues can be directly compared. This type of study will not account for any differences in inherent binding to membranes, organelles or proteins, but will measure differences in the isolated radioactivity. The

Table 3. Summary of experimental details for the evaluation of [^{125}I]IPP/[^{131}I]BMIPP/[^{123}I]DMIPP triple-labeled fatty acid mixture administered to Female Fischer rats.

	Radioiodinated fatty acid		
	(^{125}I)IPP	(^{131}I)BMIPP	(^{123}I)DMIPP
Specific activity (μCi/nmole)	2.74	0.47	1.07
μCi/rat	89	15	53
nmole/rat	32.5	32	49.5
μgm/rat	16	16	24

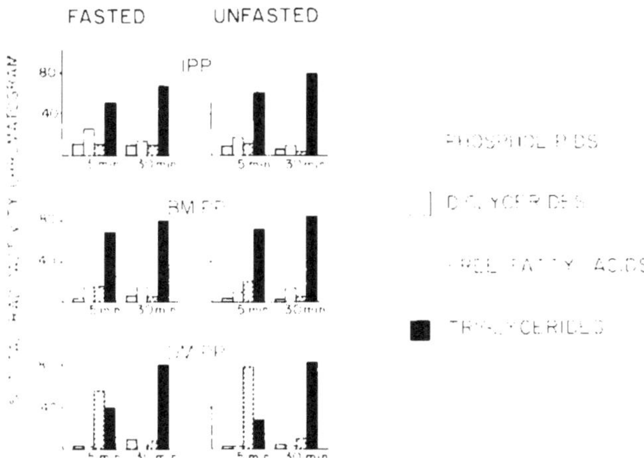

Figure 13. Comparison of the distribution of ^{125}I, ^{131}I and ^{123}I in lipid pools of heart extracts after administration of the [^{125}I]IPP/[^{131}I]BMIPP/[^{123}I]DMIPP mixture to fasted and unfasted female Fischer rats.

possibility of "competition" of the structurally-modified fatty acids for diffusion into the myocardial cells was felt to be unlikely since the effects of relative BMIPP/IPP mass ratios on biodistribution properties in rats had previously demonstrated an insignificant effect in ratios of up to 6:1 [46]. In the present experiment the mass of each fatty acid injected was very similar to eliminate any effects of possible mass differences on myocardial uptake. The details of this experiment are given in Table 3. For the triple-labeling experiments, the ^{123}I (159 keV) and ^{131}I (262 keV) photopeaks were counted simultaneously in two windows and the samples then stored in the cold until the ^{123}I contribution to the I-125 X-ray photopeak region was less than 4-5%. The samples were then counted again to determine the distribution of ^{125}I. The data from experiments with both fasted and unfasted rats are presented here. The major differences in lipid pools of the three analogues are seen at 5 min post-injection (Figure 13). At this time the relative proportion of radioactivity in the diglyceride fraction ranks in this order: IPP>BMIPP>DMIPP, whereas the relative distribution of radioactivity in the free fatty acid pool is reversed: DMIPP>BMIPP>IPP. At 30 min the majority of radioactivity (65-82%) is chromatographed with the triglyceride standard for all three analogues.

Other investigators have evaluated the myocardial lipid distribution of various radiolabeled fatty acids, including the straight chain IPP agent. Reske *et al.*[8,9] reported that 75-80% of the extractable activity from the hearts of unfasted rats injected with IPP was found in the triglyceride fraction, although no specific assay time was designated. Later reports [64] stated that in fasted rats between 45-57% of the activity was in the triglyceride fraction with approximately 10% in each of the diglyceride and free fatty acid fractions.

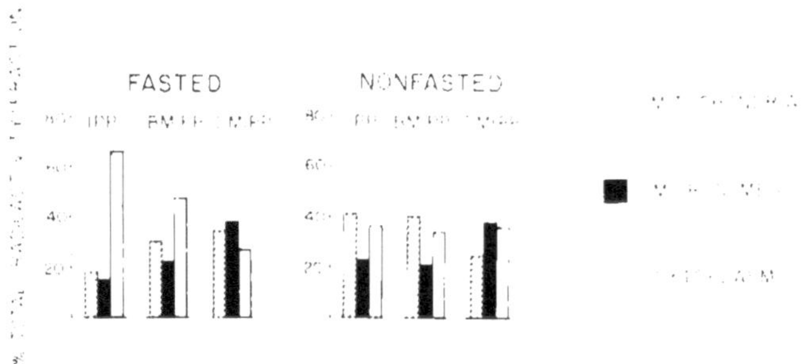

Figure 14. Distribution of radioactivity in subcellular fractions from heart homogenates 30 min after intravenous administration of either [^{125}I]IPP, [^{125}I]BMIPP or [^{123}I]DMIPP to separate groups of fasted and nonfasted female Fischer rats.

These reports compare favorably with the results reported here despite the inability to compare specific assay times. In a study by Otto *et al.* [52], terminally iodinated long chain fatty acids where n = 18 or 21 appeared to be fated primarily for triglyceride storage, whereas shorter chain fatty acids ($n \leq 15$) were subject to β-oxidation. Since the fatty acids in this study were without the phenyl moiety and were not branched, it is difficult to draw comparisons; however, it appears that the phenylpentadecanoic analogues have a chain length that would favor triglyceride storage.

To further investigate the metabolism of the 3-methyl-branched and straight chain analogues, subcellular distribution experiments were performed in independent studies with extracts of hearts excised from fasted and nonfasted rats 30 minutes after injection of the (^{125}I)labeled analogues. Comparison of the results obtained in nonfasted rats (Figure 14) shows little difference in the relative subcellular distribution of each compound at 30 minutes. In rats fasted for 24 hours, however, there are major differences in the subcellular profiles of the branched and unbranched analogues in the subcellular fractions isolated 30 minutes after injection. The IPP straight chain analogue, which shows rapid washout in the hearts of fasted rats, resulted in a proportionally greater amount of radioactivity in the cytoplasmic fraction with the corresponding proportional lower activity in the mitochondrial and microsomal fractions. Although this subcellular distribution profile of IPP obtained in fasted rats was significantly different from that observed with unfasted rats, comparison of the % dose/fraction values demonstrated similar levels of IPP in the cytoplasm. Thus, the apparent increase of radioactivity in the cytoplasm of the hearts of fasted rats is actually a proportional increase due to the loss of activity from the mitochondrial and microsomal fractions. The monomethyl-branched BMIPP analogue, which shows longer myocardial retention in vivo than IPP, showed comparatively higher percentages of radioactivity in the mitochondrial and microsomal fractions. The DMIPP dimethyl-branched analogue, which shows the longest *in vivo* myocardial retention of the three analogues, also had the

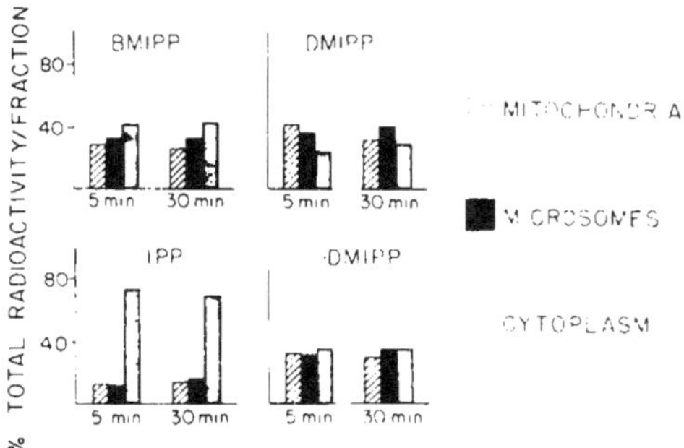

Figure 15. Comparison of the subcellular distribution of ^{125}I and ^{131}I from heart homogenates at 5 min and 30 min following the intravenous administration of either [^{131}I]IPP/[^{125}I]DMIPP or [^{131}I]BMIPP/[^{125}I]DMIPP mixtures to fasted female Fischer rats.

highest proportion of radioactivity associated with the microsomal and mitochondrial fractions. From these results and from previous studies in which the subcellular profiles of a number of fatty acids were compared, it appears that the length of retention in the hearts of fasted rats correlates with the relative proportion of radioactivity found in the mitochondrial and microsomal fractions 30 minutes after injection.

These subcellular studies were expanded to include both the 5 and 30 minutes assay periods and also lipid analysis of the subcellular fractions. Because the 3-4 day period required to complete these analyses made it impractical to use ^{123}I-labeled fatty acids, ^{131}I/^{125}I-labeled mixtures of two analogues (^{131}I)IPP/(^{125}IDMIPP and (^{131}I)BMIPP/(^{125}I)DMIPP were evaluated in fasted rats in two separate experiments. The comparative differences in the 30 minutes subcellular profiles observed in the earlier experiments were reproduced in these dual label experiments, and the subcellular distribution patterns at 5 minutes resembled those found at 30 minutes. It thus appears there are no shifts in the relative proportion of radioactivity within the subcellular fractions between 5 and 30 minutes (Figure 15). As might be expected from previously described lipid analysis of "whole hearts", however, there were differences observed in the lipid pools within these cellular fractions at the different time intervals. Lipid analysis of the pellet of the centrifugation of the crude homogenate (Figure 9) was included and may approximate the lipid profile of unfractionated heart tissue. With all cell fractions for the three analogues, there was a shift to a predominance of radioactivity in the triglyceride fraction 30 minutes after injection (Figures 16 and 17). The comparison of radioactivity lipid pools between the different cell fractions of hearts of rats injected with the same compound or the comparison of the same subcellular component of hearts with different compounds injected, however, showed a number of observable differences.

With the straight-chain IPP analogue (Figure 16), the radioactive lipid

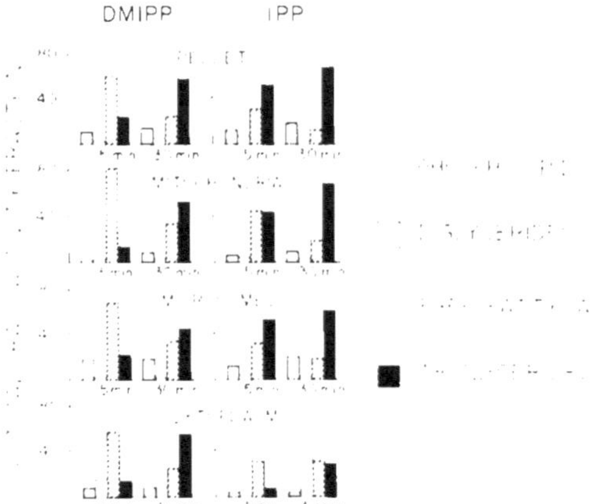

Figure 16. Distribution of radioactive lipids from the subcellular fractions of the [^{131}I]IPP/[^{125}I]DMIPP study described in Figure 15.

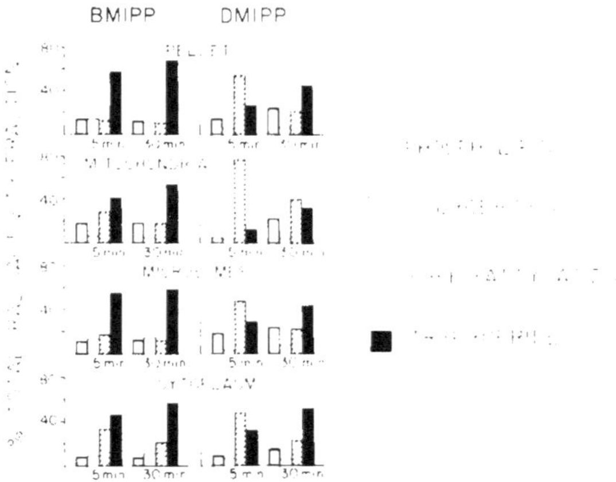

Figure 17. Distribution of radioactive lipids from the subcellular fractions of the [^{131}I]BMIPP/[^{125}I]DMIPP study described in Figure 15.

profiles of the microsomal and crude pellet fractions are quite similar, whereas the mitochondrial fraction shows a greater proportion of free fatty acid. In the cytoplasmic fraction 5 min after injection, the majority of the extractable radioactivity chromatographs with the diglyceride standard. With the monomethylbranched BMIPP analogue (Figure 17), the distribution of radioactive lipids in the microsomal fraction again resembles the crude pellet. For both the cytoplasmic and mitochondrial fractions, however, radioactivity in the free fatty acid component becomes a more predominant feature of the lipid profile particularly 5 min after injection. With DMIPP both the microsomal and cytoplasmic fractions of rat hearts injected with this dimethyl-branched fatty acid show lipid profiles similar to the crude pellet. In the mitochondrial fractions from these hearts, however, almost 80% of the extractable activity is in the form of free fatty acid.

An evaluation of the subcellular distribution profiles and the distribution of radioactive lipids extracted from the cell compounds shows distinct differences in the three analogues. Both the relative association within the mitochondrial versus the cytoplasmic fractions and the lipid profile of these two cell components appear to be the major differences that can be correlated between the structures of these analogues and the observed differences in their *in vivo* behavior. The IPP straight chain analogue shows poor myocardial *in vivo* retention and its metabolic product seem to be primarily associated with the cytoplasm where it is initially found predominantly in the diglyceride pool. At the other extreme, DMIPP shows the best myocardial retention of the three analogues and shows an early association with the mitochondria where the extractable radioactivity is almost exclusively in the free fatty acid fraction. Finally, BMIPP shows primarily equal distribution in the mitochondrial, microsomal and cytoplasmic fractions and seems to demonstrate the most rapid incorporation into triglycerides. Further analysis and identification of metabolites is being pursued. The present studies demonstrate clear differences in the myocardial metabolic basis for myocardial retention of these methyl-branched fatty acids.

The use of radioiodinated 3-methyl-branched analogues to evaluate heterogenous fatty acid uptake in hypertensive rat myocardium

The radioiodinated structurally-modified fatty acids such as (^{123}I)BMIPP and (^{123}I)DMIPP can also be potentially used to evaluate myocardial energy substrate utilization. Modified fatty acids such as 15-(p-(^{125}I)iodophenyl)-3-methyl-pentadecanoic acid (BMIPP) and 1-(^{14}C)-3-R,S-methylheptadecanoic acid (BMHDA) exhibit high myocardial extraction in rats and mice, respectively, and the myocardial residence time is much longer than palmitate. In comparative autoradiographic studies in mice, the heart to blood ratios were BMHDA (13.5 at 2 h) > palmitate (4.5 at 1 min) > BMIPP (2.3 at 5 min) > IPP (2.2 at 5 minutes).

The major role of fatty acids as substrates for myocardial metabolism suggest that these substrates may serve as a biochemical marker for early detection of any regional changes that are associated with myocardial diseases, such as hypertrophy and cardiomyopathy. Severe hypertension results in increased myocardial work which initially leads to hypertrophy and, if untreated, to heart failure [65]. In prolonged hypertension resulting from aortic stenosis, for example, the left ventricle is subjected to increased pressure load and under such circumstances the myocardium may not respond uniformly [66]. In such a situation, the relative effects on endocardium and epicardium, and on the free

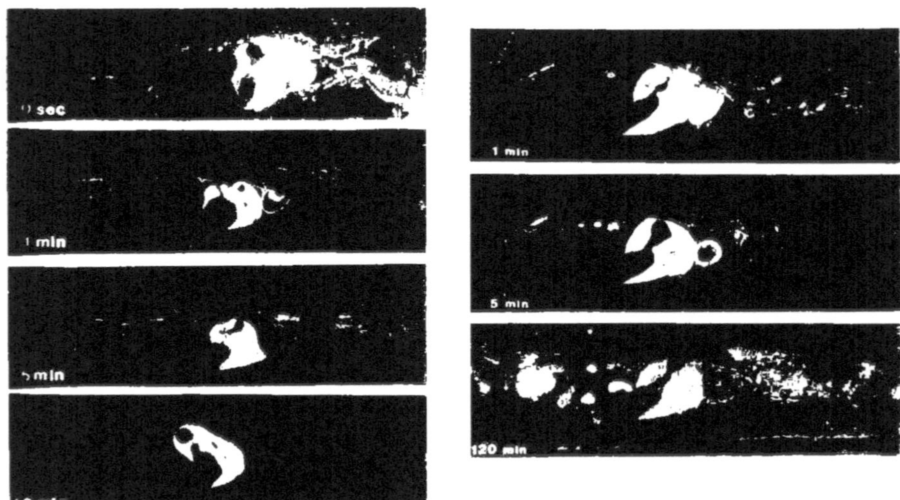

Figure 18. Wholebody autoradiographs of mice after intravenous administration of 1-[^{14}C]-palmitic acid (left panel) or 15-(p-[^{125}I]iodophenyl)pentadecanoic acid, IPP (right panel).

wall and septal region of the left ventricle may differ. A recent quantitative dual-tracer autoradiographic (ARG) study performed in a salt-induced hypertension animal model revealed an uncoupling of perfusion and substrate utilization in hypertensive myocardium [36]. Regional fatty acid and glucose utilization were studied using the branched-chain fatty acid, 1-(^{14}C)-3-R,S-methylheptadecanoic acid (1-(^{14}C)BMHDA) [45], and 2-deoxy-D-(U-^{14}C)-glucose (^{14}C)-2-DG) or (^{18}F)-2-fluoro-2-deoxy-D-glucose ((^{18}F)FDG) [67]. The regional myocardial perfusion was assessed with Tl-201-chloride. The regional distribution of perfusion (Tl-201 chloride) and fatty acid utilization (1-(^{14}C)BMHDA) were homogeneous in normotensive myocardium. Hearts from the hypertension animals showed a relatively homogeneous pattern of regional perfusion, and the utilization of fatty acid was focally decreased in the free wall and endocardium of left ventricle. The decrease in fatty acid uptake was associated with a concomitant increase in glucose utilization in the above regions. These studies demonstrated the unexpected lower fatty acid uptake in regions that exhibited normal perfusion and suggested that such differences could be assessed *in vivo* by standard imaging procedures if radioiodinated structurally-modified fatty acids behaved in the same manner.

It is quite possible that all fatty acids that show myocardial specificity will present the same heterogeneous distribution discussed above for the hypertensive Dahl rats. To detect and potentially quantitate such heterogeneous distribution in patients using either planar or single-photon computerized tomographic techniques, however, the initial distribution pattern should be "frozen" to allow adequate imaging periods. The effects of structural modifi-

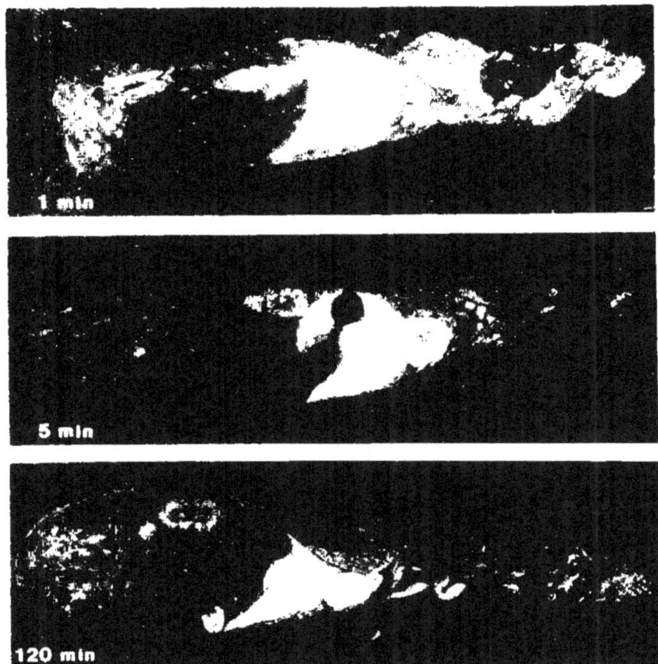

Figure 19. Wholebody autoradiographs of mice after intravenous administration of 15-(p-[^{125}I]iodophenyl)-3-R,S-methylpentadecanoic acid (BMIPP).

cations on the rate of myocardial washout using ARG studies is clearly shown in Figures 18 and 19. While the straight-chain palmitic acid and IPP analogues show rapid washout (Figure 18), the methyl-branched BMIPP analogue shows much larger retention (Figure 19). Thus, the use of radioiodinated methyl-branched fatty acids such as 15-(p-iodophenyl)-3-R,S-methylpentadecanoic acid (BMIPP) and the DMIPP dimethyl analogue were also studied in the above system. Recent dual tracer autoradiographic studies with 15-(^{131}I)BMIPP in the hearts from normotensive and hypertensive rats showed similar decreased uptake in the endocardial regions (Figure 20). These results suggest that under circumstances of persistent ventricular pressure overload and/or hypertrophy, a significant dissociation between the regional perfusion and substrate utilization occurs.

Since the DMIPP dimethyl analogue shows much longer retention and higher blood ratios than the monomethyl-BMIPP agent, biodistribution and autoradiographic studies were conducted with normotensive and hypertensive Dahl rats. For the biodistribution, groups of rats were administered 9.4 μCi each of (^{131}I)DMIPP. Six rats were used for each study. The normotensive rats had average blood pressure readings of 124.67 ± 3.77 mm Hg and the hypertensive 214.5 ± 13.91mmHg. The biodistribution data in this strain of rats are shown in

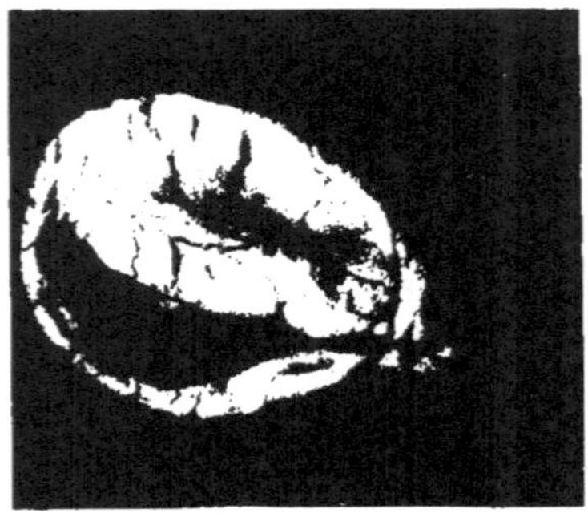
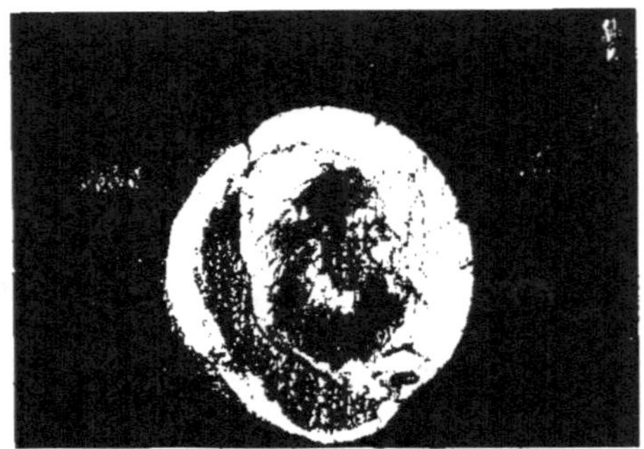

Figure 20. Autoradiographs of slices of hearts from normotensive (left) and hypertensive (right) rats 60 min after injection of [^{131}I]BMIPP. Notice heterogeneous distribution in the normotensive heart.

Table 4 and correlate well with Fischer rat data discussed in detail earlier (*vide ante*).

There is a small but significantly lower (~ 20%) myocardial concentration of the DMIPP at this time period in the hypertensive rats, and the heart: blood ratios are considerably lower. On a global basis the concentration of DMIPP in the heart and other tissue of the normotensive rats are similar. In contrast, on a regional basis the autoradiographic studies with (^{131}I)DMIPP demonstrated a homogeneous distribution in normotensive rat hearts (Figure 21) and a marked heterogeneous distribution pattern in the hypertensive rat hearts mimicking the differences described earlier for BMIPP.

Recently, the demonstration of these regional differences with a related agent, 14-(^{123}I)-3-R,S-methyltetradecanoic acid [44], have been demonstrated clinically (H.W. Strauss *et al.*, unpublished data). Studies in a patient with severe ventricular hypertrophy and in another patient with severe aortic insufficiency, but with maintained ventricular function, showed a focal zone of

Table 4. Biodistribution of [^{131}I]DMIPP in Dahl strain normotensive and hypertensive rats (t=60 min).

	Percent injected Dose/gm	
Organ	Normotensive	Hypertensive
Blood	0.132 ± 0.012	0.179 ± 0.028
Heart	2.518 ± 0.398	2.071 ± 0.469
Kidneys	0.545 ± 0.070	0.404 ± 0.085
Lungs	0.526 ± 0.036	0.513 ± 0.080
Salivary gland	0.363 ± 0.036	0.410 ± 0.089
Spleen	0.496 ± 0.059	0.446 ± 0.141
Muscle	0.178 ± 0.010	0.187 ± 0.043
Liver	2.880 ± 0.228	3.200 ± 0.554
Heart/blood	19.04 ± 2.67	11.69 ± 3.00

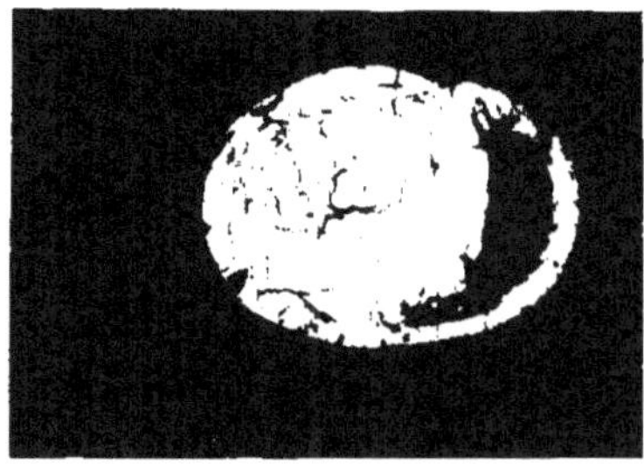
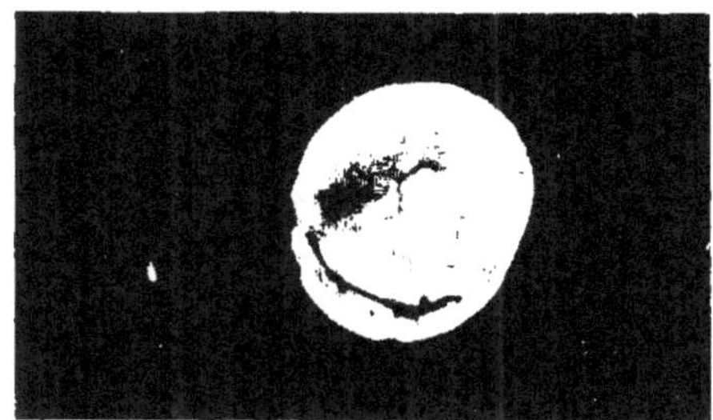

Figure 21. Autoradiographs of slices of hearts from normotensive (left) and hypertensive (right) rats 60 min after injection of [^{131}I]DMIPP. Notice decreased uptake in the endocardial regions in hypertensive myocardium.

decreased fatty acid uptake which in the former was associated with normal perfusion. In the later, however, the distributions of perfusion and fatty acid utilization were similar. These data suggest that the autoradiographic findings in hypertensive animals with ventricular hypertrophy can be observed in human subjects. It is still unclear whether this alteration in the substrate utilization is due to a defect in membrane transport, energy production/utilization or decrease in the ratio of capillaries to sarcomeres. Nonetheless, this technique could be applied in human subjects using agents labeled with gamma emitting radionuclides and SPECT systems to detect possible alterations in myocardial metabolism earlier in patients with hypertension, cardiomyopathies and related diseases, in the absence of ischemic perfusion defects.

Evaluation of the regional uptake and release rates of (^{123}I)BMIPP in normal patients and patients with single and multi-vessel coronary artery disease

Preliminary studies with (^{123}I)BMIPP have been recently conducted in a group of patients at the Department of Nuclear Medicine, University Clinic, in Vienna, Austria. Nineteen patients were evaluated who underwent coronary angiography because of the presentation of chest pain. Coronary angiography was performed using the Judkin's technique with multiple views for each coronary artery and single plane ventriculography (RAO 30°). Luminal narrowing of the coronary artery equal to or greater than 70% was described as critical. In all patients with angiographically proven coronary artery disease (CAD) thallium-201 dipyridamole stress and 4 h redistribution scintigrams were also obtained. Myocardial scintigraphy was performed with (^{123}I)BMIPP in all patients. The patients were studied fasted or at least 10 h after a light breakfast. For the (^{123}I)BMIPP studies scintigraphy was performed using a mobile gamma camera (Apex 215M, Elscint) in 15 patients and with a Large Field of View (LFOV) gamma camera (Siemens, interfaced with a dedicated computer, DEC PDP 11/34) in the remaining four patients. An all-purpose, low energy parallel-whole collimator was used in the LAO 45° projection in 14 patients and in the anterior projection in five patients. After intravenous tracer administration data were accumulated in a 64x64 word matrix for 100 min and stored in a dedicated computer (Apex, Elscint; DEC PDP 11/34). The administered dose was between 2-3 mCi (^{123}I)BMIPP in eleven patients and about 4 mCi of the agent was administered to eight patients in studies where plasma samples were analyzed to evaluate the presence of possible BMIPP catabolic products. Background corrected myocardial time-activity curves were generated, using the vena cava region as the representative of blood background. There were only minor differences in elimination parameters compared to time-activity curves generated from interpolative background corrected images.

Metabolism of BMIPP in humans

Where appropriate, the organ curves were fitted with a biexponential function or otherwise with a monoexponential function. The elimination parameters evaluated included elimination half-times in minutes of the initial and second phase. In addition, the contribution of each phase of the elimination curve was estimated by a component ratio, which was calculated by back extrapolation of each phase from the relative activity of the initial and second phase at peak activity (e.g. the activity of the initial phase at t-max/activity of the second phase at t-max).

Both plasma and urine samples from several patients were analyzed to evaluate the potential catabolism of (^{123}I)BMIPP. In ten patients blood clearance and urinary excretion for 0-2 h and 2-16 h after tracer administration were evaluated. Blood was drawn 5, 10, 15, 20, 30, 60 90 and 120 min after tracer administration. Following an initial decrease in plasma activity, with the lowest values between 15-20 min after tracer administration (5.6 $\pm$ 1.5% dose/l), there was a slight increase in ^{123}I plasma radioactivity.

In addition, to evaluate the formation of hydrophilic and lipophilic metabolites from BMIPP degradation, 0.5 ml of plasma samples were extracted with 2.5 ml chloroform/methanol (2:1 v/v). This was performed in untreated plasma samples(pH~ 7.4) and in plasma samples acidified with HCl to pH~ 2, to determine if the hydrophilic catabolites behaved as weak acids, which should be extracted into the organic phase after acidification. Following centrifugation, the resulting solid-, aqueous-, and organic phases were separated and distribution of radioactivity measured in a well-scintillation counter. By chloroform/methanol extraction of plasma samples at pH ~ 7.4 soluble catabolites were found in both the water and organic phases. Five minutes postinjection, 76.7% $\pm$ 3.9% of the radioactivity was extracted into the organic phase. The aqueous and solid phases contained 3.6% $\pm$ 1.9% and 19.8% $\pm$ 4.2%, respectively. Thereafter ^{123}I radioactivity in the aqueous phase increased to 39.1% $\pm$ 5.8% at 20 min postinjection while the organic phase decreased to 32.9% $\pm$

6.3%. In the following period, the respective relative ^{123}I radioactivity in both phases remained nearly constant. By extraction of acidified plasma samples, nearly all the aqueous radioactivity was extracted into the organic phase.

The distribution of radioactivity in the organic phase of plasma samples extracted at pH ~ 2 (n=8; t: 5 min and 90 min after injection) was further analyzed by thin layer chromatography (TLC). The organic phase was dried under a stream of nitrogen at 50°C in a water bath and subsequently redissolved in 50 μl chloroform/methanol and aliquots applied to silicagel plates (Sc 60, F 254, Fa. Merck) and separated using chloroform/acetic acid (9:1 v/v) as eluent. The distribution of radioactivity on the TLC plates was assayed by a thin layer scanner and mobility of ^{123}I radioactivity in samples compared with standards (^{123}I-BMIPP, ^{123}I-benzoic acid, ^{123}I-o-iodohippuric acid and triolein, Table 5). These analyses demonstrated a radioactive component at 5 min corresponding to BMIPP (R_f: 0.67-0.75). At 90 min, however, three radioactive peaks were seen with mean R_f values of 0.60, 0.73 and 0.89 (Table 5). These findings suggest catabolism of BMIPP by human tissues. Apart from the site where this may occur, the demonstration of catabolites other than triglycerides suggests the metabolic breakdown of this agent.

In ten patients, as mentioned before, excretion of ^{123}I radioactivity in the urine was measured 0-2 h and 2-16 h after tracer administration. Between 0-2 h and 2-16 h, 4.1% ± 0.95% and 10.5% ± 2.2% dose, respectively, were excreted. In addition, aliquots of urine excreted within 0-2 h were analyzed in a manner similar to that described for the plasma samples. Thus, extraction with chloroform/methanol was performed in untreated and acidified urine and the

Table 5. Thin-layer chromatographic analysis of ^{123}I radioactivity distribution in plasma samples after chloroform-methanol extraction (pH=2; organic phase) following intravenous administration of(^{123}I)BMIPP.

Standard	R_f values			
BMIPP	0.70 ± 0.04			
Benzoic Acid	0.59 ± 0.02			
Hippuric Acid	0.15 ± 0.01			
Triolein	0.85 ± 0.03			
	R_f values of radioactive components			
	5 min post injection		90 min post injection	
#1	0.73	0.61	0.77	0.92
#2	0.69		0.70	0.92
#3	0.67	0.67	0.84	0.96
#4	0.69		0.71	0.87
#5	0.69		0.67	0.89
#6	0.73	0.57	0.75	0.81
#7	0.75	0.60	0.80	0.91
#8	0.74	0.62	0.79	0.85

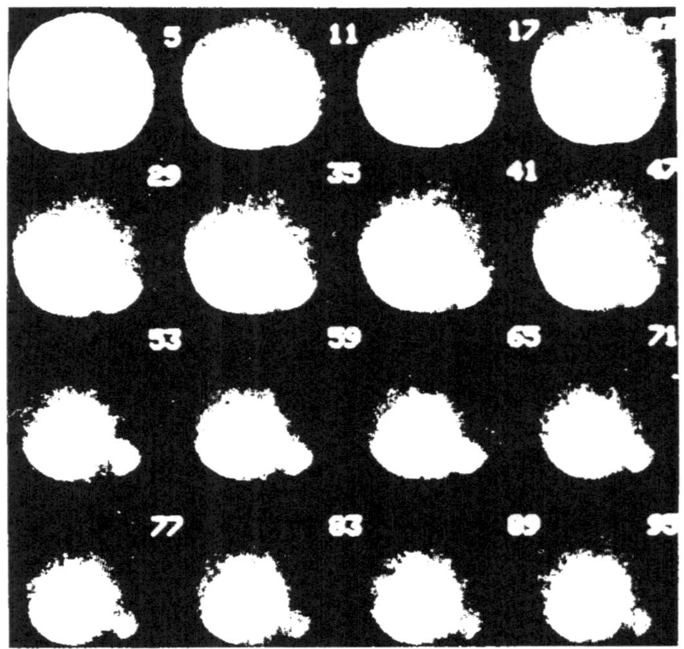

Figure 22. Serial scintigrams after i.v. injection of 3 mCi [^{123}I]BMIPP in a patient with normal coronary arteries. Each image represents the sum of five 1 min frames.

organic phase of the latter procedure was analyzed by TLC. By extraction of untreated urine with chloroform/methanol most of the radioactivity was found in the aqueous phase. Extraction of acidified urine revealed nearly equal amounts of radioactivity in the aqueous and organic phase (Table 6). By TLC fractionation a radioactive peak with an R_f value between 0.15-0.2 was found. The urine from one patient (20 μl) was analyzed by reversed phase high performance liquid chromatography. Peak identity was verified with ^{131}I orthoiodohippuric acid. The ^{123}I urine catabolite had a retention time of 2.8 min which was identical to the hippuric acid standard. Surprisingly these data demonstrate that (^{123}I)BMIPP is catabolized to material that behaves, in the TLC system used, like the glycine conjugate of 4-(^{123}I)iodobenzoic acid (hippuric acid).

Tabel 6. Summary of extraction studies of urine from patients after (^{123}I)BMIPP administration

Untreated urine	Phase	Acidified urine
86.8 ± 3.8%	aqueous	48.8 ± 3.9%
10.4 ± 3.4%	organic	48.9 ± 4.1%
3.1 ± 0.6%	solid	2.3 ± 1.2%

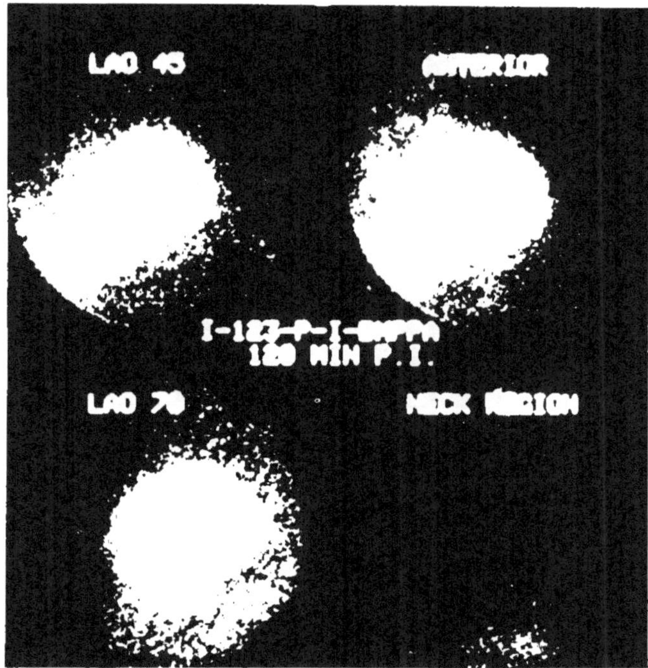

Figure 23. Uncorrected scintiphotos in a patient with three-vessel disease obtained 2 h after intravenous injection of 3 mCi [^{123}I]BMIPP. No premedication was given.

Scintigraphic findings

Four patients, three of whom had valvular heart disease, showed normal coronary arteries. The serial myocardial images obtained from one of the patients are shown in Figure 22. The heart is clearly visualized during the 95 min study period. Fifteen patients had angiographically confirmed single-vessel, double-vessel or triple-vessel disease. Coronary angiography revealed one-vessel disease in five patients. In three patients, who had previous myocardial infarction, two vessels were narrowed. In seven patients three vessels were narrowed, four of whom had suffered from a previous infarction. A typical scintiphoto of a patient with triple-vessel disease is shown in Figure 23. On the scintiphotos, reduced BMIPP uptake is clearly observed in the posterolateral (LAO 45°), posterior (LAO 70°) and in the anterior myocardial wall. The thyroid was not visualized as shown in the image of the neck region, demonstrating low in vivo deiodination of this agent, which was expected since radioiodide is stabilized by attachment to the phenyl ring.

In Figure 24, scintiphotos of a patient with two-vessel disease obtained 15 min and 40 min after tracer administration are shown. This patient had previous myocardial infarction (LAD 95%, LCX 80%). On the interpolated

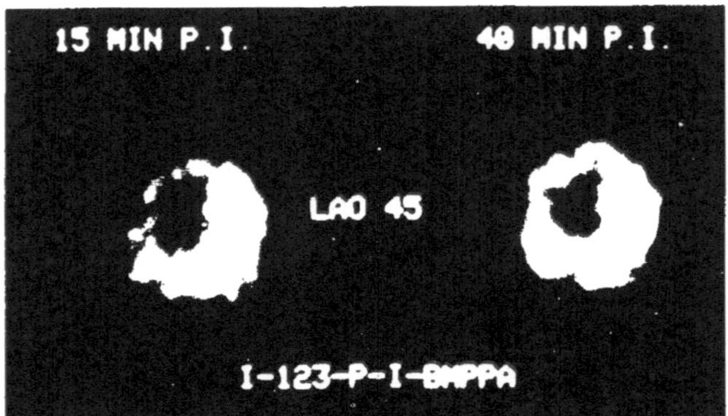

Figure 24. Myocardial images 15 and 40 min after administration of [123]IBMIPP to a patient with two-vessel disease.

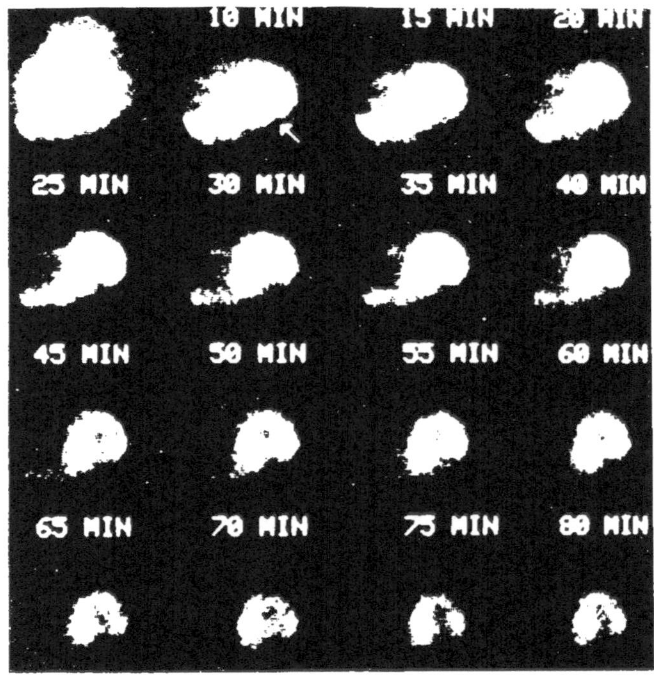

Figure 25. Serial scintigrams in a patient with three-vessel disease and previous myocardial infarction after injection of [123I]BMIPP (LAD 60%, LCX, 70%, RCA 100%). Each image represents the sum of five 1 min frames.

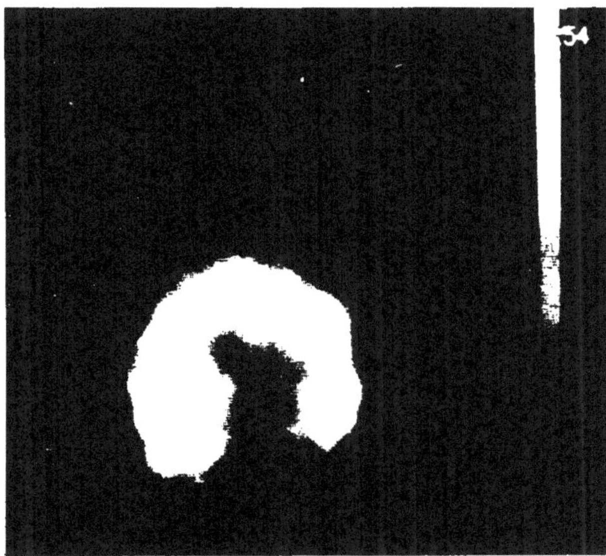

Figure 26. Interpolated background corrected image from the [^{123}I]BMIPP study of the patient described in Figure 25.

background corrected images reduced BMIPP uptake is seen in the septal wall at 15 minutes, which is less pronounced on the later image, indicating a delayed clearance of BMIPP from that region. In Figure 25, the serial images of a patient with triple-vessel desease are shown. The interpolated background corrected image (10 minutes p.i., LAO 45° view) of the patient described in Figure 25, is shown in Figure 26, and demonstrate a markedly reduced BMIPP uptake in the infarcted region (inferior) and in the postlateral wall. In the Tl-201 dipyridamole stress and redistribution scintigram, only an irreversible perfusion defect was seen in the infarcted region.

These examples demonstrate that defects in BMIPP uptake are clearly seen in infarcted as well as in noninfarcted regions supplied by stenosed vessels. By visual interpretation of scintigrams obtained at accumulation peak time regional deficits in tracer uptake were seen in 6 out of 7 infarcted regions. In the one patient with apparent normal uptake in the infarcted region the Tl-201 study also appeared normal in the respective projection (LAO 45°), but was abnormal in the others, showing an apparently reversible perfusion defect. This study was thus false negative for an infarction scar but true positive for recognizing a diseased region.

In seven regions supplied by stenosed coronary arteries but without infarction, BMIPP uptake was reduced. In six of those regions the Tl-201 dipyridamol stress redistribution scintigrams showed reversible perfusion defects, whereas in one region the Tl-201 perfusion study appeared normal. In three regions with stress induced perfusion defects in the Tl-201 study and in one region with normal Tl-201 uptake but abnormal washout the BMIPP uptake was normal. Thus, regional sensitivity was 41% for BMIPP and 53% for Tl-201 (13/32 and 17/32, respectively). In general, an abnormal uptake was seen in 11/15 CAD patients with BMIPP and in 13/15 with Tl-201, giving sensitivities of 73% and 87% respectively.

The evaluation of organ time-activity curves complemented the visual interpretation of scintigrams. The background corrected time-activity curves from heart and liver after intravenous administration of 3 mCi (^{123}I)BMIPP demonstrated a faster elimination from the liver than from the the heart. This different behaviour in organ washout of BMIPP was seen in all patients. Obviously the metabolic fate of BMIPP is different in the heart than in the liver. The respective elimination parameters from these organs are given in Table 7. In the liver the elimination behaviour of BMIPP fitted a biexponential function. However, in the heart it was monoexponential in eight patients, but biexponential in the remaining 11.

As mentioned above, a monoexponential myocardial time-activity curve was seen in eight patients (controls, n=2; 1 VD, n=1; 2 VD, n=2; 3 VD, n=3) (Table 7, upper part). The elimination half-time was prolonged from diseased regions as compared to the respective normal perfused region or the "best" region in patients with three vessel disease (Table 8). These findings were seen from regions with reduced (n=6) as well as an apparent normal BMIPP uptake, including both infarcted (n=5) and noninfarcted regions but supplied by stenosed coronary vessels (n=6).

Table 7. Elimination parameters for the heart and liver of patients after injection of [^{123}I]BMIPP

Elimination behaviour:	Heart: monoexponential in 8 patients biexponential in 11 patients Liver: biexponential in 19 patients	
Elimination parameters:	Heart	Liver
Monoexponential	n = 8	n = 0
T½ min	218.8 ± 102.5	–
range	111 – 377	
Biexponential	n = 11	n = 19
T½ I min:	13.8 ± 4.1	11.4 ± 4.4
range	7.5 – 22.9	3.9 – 22.0
T½ II min:	187.2 ± 49.8	91.5 ± 36.8
range	109 – 277	52 – 180
T½ I' min:	64.0 ± 13.0	37.5 ± 13.18
range	51 – 87	15.4 – 64.8
C-I/C-II ratio	0.34 ± 0.11	0.57 ± 0.35
range	0.18 – 0.53	0.19 – 1.65

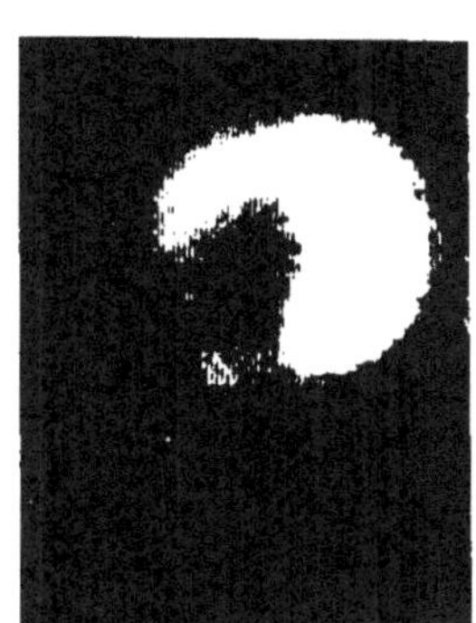

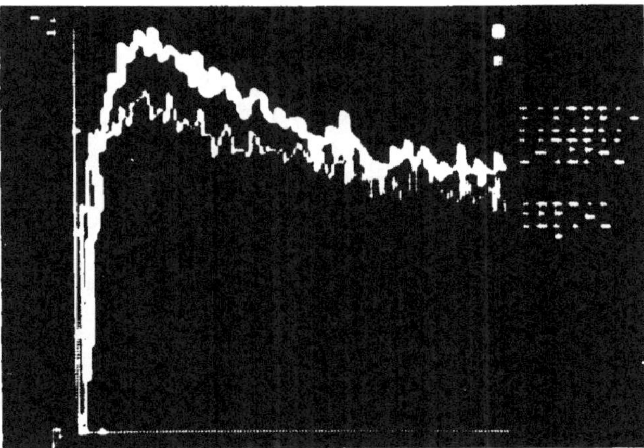

Figure 27. Time-activity curves for a patient with three-vessel disease after injection of [^{123}I]BMIPP total study period, 100 min).

In two patients with a biexponential behaviour in the normal region, the decline in myocardial activity was monoexponential in a diseased region. These included the "chronic ischemic" region in a patient with single vessel disease and an infarcted region in a patient with double vessel disease. Background (vena cava region) corrected myocardial time-activity curves, fitting a biexponential function, are given for a patient with three vessel disease and previous myocardial infarction (LAD 95%, LCX 60%, RCA 100%) in Figures 27 and 28 who showed scintigraphically a reduced BMIPP uptake in the septal and inferior (infarcted) wall. These data demonstrate a delayed washout of BMIPP from the septal region compared to the posterolateral wall. The regional myocardial elimination parameters evaluated in this subset of patients with CAD, where the myocardial time-activity curve fitted a biexponential function, are summarized in Table 9. By intraindividual comparison of normal and diseased myocardial regions significant differences were found both for the

Table 8. Myocardial elimination half-time after intravenous injection of [^{123}I]BMIPP in six patients with coronary artery disease showing a monoexponential time-activity curve

	T½ minutes
Normal region (N=6)	150.5 ± 45.6 111 – 230
"Chronic ischemic" region (N=6)	234.8 ± 107.1 140 – 407
Infarcted region (N=5)	417.6 ± 352 165 – 990

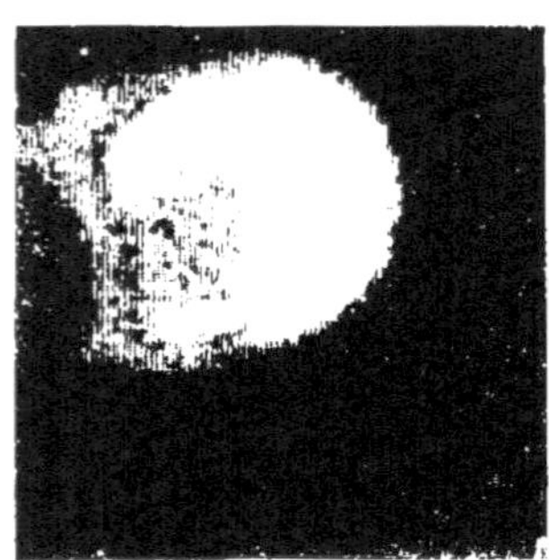

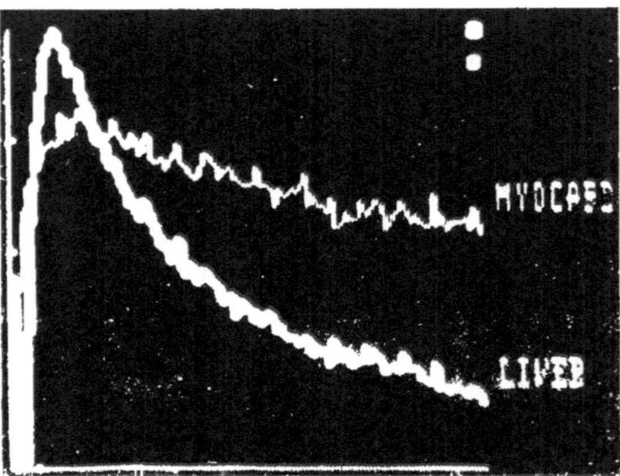

Figure 28. Comparison of the time-activity curves for heart and liver wash-out from the [^{123}I]BMIPP study of the patient shown in Figure 26 (Total study period, 100 min).

initial elimination half-time and the component ratio ($p<0.01$), being prolonged and/or reduced, respectively, from diseased regions. In all patients with CAD, including those with normal BMIPP elimination behaviour were seen. Thus, besides visual interpretation of scintigrams, the regional analysis of myocardial time-activity curves may add to the diagnostic feasibility of BMIPP for recognizing patients with heart disease. These preliminary findings appear promising, since in studies with IPP or HDA (however obtained in a greater number of patients) a regional abnormal elimination behaviour was not seen in all patients with CAD.

The availability of this new agent allowed a comparison of the absolute uptake and time-activity curves of (^{123}I)BMIPP and the linear (^{123}I)IPP

Table 9. Myocardial elimination half-time after i.v. injection of [^{123}I]BMIPP in nine patients with coronary artery disease showing a biexponential time-activity curve

Elimination parameters	Normal Region (+best vessel 3VD) (N=13)	Diseased region (N=14)
T/2 I min:	11.2 ± 4.3	19.7 ± 12.7
Range	6.7 – 18.2	9.4 – 44
T/2 II min:	153.7 ± 47.9	160.1 ± 64.2
Range	109 – 222	111 – 317
T/2 I' min:	62.4 ± 20.7	69.6 ± 22.0
Range	43 – 96	48 – 119
C-I/C-II ratio	0.36 ± 0.15	0.28 ± 0.14
Range	0.18 – 0.73	0.18 – 0.55

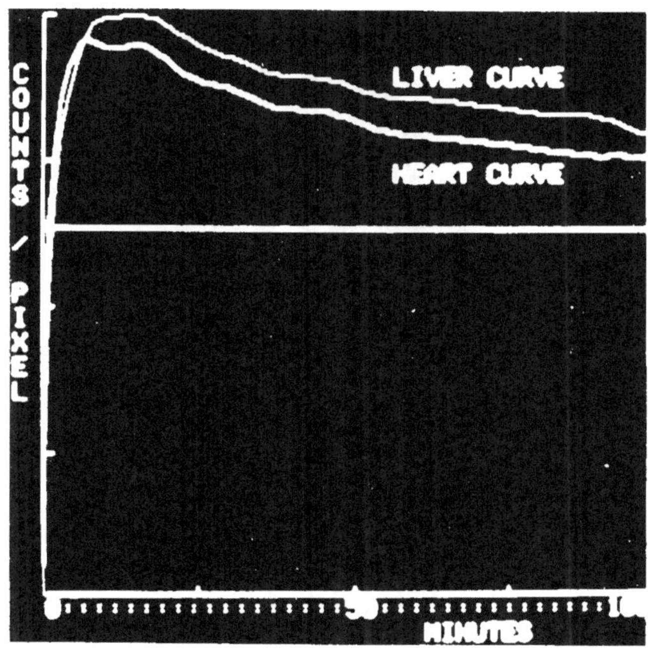

Figure 29. Typical heart and liver time-activity curve for a normal patient after injection of [^{123}I]IPP. The initial counts become negative because of the background corrections. Thus, the abscissa giving 0 counts in displayed in the upper part of the figure and the curves normalized to the ordinate become "flattened" (total study period 100 min).

straight-chain analogue which has been widely used in a much larger patient population [8-12]. Comparing the findings obtained with BMIPP to those with IPP in a similar study population (n=17; CAD: 1 VD, n=5, St.p.MI/3; 2 VD, n=3, St.p.MI/1: 3 VD, n=6, St.p.MI/2; controls, n=3) we found that peak myocardial activity occurred later with BMIPP than with IPP. Myocardial extraction, as estimated from the myocardium/background ratio, is slightly

Table 10. Comparison of [^{123}I]BMIPP and [^{123}I]IPP for myocardial scintigraphy in patients with CAD.

	BMIPP (N=19)	IPP (N=17)
T-max (min) heart	14.90 ± 3.40	10.4 ± 2.0
T-max (min) liver	8.80 ± 2.30	14.5 ± 3.3
Heart/BG at t-max	1.80 ± 0.29	1.99 ± 0.26
Heart/BG at 100 min	1.59 ± 0.26	1.24 ± 0.14
Liver/BG at t-max	2.05 ± 0.31	2.29 ± 0.29
Liver/BG at 100 min	1.45 ± 0.26	1.63 ± 0.26
% Heart	33.8 ± 12.2%	61.3 ± 6.06%
% Heart	64.6 ± 13.8%	58.7 ± 6.30%

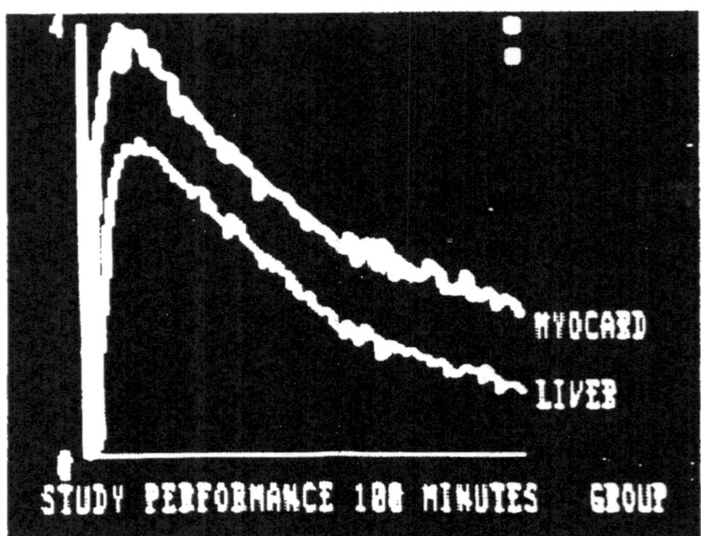

Figure 30. Time-activity curves for the heart and liver after injection of (^{123}I)IPP to a patient with normal coronary arteries (total study period, 100 min).

less for BMIPP than for IPP (Table 10). Background corrected time-activity curves of the heart and liver after intravenous injection of (^{123}I)IPP are shown in Figure 29, showing a nearly parallel activity decline from these two organs. In contrast, the background corrected time-activity curves of heart and liver after intravenous injection of (^{123}I)BMIPP show, as mentioned previously, a faster elimination from the liver than from the heart (Figure 28).

The availability of both (^{123}I)IPP and (^{123}I)BMIPP also allowed a comparison of their relative behaviour in the same patient. Studies were performed 1 week apart. Myocardial time activity curves obtained after intravenous injection of either IPP or BMIPP are compared in Figure 30. Peak activity appears higher and elimination faster in the IPP study than in the BMIPP study. The respective myocardial scintigrams of this patient (three vessel disease, LAD 70%, LCX 95%, RCA 70%) are shown in Figures 31 and 32. The interpolated background corrected images (LAO 45°) show a slightly reduced uptake in the posterolateral wall in the BMIPP study (Figure 32), whereas IPP uptake appears normal (Figure 33). This comparative evaluation of IPP and BMIPP indicates a somewhat different uptake and elimination behaviour for both tracers in various organs; the structural differences possibly implying different pathways in their metabolic usage. This is in line with findings previously given in rat experiments.

The interpretation of organ clearance curves in BMIPP studies in terms of specific metabolic pathways is not possible at this time. This lack of such a comprehensive interpretation is also encountered with other radioiodinated

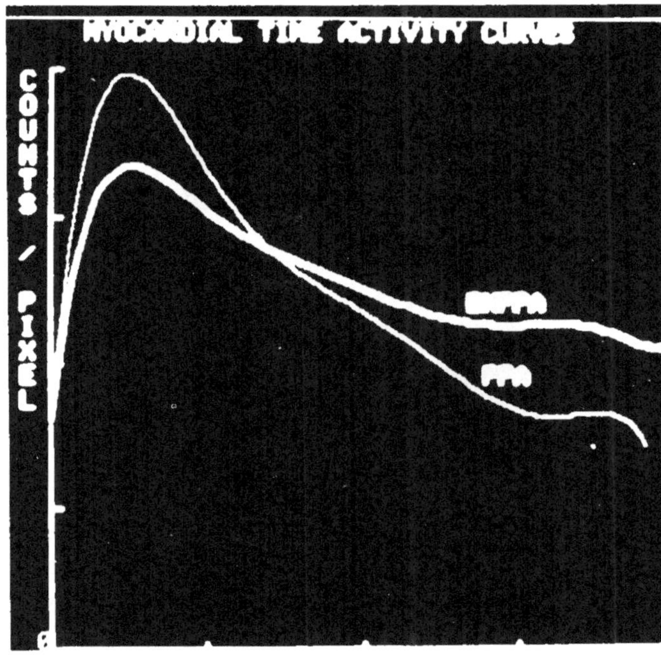

Figure 31. Comparison of the heart time-activity curves after administration of [^{123}I]IPP and (^{123}I)BMIPP to patients with three-vessel disease (total study period 100 min).

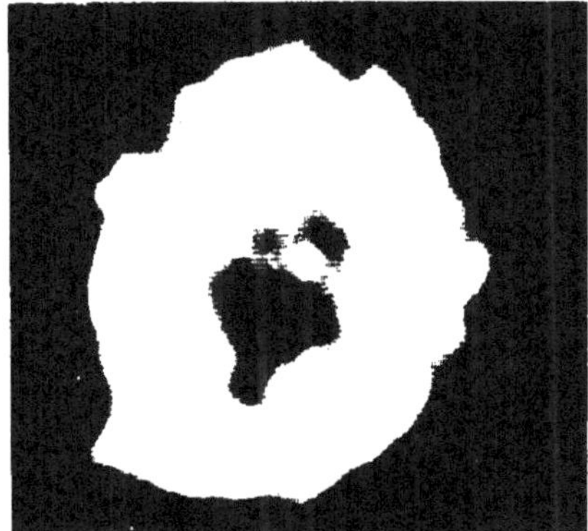

Figure 32. Interpolated background corrected image for [^{123}I]BMIPP.

fatty acid analogues. The theoretically required steps for degradation are more complex for BMIPP than for IPP (see Figure 7). Pathways for oxidative degradation of branched chain fatty acids may resemble those of branched chain amino acids, e.g. leucine. Thus an ATP dependent carboxylation may occur which is catalyzed by a biotin containing enzyme. When this mechanism is applied to BMIPP finally ^{123}I-benzoic acid will be generated as a result of

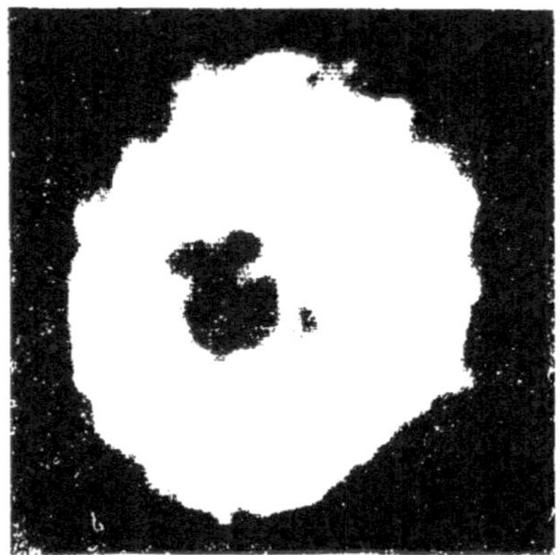

Figure 33. Interpolated background corrected image for [^{123}I]IPP.

β-oxidation. Other possibilities of BMIPP degradation may include α-oxidation, propionyl-CoA cleavage followed by β-oxidation, giving finally ^{123}I-phenylacetic acid, as described earlier (Figure 7). Possibly this complexity may be in favor for BMIPP compared to other radioiodinated fatty acid analogues, making BMIPP more susceptible for recognizing patients with heart disease. In addition, the longer myocardial retention of BMIPP may facilitate SPECT studies. However, the 3,3-dimethyl analogue appears more promising in this regard as may be assumed from animal experiments.

Acknowledgements

Research at the Oak Ridge National Laboratory was sponsored by the Office of Health and Environmental Research, U.S. Department of Energy, under contract DE-AC05840R21400 with Martin Marietta Energy Systems, Inc. Research at the Brookhaven National Laboratory was conducted in the Medical Department supported under U.S. Department of Energy Contract No. DE-AC02-7600016.

References

1. Feinendegen L F, Vyska K, Freunlieb C *et al.* (1981) Noninvasive analysis of metabolic reactions in body tissues, the case of myocardial fatty acids. Eur J Nucl Med 6: 191 - 200
2. Machulla H-J, Stoecklin G, Kupfernagel C *et al.* (1978) Comparative evaluation of fatty acids labeled with C-11, Cl-34m, Br-77, and I-123 for metabolic studies of the myocardium: Concise communication. J Nucl Med 19: 298 - 302
3. Freundlieb C, Hock A, Vyska K *et al.* (1980) Myocardial imaging and metabolic studies with 17-(^{123}I)iodoheptadecanoic acid. J Nucl Med 21: 1043 - 1050

4. van der Wall E E, Heidendal G A K, den Hollander W *et al.* (1981) Metabolic myocardial imaging with ^{123}I-labeled heptadecanoic acid in patients with angina pectoris. Eur J Nucl Med 6: 391 - 396
5. van der Wall E E, den Hollander W, Heidendal G A K *et al.* (1981) Dynamic myocardial scintigraphy with ^{123}I-labeled free fatty acids in patients with myocardial infarction. Eur J Nucl Med 6: 383 - 389
5. Dudczak R, Kletter K, Frischauf H, Schmolinger R, Derfler K, Losert U.(1982) Myocardial turnover rates of I-123-heptade canoic acid (HDA) and (pIPPA). Rad Isot Klin und Forschung 15: 685 - 696
7. Machulla H-J, Marsmann M, Dutschka K (1980) Biochemical concept and synthesis of a radioiodinated phenyl fatty acid for in vivo metabolic studies of the myocardium. Eur J Nucl Med 5: 171 - 173
8. Reske S N, Machulla H-J, Winkler C (1982) Metabolism of 15-p-(I-123)-phenyl)pentadecanoic acid (IP) in hearts of rats. J Nucl Med 23: P10
9. Reske S N, Simon H, Machulla H-J, Biersak H J *et al.* (1982) Myocardial turnover of p-(I-123-phenyl)-pentadecanoic acid (IP) in patients with CAD. J Nucl Med 23: P34
10. Dudczak R, Hofer R (1983) Myocardial scintigraphy with ^{123}I-labeled fatty acids. Summary of round table discussion. J Radioanalyt Chem 79: 329 - 336
11. Dudczak R, Schmoliner R, Kletter K *et al.* (1983) Clinical evaluation of ^{123}I-labeled p-phenylpentadecanoic acid (p-IPPA) for myocardial scintigraphy. J Nucl Med All Sci 27: 267 - 279
12. Dudczak R (1983) Myokardszintigraphie mit jod-123-markierten Fettsauren. Wien Klin Wochenschr 95: 4 - 35
13. Dudczak R, Kletter K, Frischauf H *et al.* (1984) The use of ^{123}I-labeled heptadecanoic acid (HDA) as metabolic tracer: Preliminary report. Eur J Nucl Med 9: 81 - 85
14. Höck A, Freundlieb C, Vyska K *et al.* (1983) Myocardial imaging and metabolic studies with [17-(^{123}I)]iodoheptadecanoic acid in patients with idiopathic congestive cardiomyopathy. J Nucl Med 24: 22 - 28
15. Bing R J, Sigel A, Unger J *et al.* (1954) Metabolism of the human heart. Am J Med 16: 504 - 515
16. Ballard F B, Danforth W H, Naegel S *et al.* (1960) Myocardial metabolism of fatty acids. J Clin Invest 39: 717 - 723
17. Evans J R, Gunton R W, Baker R G *et al.* (1965) Use of radioiodinated fatty acid for photoscans of the heart. Circ Res 16: 1 - 10
18. Gunton R W, Evans J R, Baker R G *et al.* (1965) Demonstration of myocardial infarction by photoscans of the heart in man. Am J Cardiol 16: 482 - 487
19. Poe N D (1977) Rationale and radiopharmaceuticals for myocardial imaging. Semin Nucl Med 7: 7 - 14
20. Poe N D, Robinson G D, Zielinski F W *et al.* (1977) Myocardial imaging with I-123-hexadecenoic acid. Radiology 124: 419 - 424
21. Poe N D, Eber L M, Normann A S *et al.* (1977) Myocardial images in nonacute coronary and noncoronary heart diseases. J Nucl Med 18: 18 - 23
22. Robinson G D (1977) Synthesis of 123-I-16-iodo-9-hexadecenoic acid and derivatives for use as myocardial perfusion imaging agents. Int J Appl Rad Isot 28: 149 - 156
23. Weiss E S, Hoffman E J, Phelps M E *et al.* (1976) External detection and visualization of myocardial ischemia with ^{11}C-substrates in vivo and in vitro. Circ Res 39: 24 - 32
24. Schön H R, Schelbert H R, Robinson G *et al.* (1982) C-11 labeled palmitic acid for non-invasive evaluation of regional myocardial fatty acid metabolism with positron-computed tomography. Am Heart J 103: 532 - 547
25. Robinson C D, Lee A W (1975) Radioiodinated fatty acids for heart imaging: Iodine monochloride addition compared with iodine replacement labeling. J Nucl Med 16: 17 - 21
26. Okada R D, Elmaleh D E, Werre G S *et al.* (1983) Myocardial kinetics of I-123-labeled 16-hexadecanoic acid. Eur J Nucl Med 8: 211 - 217

27. Elmaleh D R, Knapp F F Jr, Yasuda T *et al.* (1981) Myocardial imaging with 9-[Te-123]m-telluraheptadecanoic acid. J Nucl Med 22: 994 - 999
28. Knapp F F Jr, Ambrose K R, Callahan A P *et al.* (1979) Tellurium-123m-labeled isosteres of palmitoleic and oleic acids show high myocardial uptake, Radiopharmaceuticals, Vol II. New York: Society of Nuclear Medicine
29. Knapp F F Jr, Ambrose K R, Callahan A P *et al.* (1981) Effects of chain length and tellurium position on the myocardial uptake of Te-123m fatty acids. J Nucl Med 22: 988 - 993
30. Knapp F F Jr, Goodman M M, Callahan A P *et al.* (1983) New myocardial imaging agents: stabilization of radioiodine as a terminal vinyl iodide moiety as tellurium fatty acids. J Med Chem 26: 1293 - 1300
31. Knapp F F Jr, Goodman M M. The design and biological properties of iodine-123-labeled β-methyl-branched fatty acids. Eur Heart (1985) 6 (Suppl B): 71 - 83
32. Goodman M M, Knapp F F Jr, Callahan A P *et al.* (1982) Synthesis and biological evaluation of 17-(^{131}I)iodo-9-telluraheptadecanoic acid, a potential myocardial imaging agent. J Med Chem 25: 613 - 618
33. Okada R D, Knapp F F Jr, Elmaleh D R *et al.* (1982) Tellurium-123m-labeled-9-tellurahep-tadecanoic acid: a possible cardiac imaging agent. Circulation 65: 305 - 310
34. Bianco J A, Pape L A, Alpert J S, Zheng M, Hnatowich D, Goodman M M, Knapp F F Jr (1984) Accumulation of radioiodinated 15-(p-iodophenyl)-6-tellurapentadecanoic acid in ischemic myocardium during acute coronary occlusion and reperfusion. J Am Coll Cardiol 4: 80 - 87
35. Yonekura Y, Tamaki N, Torizuka K *et al.* (1983) Quantitative autoradiographic measurement of regional myocardial substrate uptake in hypertensive rats. J Nucl Med (Abstr) 24: P24
36. Yonekura Y, Brill A B, Som P, Yamamoto K, Srivastava S C, Iwai J, Elmaleh D R, Livni E, Strauss H W, Goodman M M, Knapp F F Jr (1985) Regional myocardial substrate uptake in hypertensive rats: a quantitative autoradiographic measurement. Science 227: 1494 - 1496
37. Yamamato K, Som P, Brill A B (1984) Comparative dual tracer studies of β-methyl-(l-C-14)-heptadecanoic acid and 15-p-(I-131)iodophenyl-β-mehtylpentadecanoic acid (BMPDA) in hypertensive rats. J Nucl Med (Abstr) 25: P31
38. Goodman M M, Kirsch G, Knapp F F Jr (1982) Synthesis of radioiodinated ω-p-(iodo-phenyl)-substituted methyl-branched long-chain fatty acids. J Labeled Compd Radiopharm 19: 1316 - 1318
39. Goodman M M, Knapp F F Jr, Callahan A P, Ferren L A (1982) A new, well-retained myocardial imaging agent: radioiodinated 15-(p-iodophenyl)-6-tellurapentadecanoic acid. J Nucl Med 23: 904 - 908
40. Goodman M M, Kirsch G, Knapp F F Jr (1984) Synthesis and evaluation of radioiodinated terminal p-iodophenyl-substituted α- and β-methyl-branched fatty acids. J Med Chem 27: 390 - 397
41. Goodman M M, Knapp F F Jr, Elmaleh D R, Strauss H W (1984) New myocardial imaging agents: synthesis of 15-(p-iodophenyl)-3-(R,S)-methylpentadecanoic acid by decomposition of a 3,3-(1,5-pentanediyl)triazene precursor. J Org Chem 49: 2322 - 2325
42. Elmaleh D R, Livni E, Levy S *et al.* (1982) Radioiodinated beta methyl omega-phenyltetrade-canoic acid (BMTPA): a potential new agent for studies of myocardial fatty acid (FA) metabolism. J Nucl Med (Abstr) 23: P103-P104
43. Livni E, Elmaleh D R, Levy S *et al.* (1982) Beta-methyl (1-^{11}C)heptadecanoic acid: a new myocardial metabolic tracer for positron emission tomography. J Nucl Med 23: 169 - 175
44. Livni E, Elmaleh D R, Schluederberg J *et al.* (1982) A potential new agent for studies of myocardial fatty acid metabolism: ^{131}I-ω-iodophenyl-β-mehtyltetradecanoic acid. In: Nuclear Medicine and Biology Advances, Vol 2. New York: Pergamon, pp 1684 - 1686
45. Chien K R, Han A, White J, Kulkarni P (1983) In vivo esterification of a synthetic ^{125}I-labeled fatty acid into cardiac glycolipids. Am J Physiol 254 (Heart Circ Physiol) H693-H697

46. Knapp F F Jr, Srivastava P C, Callahan A P *et al.* (1984) Effect of tellurium position on the myocardial uptake of radioiodinated 18-iodotellura-17-octadecanoic acid analogues. J Med Chem 27: 57 - 63
47. Bergstrom S, Borgstrom B, Tryding N (1954) Intestinal absorption and metabolism of 2:2-dimethylstearic acid in the rat. Biochem J 58: 604 - 608
48. Tryding N (1957) Intestinal absorption and metabolism of 2,2-dimethylstearic acids in man. Ark Kemi 11: 307 - 312
49. Tryding N, Westoo G (1957) On the metabolism of 2,2-dimethyl-nonodecanoic acid in man. Ark Kemi 11: 313 - 316
50. Goodman D S, Steinberg D (1958) Studies of the metabolism of 3,3-dimethylphenyl-myristic acid, a nonoxidizable fatty acid analogue. J Biol Chem 233: 1066 - 1071
51. Otto C A, Brown L E, Wieland D M (1981) Structure-distribution study of I-123-ω-iodo fatty acids. J Labeled Cpd Radiopharm 18: 43 - 44
52. Otto C A, Brown L E, Wieland D M *et al.* (1981) Radioiodinated fatty acids for myocardial imaging: effects of chain length. J Nucl Med 22: 613 - 618
53. Okada R D, Elmaleh D R, Weisse G S *et al.* (1983) Myocardial kinetics of ^{123}I-labeled-16-hexadecanoic acid. Eur J Nucl Med 8: 211 - 217
54. Kloster G, Stocklin G (1982) Determination of the rate determining step in halofatty acid turnover in the heart. In: Radioaktive Isotope in Klinik und Forschung Band 15, Verlag H Egermann, Wien pp 235 - 241
55. Kloster G, Stocklin G, Smith E F *et al.* (1984) ω-halofatty acids: a probe for mitochondrial membrane integrity — in vitro investigations in normal and ischemic myocardium. Eur J Nucl Med 9: 305 - 311
56. Visser F C, Westera G, van Eenige M J *et al.* (1985) The myocardial elimination rate of radioiodinated heptadecanoic acid. Eur J Nucl Med 10: 118 - 122
57. Murad S, Kishimoto Y (1975) α-Hydroxylation of lignoceric acid to cerebronic acid during brain development. J Biol Chem 250(15): 5841 - 5846
58. Hajra A K, Radin N S (1963) In vivo conversion of labeled fatty acids to sphingolipid fatty acids in rat brain. J Lipid Res 4: 448 - 453
59. Steinberg D, Herndon J H, Unlendorf B W, Mize C E, Avigan J, Milne G W A (1967) Refsum's disease: Nature of the enzyme defect. Science 156: 1740 - 1742
60. Steinberg D, Mize C E, Avigan J (1967) Studies on the metabolic error in Refsum's disease. J Clin Invest 46: 313 - 322
61. Steinberg D, Vroom F Q, Engel W K, Cammermeyer J, Mize C E, Avigan J (1967) Refsum's disease: A recently characterized lipidosis involving the central nervous systems. Ann Intern Med 66: 393 - 395
62. Steinberg D (1972) Phytanic acid storage disease: Refsum's disease In: Stanbury J B, Wyngaarden J B, Fredrickson D S (eds) The metabolic basis of inherited disease. New York: McGraw-Hill, pp 833 - 853
63. Folch J, Lees M, Stanley G H S (1957) A simple method for the isolation and purification of total lipids from animal tissues. J Biol Chem 226: 497 - 509
64. Reske S N, Sauer W, Machulla H-J *et al.* (1984) 15-(p-(^{123}I)iodophenylpentadecanoic acid as a tracer lipid metabolism-comparison with (1-^{14}C)palmitic acid in murine tissues. J Nucl Med 25: 1335 - 1342
65. Braunwald E, Ross J, Sonnenblick E H (1976) Mechanisms of contraction of the normal and failing heart. Boston: Little Brown and Company
66. Groette G J, Strauss H W *et al.* (1979) The influence of left ventricular volume and wall motion on myocardial images. Circulation 59: 1172 - 1177
67. Fowler J S, MacGregor R R, Wolf A P *et al.* (1981) A shielder synthesis system for production of 2-deoxy-2[^{18}F]fluoro-D-glucose. J Nucl Med 22: 276 - 380
68. Poe N D, Robinson G D, Graham L S *et al.* (1976) Experimental basis for myocardial imaging with ^{123}I labeled hexadecanoic acid. J Nucl Med 17: 1077 - 1082

10. Progress in cardiac positron emission tomography with emphasis on carbon-11 labeled palmitate and oxygen-15 labeled water

K.A.A. FOX, R.M. KNABB, S.R. BERGMANN and B.E. SOBEL

Introduction

Although specific biochemical abnormalities undoubtedly underlie many cardiac disorders, most noninvasive diagnostic modalities delineate anatomic and functional manifestations of such disorder rather than their underlying mechanisms. Thus, echocardiography, radionuclide ventriculography, scintigraphy, angiography, X-ray computer assisted tomography, and magnetic resonance proton imaging (MRI) define altered cardiac and coronary arterial anatomy, structure, and function in disease states but not their underlying biochemical derangements. The diversity of myocardial histopathological responses to injury is limited. In consequence, anatomic or functional descriptions do not necessarily reflect the diversity of the underlying processes. Cardiac positron emission tomography (PET) is being developed in part to assess the biochemical processes which underlie such disorders.

Positron emission tomography permits quantitative characterization of the disposition of labeled substrates and tracers employed for delineation of intermediary metabolism and myocardial perfusion. Interpretations are dependent upon the accuracy of quantitative recovery of counts attributable to the tracer and appropriate selection of tracer kinetic models employed to characterize perfusion and metabolism. This discussion reviews the extent to which objectives of PET have been attained with respect to myocardial metabolism. In view of the intimate relationships between substrate utilization and myocardial perfusion, assessment of both will be discussed with respect to experimental and clinical tomographic applications. Our review will focus on the assessment of ischemic and reperfused myocardium with ^{11}C-labeled fatty acids and with ^{15}O-labeled water. Complexities encountered in the quantification of specific components of myocardial metabolism based upon external determinations of clearance of the radiotracers are substantial. Although progress has been made with respect to instrumentation, count recovery, and rapidity of data acquisition, the resolution of events with both high temporal flux and with respect to respiratory and cardiac motion is difficult. Nevertheless, considerable amounts of information with practical clinical value can be obtained from cardiac tomography with tracers of myocardial metabolism and perfusion.

Clinical rationale

The need for external determination of the impact of interventions on myocardium is expecially apparent in the assessment of the extent of myocardial infarction and its limitation. Examples include evaluation of the impact of pharmacologic and thrombolytic interventions on the ischemic myocardium. Positron emission tomographic studies with labeled fatty acids permit quantification of myocardium at risk for necrosis [1-4] and the volume of myocardium subjected to hypoperfusion [5-12]. An approach combining both improves sensitivity by using the patient as his own control. Such an approach should help to define the efficacy of potentially beneficial therapeutic regimens prior to implementation of large scale, randomized, and unfortunately expensive clinical trials. Thus, tomography studies of clinically defined subgroups may provide a cost-effective basis for selection and design of large, multicenter studies with conventional clinical endpoints.

The capabilities of PET provide an excellent opportunity for the study of integrated metabolism *in vivo*. Sequential analyses of tissue *in vitro* provide information relating to specific metabolic interactions at a given time. Analyses *in vitro* are often restricted to studies in experimental animals. They require disruption of the tissue and dissociation of ultrastructural interrelationships influencing numerous enzyme systems. In contrast, PET delineates net effects of myocardial processing of labeled substrates or tracers rather than individual biochemical reactions. However, with substrate analogs or inhibitors of specific pathway insight can be gained regarding individual components of myocardial metabolism *in vivo*. Within constraints required by radiation dosage limits, tomographic studies permit repeated examinations of the same individual throughout the time course of a disease process.

Positron tomography facilitates assessment not only of persistent abnormalities of perfusion and metabolism but also of stress induced augmentation of coronary flow or cardiac work. Subcritical coronary stenoses do not alter flow under resting conditions, but myocardium in their region of supply may manifest signs of ischemia as a result of increased oxygen demand. The physiological impact of such stenoses has been assessed tomographically with dipyridamole-induced hyperemia [13-15]. Detection and sequential assessment of occult coronary disease has been accomplished [11]. Tomographic characterization of metabolism and perfusion associated with cardiomyopathies has already proven diagnostically useful [16-18] with inhomogeneities of substrate utilization not evident by anatomic imaging or analysis of biopsies.

Recent identification and differentiation of myocardial ischemia and infarction from normal tissue have been accomplished with ^{18}F-2-fluoro-deoxyglucose and ^{13}N-ammonia. The observations made suggest that ischemic but still viable myocardium can be differentiated from myocardium undergoing infarction [4].

Historical perspective

Although Dirac (1930) postulated the existence of positively charged electrons, i.e. positrons [19], and their existence was confirmed in the 1930s, potential biological applications involving these subatomic particles did not become apparent until the 1950s. In 1953 Brownell and Sweet recognized that the locus of a positron-emitting radionuclide within tissue could be defined precisely and accurately because of the nature of the radiation emitted [20]. Such radiation (annihilation radiation) occurs when an emitted positron interacts with an electron to yield two photons emitted at an angle of almost 180°.

As a result of pioneering studies of Brownell and Sweet and the development of a prototype imaging device employing coincidence circuitry in the Brookhaven National Laboratory in 1962 [21], positron tomography developed rapidly in conjunction with an increased availability of cyclotrons used to produce the short half-life, positron emitting radionuclides. Advances in computer technology and instrumentation soon permitted rapid and accurate quantification of the distribution of positron emitting radionuclides within tissue. However, despite considerable progress in the noninvasive determination of distributions of tracer in organs of interest, much remains to be learned with respect to interpretation of the complex biological behavior of the tracers and the factors influencing quantitative delineation of the distribution of radioactivity within the beating heart *in vivo*.

Characteristics of positron emission tomographic instrumentation

Positron emission tomographic systems can be regarded as devices designed for noninvasive tissue autoradiography (Figure 1). The simplest forms consist of pairs of scintillation detectors that scan an object of interest from a large number of angles of view. The detection of radiation photons with coincident circuits occurs only when both detectors in a pair sense annihilation photons within a predetermined time window [22,23].

Recent advances in plastic scintillation crystals and photomultipliers as well as improvements in coincidence detection circuitry have made it feasible to measure, with considerable accuracy, the time difference between the arrival of each of the two photons at the opposing detectors [24-27]. Tomography incorporating time-of-flight correction takes account of the very small differences in arrival time of the two annihilation photons in each pair. Because the photons propagate at the speed of light, a 7.5 cm spatial resolution requires measurement of a 500 picosecond time differential. The capability to resolve

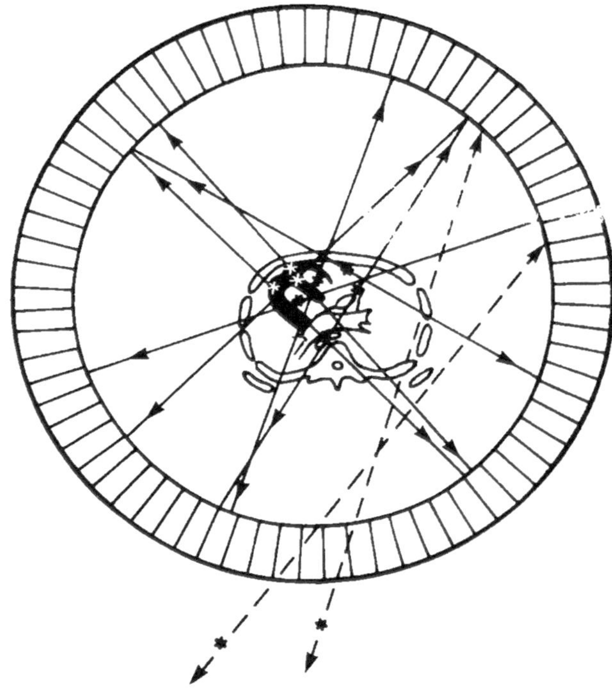

Figure 1. Schematic depicition of a ring of detectors from a positron emission tomography, including a cross section of the thorax and heart in the plane of the mitral valve apparatus. Positrons are emitted from radiotracer within the heart, the blood pool and extracardiac structures. Annihilation of positrons results in emission of a pair of 511 keV photons at an angulation of 180°. Events which occur within the field of view activate a pair of opposing detectors if they arrive within a narrowly defined time interval (i.e. 500 picoseconds), thus providing electronic collimation by localizing the event along the line between that detector pair (solid lines). Extraneous activity is rejected because only a single detector is activated within the coincidence resolving time (broken lines). In practice, tomographs may be composed of multiple rings of adjacent detectors allowing visualization of a larger region axially and permitting reconstruction of images into transverse, sagittal, or coronal planes.

such time intervals has been acquired only recently for complete systems [25,27].

A typical tomographic instrument consists of series of rings of detectors arranged in a circular or other arrays coupled with the electronic circuitry necessary for a recording and timing acquisition of the data. Annihilation events that occur outside the defined volume interrogated by each pair of detectors are not recorded (Figure 1). The spatial resolution that can be achieved depends in part upon the aperture of the detectors [28]. It is limited by the distance traveled by positrons in tissue (1 to 6 mm) (path length) prior to annihilation. Furthermore, annihilation photons are not emitted at exactly 180° from each other [29]. To maximize information, each detector is operated in coincidence with multiple opposing detectors thus providing numerous coincidence lines through an imaged object. Cross coincidences between arrays are often used to increase the number of reconstructed planes. The detector array may be rotated around the imaged object to increase the number of coincident lines acquired because the fidelity of a reconstruction to the actual distribution of positron-emitting radionuclides within an imaged object depends upon the number of projections obtained [25,30-32]. Coincident data are stored and processed in a digital computer system with correction for attenuation and physical decay of radioactivity as a function of time. The appreciable attenuation that occurs despite the relatively high energy of annihilation photons can be compensated by employing attenuation scanning by means of an external source of positrons [32].

Significant progress has been made with regard to the implementation of reconstruction algorithms for tomographically derived information [33,34]. Calibration of the instrumentation is generally achieved by imaging appropriately designed phantoms containing known amounts of radioactivity [35].

With current instrumentation, spatial resolution is in the order of 8 mm. For cardiac imaging, tomographic quantification of the distribution of tracers is limited by several physical considerations including the influence of cardiac and respiratory motion, spillover of radioactivity, and partial volume effects [36-40]. Because of cardiac and respiratory motion, integrated data acquisition results in apparent dispersion of loci of radioactivity commensurate with the movement of the object. Cardiac gating and breath-holding or respiratory synchronization of tomography can be employed, but such approaches decrease the amount of information that can be obtained during a given scan interval.

Spillover of radioactivity from adjacent regions of tissue requires correction. This is particularly important when blood pool activity is high or when descrete segments of an organ of interest contain low activity in comparison with adjacent segments. The influence of blood pool activity and spillover can be compensated by methods employing blood pool subtraction [9,40].

Partial volume effects may have a significant influence on image reconstruction [36,38,40-42]. When the dimensions of an imaged object are less than at least twice the absolute spatial resolution of the instrument, count recovery decreases as a function of the dimensions of the imaged object [36]. Thus, for a full width half-maximum resolution of 8 mm (the minimum distance required to resolve two adjacent lines with half-maximal efficiency) an object size greater than 16 mm is required to avoid the need for correction for partial volume effects. Accordingly, imaging of the left ventricular wall in man requires corrections for wall thickness. Average wall thickness measurements may suffice for some applications. More exact determination with CT, echocardiography, or MRI is possible. Both CT and MRI can define cardiac anatomy per se with spatial resolution far superior to that obtainable by positron tomography.

In contrast to positron emission tomography, single photon emission computed systems (SPECT) are limited by the variable attenuation of the energy associated with the emitted photons as a function of the distance between the emitting source and the detector. In addition, with single photon imaging devices spatial resolution is a function of the depth of the emitter within the tissue in relation to the locus of the detector [30,31]. In contrast, a fundamental property of positron emission tomographic devices permits the detection of the source of the radiotracer by means of electronic columnation. Coincidence mode detection results in constant spatial resolution regardless of the locus of the emitting radiation with respect to the detectors [30].

Characteristics of tracers employed for cardiac positron emission tomography

Positrons have a mass comparable to that of electrons but a positive charge ($\beta+$). They are products of the decay of radioisotopes such as carbon-11, oxygen-15, nitrogen-13, or fluorine-18. The process of decay leads to release of a positron-neutrino pair. When the kinetic energy of the positron declines substantially, as a result of interactions with matter, the particle interacts with an electron resulting in the annihilation of both and the conversion of their mass into two photons of energy. The two gamma photons leave the site of interaction in opposite directions. Each has an energy of 511 keV. Positron emission can therefore be detected by pairs of crystal scintillation detectors 180° apart, with a field of view between them providing electronic columnation. In contrast, the neutrino is undetected. If a point source of positron-emitting material is moved within the field of view between any two such detectors, the court rate remains virtually unchanged because the algebraic sum of the combined attenuation of the two photons sensed by each detector remains constant. If the path lengths of a pair of photons are a and b, attenuation is determined by $e^{-\mu(a+b)}$ and thus depends on the total length of the absorber (a+b) and μ, the linear attenuation coefficient for 511 keV photons characteristic of each material.

The short radioactive half-life of many of the positron-emitting radionuclides permits sequential evaluations and avoids high radiation burdens for patients. Rubidium-82 (^{82}Rb) ($t_{1/2}$=78 s), oxygen-15 (^{15}O) ($t_{1/2}$=2.1 min), nitrogen-13 (^{13}N) ($t_{1/2}$=10 min), carbon-11 (^{11}C) ($t_{1/2}$=20.4 min), and fluorine-18 (^{18}F) ($t_{1/2}$=110 min) exhibit chemical and physical properties that make them particularly attractive for use in positron tomography. The radionuclides ^{11}C, ^{15}O, ^{13}N are chemically indistinguishable from their nonradioactive counterparts in physiological substrates used by the heart and can be incorporated into substrates that participate in a physiologically representative fashion in metabolic processes. Their short radioactive half-lives permit sequential evaluations of both perfusion and metabolism in the same subject. They are particularly useful for serial studies required for evaluation of transient phenomena. However, many tracers with short physical half-lives require a cyclotron on-site for production.

Generator-produced radionuclides including gallium-68 ($t_{1/2}$=68 min) and rubidium-82 ($t_{1/2}$=78 s) have been used for estimation of myocardial blood flow. Such radionuclides may be coupled in lipid or albumin complexes [5,9,43] or used in isolation [10,11,44-46]. Their use provides potential advantages with respect to cost and convenience but their suitability for differentiation of abnormalities of perfusion and metabolism has been questioned [7,45,46].

Assessment of myocardial perfusion with positron emission tomography

Accurate quantification of regional myocardial perfusion by means of positron tomography requires not only that the spatial distribution of tracer be measured accurately but also that the biological behavior of the tracer fulfills the assumptions inherent in the mathematical models upon which interpretations are based. Limitations on the quantitative measurement of regional myocardial blood flow are imposed by constraints affecting accurate count recovery and constraints relating to application of the models and the biological behavior of the tracer.

Tracers for assessment of perfusion can be categorized into three groups, each of which is governed by a different set of tracer kinetic assumptions. The extent to which the assumptions concerning the behavior of a tracer satisfy the mathematical modeling requirements varies within and between classes.

One class is epitomized by radiolabeled microspheres. Assumptions underlying their use are that microspheres in arterial blood give rise to an organ distribution of uniformly mixed labeled particles in accordance with blood flow to each organ because of trapping of the spheres in arteriolar or capillary beds [47]. The microsphere approach provides a reference standard when invasive tissue analysis is possible in experimental studies. In practice, 9 to 15 micron spheres are trapped almost completely in a single vascular transit. Their distribution in most tissues is an accurate reflection of regional perfusion. Although direct analysis of the distribution of tracer in samples of tissue is utilized in experimental animals, it is not applicable to patients. However, PET permits an "autoradiographic" measurement potentially applicable *in vivo*. The feasibility of tomographic assessment of perfusion with the use of positron emitting microspheres has been well documented [6,48].

Gallium-68 has been used to label macroaggregates of albumin somewhat analogous to microspheres for quantification of regional myocardial blood flow in experimental animals (Figure 2). Tomographic measurement of flow corresponds closely with results obtained by quantification of conventional gamma emitting microspheres in samples of tissue assayed *in vitro*. Recently, carbon-11 has been covalently bound to albumin microspheres and used to measure regional myocardial blood flow tomographically in animals and in

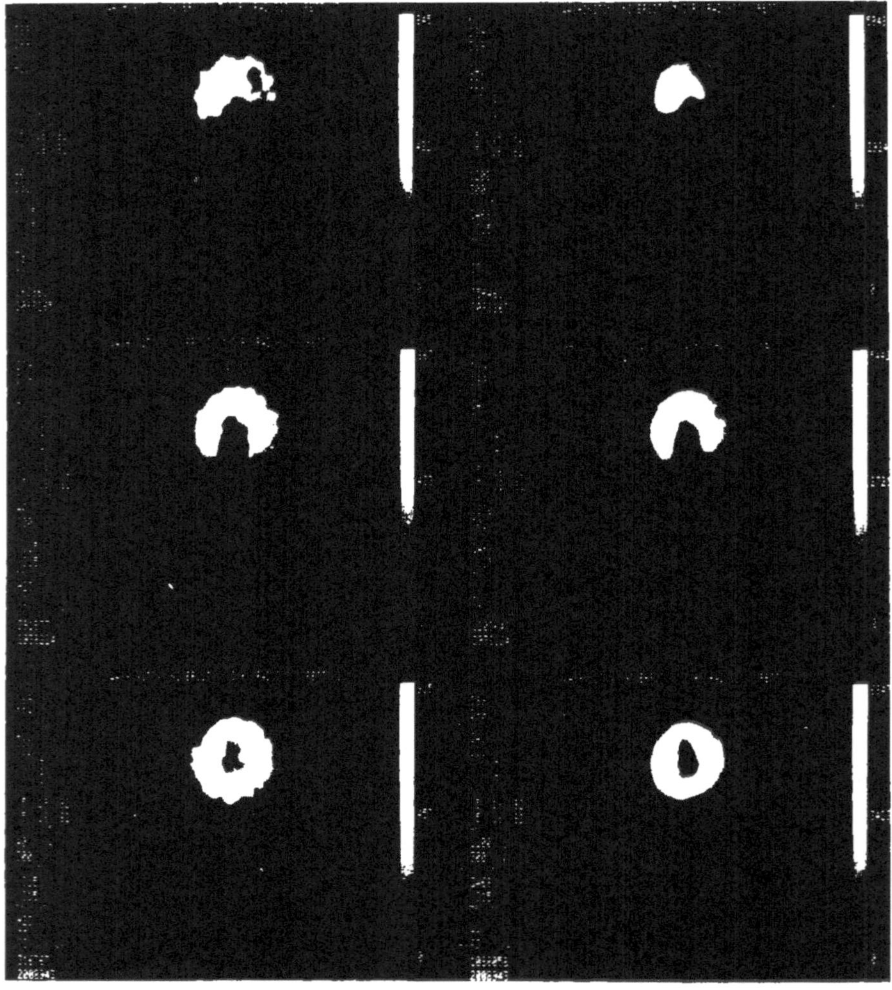

Figure 2. Tomograms from three adjacent planes through the ventricle of a normal dog. $H_2{}^{15}O$ distribution, corrected for vascular tracer with $C^{15}O$ as described in the text, is depicted on the left, and ^{68}Gallium-microsphere distribution on the right. In each image, anterior myocardium is to the top, lateral wall to the left, and intraventricular septum to the right (i.e. as viewed from above). The much thinner right ventricle is not clearly defined (upper panels), and activity does not accumulate in the mitral valve region which is located posteriorly in the middle pair of images.

man [6,49]. The limitations of this approach include the need for administration of tracer via left atrium or left ventricle and the potential hazards of administration of particulate material into the coronary circulation supplying myocardium in which perfusion may be compromised already. Nevertheless, adverse effects of such administration have not been evident clinically. Additional potential constraints relate to alterations in the distribution of microspheres with ischemia [50] or when microvascular damage is present as may pertain with ischemia followed by reperfusion.

A second approach for the measurement of myocardial blood flow and one that has been applied extensively in clinical studies is the fractional distribution method originally proposed by Sapirstein. It is based on the assumption that an intravenously administered radiopharmaceutical, usually a monovalent cation, is taken up and released by cells throughout the organism in a consistent fashion with extraction independent of regional flow or metabolic status of the tissue [50,51]. The spatial distribution and regional accumulation in tissue of the cation after intravenous injection is a function of blood flow. Most radiopharmaceuticals employed for determinations based on this type of analysis are potassium analogs. Thallium-201 (^{201}Tl) is the most common radioisotope for assessment of myocardial perfusion scintigraphically. Positron-emitting potassium analogs used for tomographic assessment of perfusion include isotopes of rubidium and potassium (^{82}Rb, ^{81}Rb, and ^{43}K) and nitrogen-13-labeled ammonia (employed in the form of $^{13}NH_4^+$).

Application of the fractional distribution method is relatively straightforward and requires only intravenous injection of tracer. However, the tracers used exhibit serious limitations for quantitative estimates of myocardial blood flow. Unfortunately, the biological behavior of the single photon and positron-emitting tracers used do not fulfill the assumptions entailed in use of the method [50-52]. The first pass extraction is not consistent with respect to flow but rather inversely related to flow because transmembrane cellular transport of the cations is a function of residence time of the tracer in the capillary bed [44,53,54]. For most of the tracers used, myocardial sequestration varies as a function of flow and as a function of the metabolic status of the myocardium [46,55,56]. Methods have been proposed for use of ^{82}Rb with the tissue content of rubidium corrected for the variation of extraction fraction on a regional basis. However, accurate assessment of regional or pixel by pixel extraction fraction for a tracer with very rapid vascular transit presents substantial problems.

Limitations related to variable myocardial extraction of ^{13}N labeled ammonia have been characterized extensively. Although perfusion has been evaluated with positron emitting radiotracers such as ^{82}Rb and $^{13}NH_3^+$, accurate quantification of regional perfusion with these moieties has been elusive. Nevertheless, valuable clinical information has been obtained including determination of extraction of labeled metabolic substrates with reference to estimates of perfusion. In addition, alterations of perfusion and regional metabolism in response to pharmacological vasodilator stress may be used to assess severity of coronary artery disease [13,14,57]. The relationship between abnormalities of extraction of ^{13}N ammonia and changes in accumulation of deoxyglucose may provide descriptors of viable but transiently ischemic myocardium [4].

A third means for measurement of myocardial blood flow employs diffusible tracers. It is based upon an approach developed by Kety and Schmidt [58-61] described first in 1955 and applied initially to measurement of cerebral blood flow. The mathematical model employed describes the exchange of an inert diffusible tracer across the capillary tissue interface and between vascular and tissue compartments. It represents an extension of the Fick principle. Myocardial blood flow can be calculated from analysis of the clearance of radioactivity from the heart with a corollary of the Kety-Schmidt model.

$$Q = K\lambda W/D$$

where Q = myocardial blood flow (ml/100 g/min)
K = myocardial tracer disappearance rate constant
λ = tracer tissue: blood partition coeffient
W = weight of the myocardium
D = specific gravity of myocardium

However, most presently available positron tomographic systems are not able to acquire data sufficiently rapidly (i.e. every 1-2 seconds) to fulfill the counting statistic requirements for practical use of this method for cardiac tomography.

Because of these limitations, alternative methods for estimating myocardial blood flow have been developed for use with diffusible tracers employing equilibrium imaging [62-64]. Although equilibrium approaches have advangeges with respect to steady-state imaging systems and require only relatively slow speed instruments, disadvantages include distortion attributable to high vascular pool radioactivity and potentially high radiation burdens for patients. Estimates of flow with such methods are sensitive to measurement errors affecting assay of arterial tracer activity and assay of the concentration of tracer in regions of interest. At equilibrium, differences between the activity in the two compartments are small. Large changes in flow may be reflected by only modest changes in the concentration of the tracer within the myocardium.

In studies from our laboratory, a constant infusion technique was modified by employing exponentially increasing infusions of ^{11}C-butanol or $H_2{}^{15}O$ to decrease the time required for attainment of an approximation of equilibrium and estimation of flow. The method provides determinations of flow which are relatively insensitive to measurement errors. It has been used successfully in isolated perfused hearts and in intact dogs [65,66]. However, for studies *in vivo*, the high concentrations of circulating tracer in the left ventricular cavity result in substantial spillover of radioactivity in blood to pixels corresponding to myocardium, and the radiation burden is appreciable.

The development of tomographic instrumentation with the capability of acquiring data within short intervals (i.e. 10 s intervals), permitted application of a modification of a method of estimating flow based originally on the method of Freygang and Sokoloff [67]. In the original applications tracers were infused intravenously at a constant rate. Simultaneous arterial sampling was used to define the input function of radioactivity. Autoradiography of the brain was performed after completion of studies in experimental animals. In keeping with principles underlying autoradiography, regional myocardial blood flow could be calculated from the following equation [67]:

$$C(T) = \lambda k \int_{o}^{t} Ca(t)e^{-kt}dt$$

where: $C(T)$ = the concentration of tracer in tissue
λ = tissue/blood partition coefficient
k = mF/λ, where $m = 1\text{-}e^{(-PS/F)}$
F = flow
PS = permeability-surface area product
Ca = the concentration of tracer in arterial blood as a function of time, t
t = time after injection

Positron emission tomography permits the use of a modification of this approach, (an "autoradiographic" method) *in vivo*. However, tomographic instrumentation can not provide instantaneous temporal resolution. Thus tomograms acquired represent integral values for radioactivity over 20 or 40 seconds intervals. Judging from results of computer simulations, integration of the operational equation does not invalidate the use of this technique for determination of flow *in vivo* [68]. The input function can be determined from frequent arterial sampling or tomographically by assessing tracer activity in cardiac chamber blood pools with co-calibration. Values for the tissue to blood partition coefficients must be determined independently. The assumptions entailed include: 1) the uptake of tracer in tissue is flow dependent and not diffusion limited; 2) no significant arterio-venous shunts are present; 3) the solubility of tracer is constant; and 4) flow is constant and homogeneous throughout the sampled region of interest during the data acquisition interval. We have shown that limitations to free diffusion of water in myocardium are modest, constant, and not altered by changes in flow [9]. Although more than 97% of nine micron microspheres are trapped during a single capillary transit through myocardium, diffusional shunting of H_2O cannot be excluded [67-71]. However, single pass extraction of $H_2{}^{15}O$ was found to be invariant over a wide range of flow [9].

The applicability of assumptions of homogeneity of flow depends in part upon the size of the regions of interest interrogated. Adaptation of the "autoradiographic" method described for PET may introduce errors related to limited spatial resolution of the instrument, partial volume and motion effects, and spillover. However, when we evaluated the tissue autoradiographic method with $H_2{}^{15}O$ for measurement of myocardial blood flow, we observed a close correlation between results obtained with microspheres in open chest

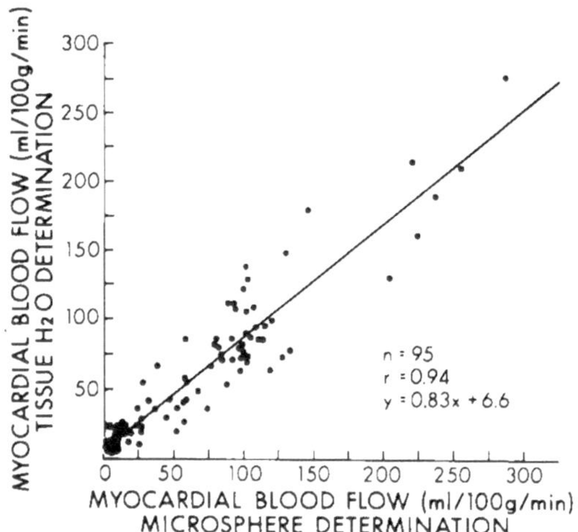

Figure 3. Correspondence between myocardial blood flow assessed with oxygen-15 water and radiolabeled microspheres determined invasively. The data, obtained from nine dogs pertain to normal and infarcted myocardium. In four animals flow was augmented with dipyridamole. A close correlation is demonstrated between flow measurements obtained with $H_2{}^{15}O$ and with the microsphere technique (reproduced with the permission of the American Heart Association, Inc., [9]).

dogs (Figure 3). In addition we demonstrated the utility of the approach for cardiac positron emission tomography [9].

In open chest dogs the single pass extraction of $H_2{}^{15}O$ by the heart averaged $96 \pm 5\%$ at flows of 80 to 100 ml/100 g/min and did not differ significantly over a wide range of flows (from 12 to 300 ml/100 g/min). Because the extraction fraction was high and consistent, the extraction of tracer appeared to be flow limited rather than diffusion limited over the ranges of flow studied. Thus, the tracer should provide a good index of flow *in vivo*. The underlying assumptions were tested initially in open chest dogs given a 60 s intravenous infusion of $H_2{}^{15}O$ (Figure 3). $H_2{}^{15}O$ content was measured directly by analysis of tissue. Regional flow was calculated by direct application of the tissue autoradiographic method. Flows determined in this way correlated closely with flows measured with the radiolabeled microsphere technique (Figure 3).

Experiments were performed in which the tissue autoradiographic method was employed with positron tomography in intact animals. Before regional tissue $H_2{}^{15}O$ activity could be determined from images of myocardium, correction was required for contributions from intravascular tracer as well as spillover of activity from the cardiac chamber blood pool into myocardium. A method was developed with oxygen-15 labeled carbon monoxide ($C^{15}O$) given by inhalation [9]. This tracer binds avidly to red blood cells in the blood pool. Blood pool $H_2{}^{15}O$ activity can be calculated and subtracted by the computer on a pixel by pixel basis to yield an image representing the distribution of $H_2{}^{15}O$ in tissue (Figure 4). Extravascular, or tissue $H_2{}^{15}O$ is appreciated as the difference

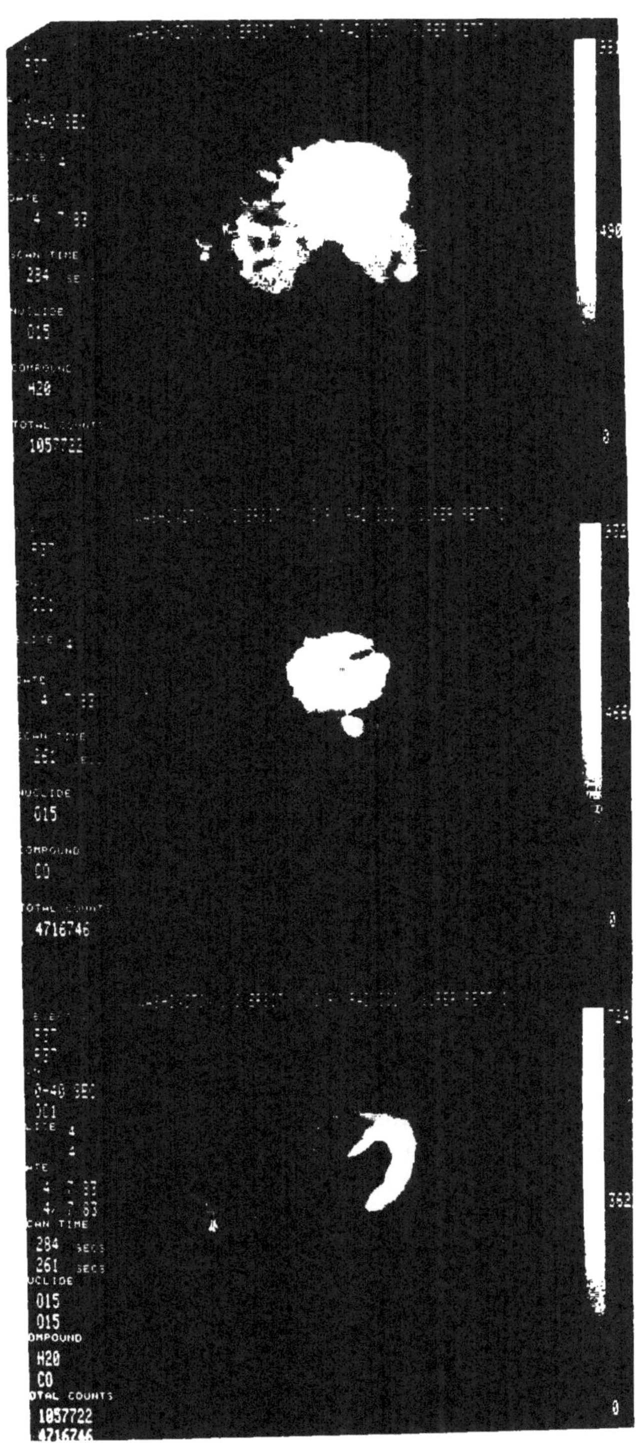

284
015
H20
1057722
015
CO
4716746
284
261
015
015
H20
CO
1057722

Figure 4.

between total $H_2{}^{15}O$ in each pixel and $H_2{}^{15}O$ activity attributable to that in the blood pool. Blood pool activity is computed as the product of $C^{15}O$ counts in a pixel multiplied by a scale factor equal to the ratio of $H_2{}^{15}O$ counts in the blood divided by $C^{15}O$ counts in the blood. This ratio can be determined tomographically from a region of interest in the center of the left ventricular blood pool (Figure 4).

The short physical half-life of ^{15}O allows sequential collection of $H_2{}^{15}O$ and $C^{15}O$ images within approximately ten minutes because counts from the first ^{15}O study approach background after five half-lives.

Results obtained with PET indicated that the $H_2{}^{15}O$ determinations of flow correlated closely with those obtained tomographically with ^{68}Ga macro-aggregated albumin microspheres (Figure 2). The instrumentation available at the time the validation studies were performed did not permit gating with respect to the cardiac cycle. Thus, relative rather than absolute measurements of flow were acquired. Within these qualifications, the distribution of $H_2{}^{15}O$ determined tomographically accurately reflected tissue perfusion.

In subsequent studies, Huang *et al.* demonstrated the feasibility of determination of myocardial blood flow with a more prolonged infusion of $H_2{}^{15}O$ tracer. Tomographic determinations of flow *in vivo* correlated closely with measurements with microspheres [12].

Results from our laboratory demonstrated the utility of applying the $H_2{}^{15}O$ technique for delineation of myocardial ischemia and reperfusion in acute and chronic derangements [9,72,73]. In addition, the functional impact of subcritical coronary arterial stenoses on myocardial perfusion was definable with this approach before and after pharmacologically induced vasodilatory stress [15] (Figure 5). As illustrated in Figure 5, the technique developed permits determination of the impact of a subcritical coronary stenosis on myocardial perfusion even when no perfusion defect is present at rest. In contrast, angiographic criteria define the distribution of the coronary stenoses and collaterals without directly characterizing the functional impact of the summation of these phenomena on myocardial perfusion [74]. Accordingly, clinical assessment of the significance of coronary arterial abnormalities are likely to ultimately require consideration not only of angiographic data but also estimates of regional perfusion and factors potentially modifying extraction or clearance of radiolabeled tracers.

←

Figure 4. Tomograms obtained in one midventricular plane of a human subject. The top image shows the distribution of $H_2{}^{15}O$ in blood as well as tissue. The middle image was obtained separately after inhalation of $C^{15}O$ and thus depicts only the blood pool. The resulting subtracted image of extravascular $H_2{}^{15}O$ distribution is shown in the lower image. In these tomograms myocardium is depicted as viewed from below.

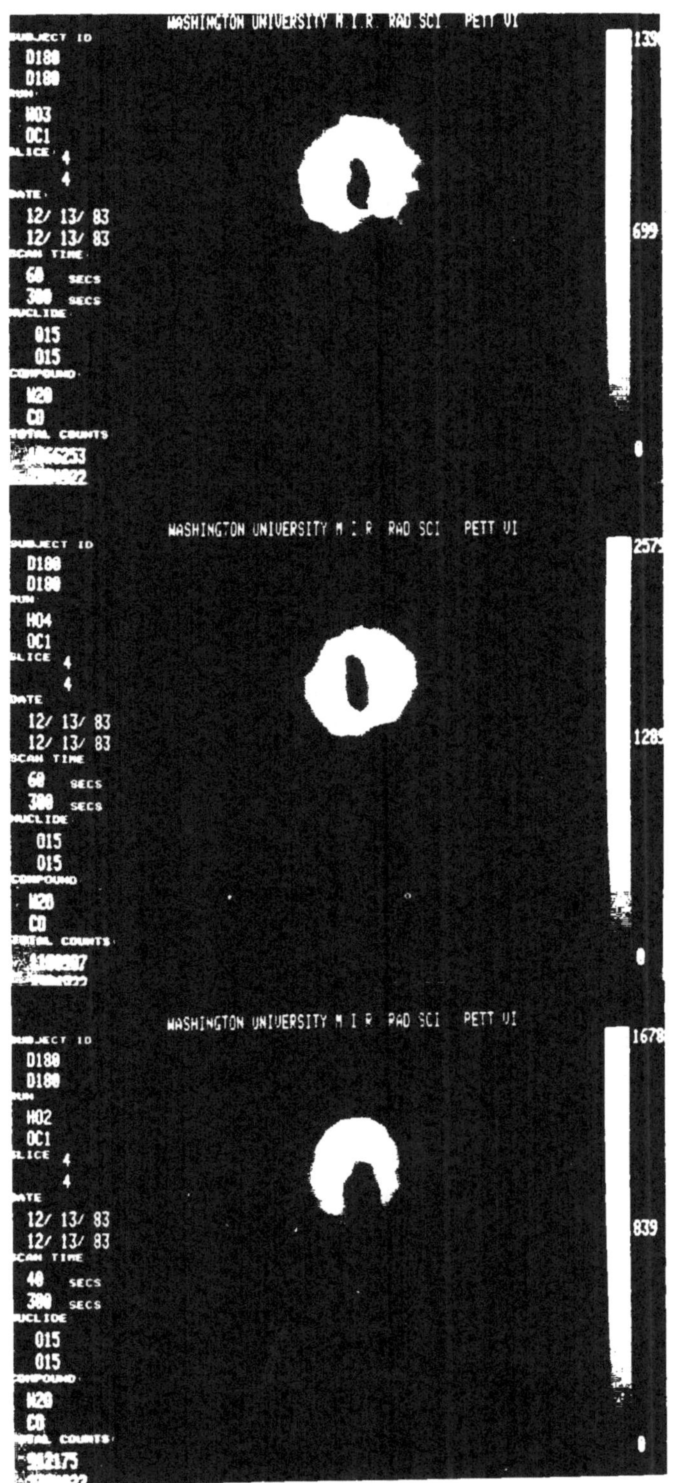
WASHINGTON UNIVERSITY M.I.R. RAD SCI PETT VI
SUBJECT ID
D180
D180
RUN
H03
OC1
SLICE
4
4
DATE
12/ 13/ 83
12/ 13/ 83
SCAN TIME
60 SECS
300 SECS
NUCLIDE
015
015
COMPOUND
H20
CO
TOTAL COUNTS
699
0
WASHINGTON UNIVERSITY M.I.R. RAD SCI PETT VI
SUBJECT ID
D180
D180
RUN
H04
OC1
SLICE
4
4
DATE
12/ 13/ 83
12/ 13/ 83
SCAN TIME
60 SECS
300 SECS
NUCLIDE
015
015
COMPOUND
H20
CO
TOTAL COUNTS
0
WASHINGTON UNIVERSITY M.I.R. RAD SCI PETT VI
SUBJECT ID
D180
D180
RUN
H02
OC1
SLICE
4
4
DATE
12/ 13/ 83
12/ 13/ 83
SCAN TIME
40 SECS
300 SECS
NUCLIDE
015
015
COMPOUND
H20
CO
TOTAL COUNTS
839
0

Figure 5.

Cardiac positron tomography with tracers of metabolism

The spatial distribution of labeled substrate in myocardium is determined by the temporally dependent fate of each of the labeled components of the metabolized radiotracer. Tracers used to assess myocardial metabolism can be categorized as labeled substrates and labeled substrate analogs [23,29,75-79]. The former include ^{11}C-labeled fatty acids such as 1-^{11}C-palmitate [1,3,16,80-91]. Some studies have been performed with ^{11}C-glucose [81], pyruvate [92], lactate [93], acetate [94], and amino acids [95,96]. Substrate analogs such as fluorine-labeled deoxyglucose [4,97-101] or ^{11}C-beta-methyl-heptadecanoic acid [102,103] may offer advantages with respect to interpretation of the tissue extraction in the absence of significant oxidation of tracer.

The use of ^{15}O labeled hemoglobin is attractive for characterization of overall oxidative metabolism, and results of initial studies in open chest animals have been encouraging [104]. However, for use in intact animals and patients serious limitations are encountered with respect to count recovery and spillover restricting the utility for cardiac tomography of the oxygen single breath inhalation technique. For studies of brain, cardiac and respiratory gating are not needed, and spillover from the lung does not present a problem [105,106].

Equilibrium methods have been used for determination of myocardial oxygen utilization, but the problems of high blood and lung to tissue spillover have hampered interpretation. Because of the short half-life of ^{15}O, characterization of utilization of ^{15}O oxygen is particularly challenging. Tomographic detection does not differentiate ^{15}O oxygen from the $H_2{}^{15}O$ derived from oxidation. Thus, corrections for radiolabeled water of metabolism are needed.

Some tracers such as rubidium-82 and ^{13}N-ammonia exhibit biological characteristics partly dependent upon myocardial viability and metabolism and partly dependent on flow and residence time [44-46,55]. Although such tracers have been employed for estimation of myocardial perfusion, their limitations with respect to quantification of perfusion have been demonstrated [44-46,56,107-109]. Thus, although ^{82}Rb has been employed as a tracer of myocardial perfusion, others have employed it to determine "an index of viability of the myocardium" [11].

←

Figure 5. Midventricular tomograms from a single plane of a dog with a 70% diameter stenosis of the left anterior descending coronary artery. Images represent tissue $H_2{}^{15}O$ activity and are corrected for vascular tracer with the use of $C^{15}O$. The uppermost image was obtained under baseline conditions and reflects relatively homogeneous perfusion (mitral valve apparatus appears posteriorly in this plane). The middle image was obtained after administration of the coronary vasodilator dipyridamole. A relative defect in perfusion is apparent since the hyperemia in the normal region was much greater than in the anterior region supplied by the stenosed vessel. Actual blood flow was increased four-fold in the normal regions and two-fold in post-stenotic zones (confirmed with microspheres). The lower image was obtained immediately after occlusion and reperfusion of the stenotic artery and demonstrates hyperemia in the poststenotic zone. This finding is consistent with the presence of a noncritical stenosis.

Development and validation of appropriate tracer kinetic models for interpretation of results with labeled substrates have been difficult. However, recently, progress has been considerable [41,80,83-87,110].

Fatty acid metabolism in normoxic or ischemic myocardium

Under physiological conditions, the heart preferentially oxidizes fatty acids to meet its energy requirements. Metabolism of nonesterified fatty acid (NEFA) accounts for 40 to 80% of total energy production by the heart [75,111-113]. Accordingly, tomographic characterization of metabolism of this substrate is of particular interest.

Palmitate (16:0) comprises 25 to 30% of circulating fatty acid. Its oxidation accounts for up to 50% of overall myocardial energy production under normoxic conditions [87,113]. NEFA is bound to albumin in the circulation but is in equilibrium with small quantities of unbound NEFA (Figure 6). Its extraction by the myocardium is influenced by the concentration of NEFA in the arterial blood, the fatty acid to albumin ratio, and the myocardial affinity for individual fatty acids species as a function of chain length and saturation. Oxygenation of tissue and hormonal environment exert marked influences on fatty acid extraction and utilization [75,111, 112,114].

Mechanisms responsible for transport of fatty acids from the blood to the myocyte are controversial [75,110-115]. Passive diffusion is pivotal. However, active transport may play a significant role [116]. Transfer of the fatty acid across the sarcolemma is influenced by the equilibrium between free NEFA and NEFA bound to albumin in interstitial fluid and the binding of NEFA to intracellular fatty acid binding protein (Figure 6) [110,117-119]. Aggregation of fatty acid binding protein may influence the activity of membrane bound enzyme systems associated with metabolism of NEFA [118,119]. By regulating cytosolic concentrations of fatty acid and directly influencing the concentration of free co-enzyme A, binding proteins may modulate both microsomal esterification and mitochondrial β-oxidation of fatty acid. Fatty acids may back-diffuse to extracellular fluid without undergoing metabolic alterations (Figure 6) [80]. Alternatively, they may be thioesterified intracellularly to fatty acid-CoA esters (acyl-CoA). Thioesterification is mediated by an acyl-CoA synthetase located on the outer mitochondrial membrane. Activity of this enzyme is modulated through inhibition by AMP, inorganic phosphate, acyl-CoA and substrate availability, in turn influenced by protein binding. Fatty acid thioesters can undergo β-oxidation after transport into mitochondria via interconversions involving carnitine. Alternatively, they may be incorporated into triglycerides or phospolipids (Figure 6) [75,80,111,112,115,120].

Under physiologic conditions sufficient oxygen is available for oxidation of the reduced adenine nucleotides $FADH_2$ and NADH. In ischemic myocardium

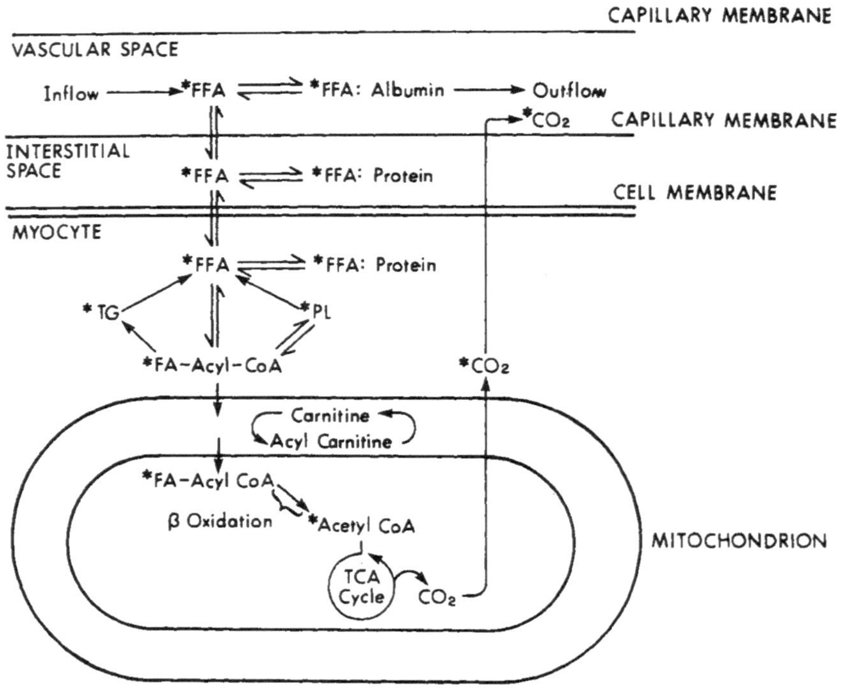

Figure 6. Diagrammatic representation of the distribution of labeled fatty acid (* denotes label). Free fatty acid (FFA) which is not bound to albumin can leave the vascular space and transverse the capillary endothelium. Interstitial free fatty acid is in equilibrium with FFA associated with binding proteins. Both passive diffusion and active transport may contribute to entry into myocardial cells, where free fatty acid is also in equilibrium with binding proteins. Free fatty acid can diffuse back into the interstitial space, or undergo thioesterification with coenzyme A (FA-Acyl-CoA). Labeled fatty acid can be incorporated into triglycerides or phospholipids or carried across the mitochondrial membrane via the carnitine shuttle. Beta-oxidation yields shorter chain fatty acyl CoA, and acetyl CoA, which is oxidized via the tricarboxylic acid (TCA) cycle. Labeled carbon dioxide from the TCA cycle can diffuse across the cell and interstitial space and into the vascular compartment.

$FADH_2$ and NADH accumulate inhibiting β-oxidation and diminishing the rate of formation of acetyl CoA. Availability of pyruvate is limited because of increased metabolism of pyruvate to lactate under anaerobic conditions [75,111-114]. In addition, several enzymes involved in intermediary metabolism of carbohydrates are inhibited by lactate or hydrogen ion that accumulate with hypoxia or by increases in the $NADH/NAD^+$ ratio. Structural and functional abnormalities possibly mediated by generation of free radicals in ischemic tissue may reflect lipid peroxidation and may be associated with exacerbations of impairment of intermediary metabolism. The increase in intracellular free fatty acids with ischemia [120] coupled with accumulation of alpha-glycerophospate because of increase anaerobic glycolytic flux result in the shunting of fatty acid into triglycerides with subsequent augmentation of the neutral lipid pool size.

Increase in long-chain acyl CoA and acyl-carnitine are seen with ischemia in isolated hearts and in hearts of experimental animals *in vivo* [121-124]. The increase in acyl CoA occurs almost exlusively in mitochondria. Long-chain acyl-carnitine accumulates predominantly in the cytosol [124]. Inhibition of β-oxidation results in accumulation of intermediated including β-hydroxy-palmitate and stearate [125-127]. Unsaturated intermediates may exert profound and deleterious effects on membranes and membrane-associated enzyme systems [124,128]. Long-chain acyl CoA and acyl carnitine are amphipathic metabolites capable of interacting with and disrupting membranes and hence contributing to electrophysiologic derangements associated with ischemia [124].

Kinetics of labeled fatty acids

The kinetics of labeled palmitate have been characterized in myocardium under normoxic and ischemic conditions [80-91]. Independent control of myocardial work and of substrate utilization are possible in isolated perfused hearts [87]. With the use of such preparations the time-activity curve for clearance of the ^{11}C-activity from myocardium exhibits three main components [81-85]. Extraction and clearance of ^{11}C-palmitate has been characterized in open chest animal studies [80,85,86] and analogous findings have been obtained recently in clinical tomographic studies [3,16,89].

The first component of the tracer time-activity curve reflects vascular transit of non-extracted tracer (Figure 7). The second reflects primarily β-oxidation of the fatty acid [80,82,83,85,86]. During the third phase clearance of tracer is low, consistent with prior incorporation and slow turnover of the radiolabel in triglyceride and phospholipid pools [80]. After vascular transit of non-extracted tracer, the rate of clearance of ^{11}C-activity is diminished from ischemic myocardium consistent with reduced β-oxidation, incorporation of some tracer into the triglyceride pool, and slow turnover of neutral and phospholipid pools [80]. However, interpretations are complex because efflux of non-metabolized fatty acid from ischemic or hypoxic myocardium contributes substantially to the net removal of radioactivity from myocardium [80]. Definitive interpretation of tracer kinetics requires differentiation of the fate of label residing in individual lipid fractions. We have examined the fractional distribution of radiotracer from lipid components in association with externally determined clearance and directly measured arterio-venous extraction of each substrate [80]. Results indicate that despite back-diffusion of non-metabolized tracer, net clearance is diminished with ischemia or hypoxia as a consequence of increased incorporation of labeled fatty acid into lipid pools with slow turnover rates [80]

To determine whether decreased utilization of substrate in ischemic myo-

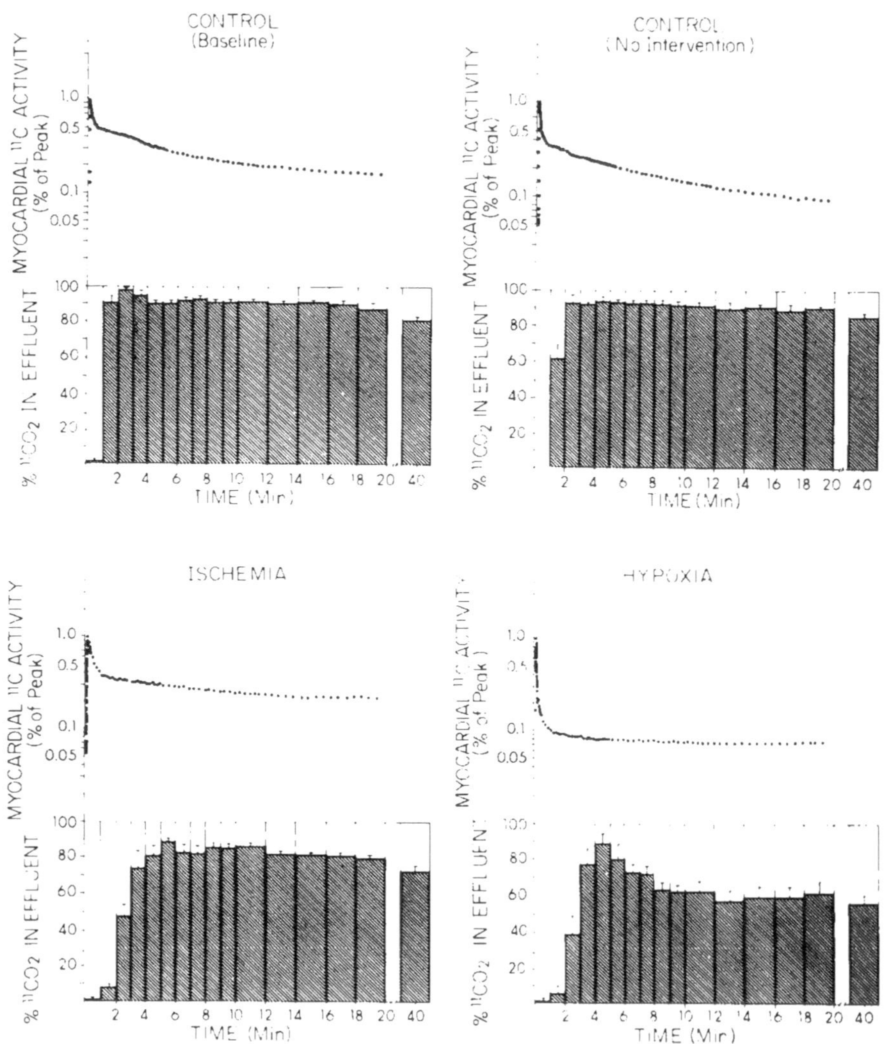

Figure 7. Myocardial ^{11}C time-activity curves obtained with high temporal resolution from one dog under baseline (upper left) and later under control conditions with no intervention (upper right); from another animal with ischemic perfusion (lower left); and from a third animal with hypoxic perfusion (lower right). Myocardial radioactivity is corrected for isotope decay and normalized with peak counts set equal to 1.0. The time-activity curves can be divided into a very early component of vascular transit, and early and late components of the clearance of tissue radioactivity. The histogram corresponding with each portion of the time-activity curve indicates, for the entire group, the respective proportions of the effluent constituted by $^{11}CO_2$ (cross-hatched bars ± SE) and back-diffusion of unaltered ^{11}C-palmitate (open bars). With ischemia or hypoxia the onset of β-oxidation of the tracer is delayed and the fraction of tracer metabolized to $^{11}CO_2$ is diminished. Net tissue extraction of ^{11}C-palmitate (extraction fraction x flow) is diminished with ischemia or hypoxia, and the rate of clearance of activity is reduced substantially despite back-diffusion of unaltered tracer (reproduced with permission of the American Heart Association, Inc., [80]).

cardium is a reflection simply of decreased supply as a result of low flow, we utilized isolated perfused rabbit hearts [87]. Flow was reduced but myocardial oxygen consumption and work were maintained constant by continuous adjustment of left ventricular end-diastolic pressure and heart rate. Overall utilization of palmitate remained constant despite decreased delivery of substrate. Thus, despite a decrease in perfusion of 50 to 75%, myocardial extraction of delivered substrate increased such that net utilization remained constant. Further reduction of perfusion resulted in mechanical decompensation and an abrupt and dramatic decline of substrate utilization. Utilization of glucose and production of lactate remained constant over the ranges of perfusion studied. Thus, oxygen delivery was not limiting when external work declined.

Reduced flow *in vivo* is generally associated with decreased cardiac work, and accordingly, with decreased metabolic demand. However, the results obtained *in vitro* indicate that when impaired extraction of substrate is seen with low flow *in vivo*, a decrease in extraction of fatty acid can be considered to reflect depressed myocardial metabolism rather than simply decreased delivery of substrate [84,87].

In several studies [81,82] the extraction and clearance of labeled fatty acid were assessed in isolated perfused hearts. Tracer radioactivity was measured with a pair of columnated sodium iodide detectors. Substrate utilization was controlled while clearance of tracer activity was characterized by coincidence detection. The detection system recorded global activity from isolated hearts. It served, in a sense, as a simple model of two probe "tomography". The slope of the time-acitivity curve was related qualitatively to work of the left ventricle and to oxygen consumption measured directly. Under conditions of low flow, net extraction of ^{11}C-fatty acid decreased markedly. This decrease provided a foundation for detection of ischemia *in vivo* [81]. However, as shown in subsequent studies, the correlation between ^{11}C-palmitate clearance and $M\dot{V}O_2$ is not close because of the influence of washout of nonmetabolized tracer [80]. Thus, $M\dot{V}O_2$ cannot be extrapolated directly from the slope of clearance of the fatty acid time-activity curve.

To determine whether the observed decreases in clearance of ^{11}C-palmitate from ischemic myocardium were attributable simply to low flow or whether they reflected metabolic consequences of hypoxia as well, we performed additinal studies in open chest dogs [80,84]. Hearts were perfused by an extracorporeal circuit. The kinetics of uptake and clearance of ^{11}C-palmitate were evaluated after intracoronary bolus injections of tracer. The clearance of extracted ^{11}C-palmitate during the early phase (3 to 7 min after injection of tracer) was decreased by 61% when the coronary arterial flow was reduced to 36% of control. However, when flow was maintained constant but perfusion was implemented with hypoxic rather than normoxic blood, the clearance of tracer was reduced by 52% [84]. Thus, with flow held constant but the supply of oxygen limited, the clearance of tracer was altered. Accordingly, metabolic manifestations of impaired oxygenation could be differentiated from changes in tracer kinetics reflecting low flow per se.

Despite either reduction of flow or delivery of oxygen, myocardium continues to extract fatty acid. However, net extraction and metabolism of fatty acid is markedly reduced in comparison to the case in normal tissue. Under control conditions, 90 to 95% of extracted fatty acid is metabolized to $^{11}CO_2$ (80) (Figure 7). With either ischemia or hypoxia, the proportion of ^{11}C-palmitate oxidized to $^{11}CO_2$ decreases, and back-diffusion of initally extracted ^{11}C-palmitate increases. Almost 50% of total clearance of radiotracer from myocardium is accounted for by efflux of nonmetabolized tracer under conditions of hypoxia or ischemia (Figure 7). Thus, estimates of the extent of oxidative metabolism based solely upon the slope of the clearance curve substantially exceed actual rates of β-oxidation. Nevertheless, despite the contribution of back diffusion of non-extracted fatty acid, overall clearance of tracer is diminished with ischemia. These observations are consistent with the demonstration of increased incorporation in hypoxic tissue of fatty acid into triglyceride and reduced turnover of this lipid pool. Because of differential rates of clearance from normoxic and ischemic myocardium, net differences in residual activity are minimized as the interval after injection of tracer becomes prolonged. Thus, in order to appropriately characterize the extent of extraction and clearance of tracer from myocardium, PET systems with high temporal resolution are required.

The following approaches may be useful in providing unambiguous interpretation of rates of clearance of tracer: (1) positron-emission tomography with rapid data acquisition, correction for partial volume effect, spillover, and gating to the cardiac cycle to permit accurate determination of net fatty acid extraction in brief intervals early after administration of tracer. Conditions can be selected to minimize the cumulative effects of back diffusion and the disparate rates of clearance from ischemic compared with normal zones; (2) use of instrumentation with high temporal resolution to permit estimation of extraction from the measured input function of the tracer; and (3) comparisons of the extraction and clearance of ^{11}C-palmitate with respect to extraction of ^{11}C-palmitate analogs trapped by the myocardium without undergoing oxidation during the data acquisition interval to provide independent indexes of the extent of back diffusion under specified conditions.

The decrease in the disappearance rate of ^{11}C-palmitate radioactivity from ischemic myocardium in animals suggests that analogous changes will be detectable in patients evaluated with PET. However, radioactivity detected in a given region of myocardium reflects not only activity associated with ^{11}C-palmitate but also activity associated with $^{11}CO_2$ and other metabolic intermediates. Myocardial clearance of tracer reflects not only the washout of labeled metabolites during the imaging interval but also back-diffusion of tracer neither trapped nor metabolized after initial extraction.

Quantification of the contributions of $^{11}CO_2$ and efflux of ^{11}C-palmitate

Interpretation of the fate of the radioactive label derived form 1-^{11}C-palmitate can be enhanced by considering the following [80]:

$$^{11}C(Tp) + {}^{11}C(R) = 100\%$$

where: $^{11}C(Tp)$ = throughput of ^{11}C activity (%)
$^{11}C(R)$ = ^{11}C activity retained in tissue (%) on first pass.
At time t':

$$^{11}C(R)t - {}^{11}C(R)t' = F \int_{t}^{t'} ({}^{11}C(CO_2) + {}^{11}C(P)) \, . \, dt$$

where: $^{11}C(CO_2)$, $^{11}C(P)$ are the concentrations of ^{11}C activity in the efflux, measured as $^{11}CO_2$ or ^{11}C-palmitate from time t to time t', (shown to be the only forms of tracer in the effluent); and $^{11}C(R)t'$ = residue of ^{11}C activity in tissue at time t' (as FFA, phospholipids, triglycerides and with small components of mono and diglycerides); F = flow (ml/100 g/min).

The relevant equations are depicted graphically in Figure 8. Although tomography can delineate the spatial distribution of the radiotracer, it cannot define uniquely the metabolic form in which tracer resides. Thus, appropriate interpretation of static or dynamic displays requires independent determination of the rate of turnover of metabolites and specific radioactivity within precursor pools in which the tracer resides.

Corroboration of clinical and experimental studies

Despite the complexities encountered in attempting to obtain quantitative information characterizing metabolism from tomographic studies with labeled fatty acids, useful clinical insights have been gained [3,16,88,89,93,130-132]. In initial tomographic studies of myocardial infarction performed in our laboratory in 1976, accumulation of ^{11}C-palmitate was detected with a single slice tomographic instrument [1]. ^{11}C-palmitate in myocardium was homogeneous [88,89]. However, as demonstrated in dogs subjected to coronary ligation, infarction results in transmural reduction of incorporation of ^{11}C-palmitate. Diminution of the accumulation of ^{11}C-palmitate detectable tomographically correlated closely (r=0.93) with depletion of myocardial creatine kinase [1], an independent criterion of irreversible injury, and with infarct size characterized histologically. In clinical studies ^{11}C-palmitate was employed successfully for estimation of infarct size [88,89]. Tomographic estimates obtainable within 15 to 30 min correlated closely with enzymatic estimates of infarct size based upon analysis of plasma creatine kinase curves acquired over the ensuing 48 to 72 h

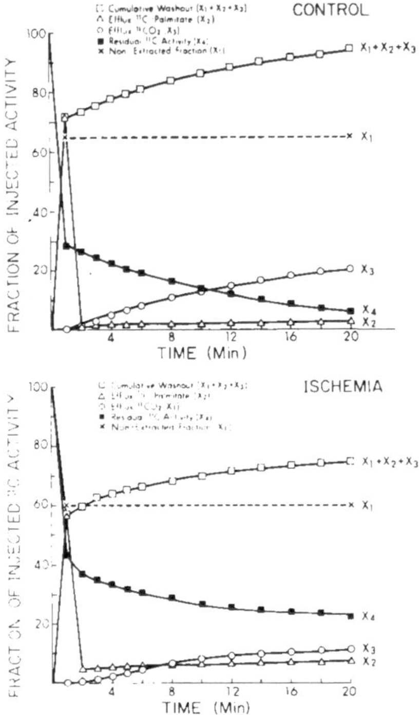

Figure 8. The fate of tracer after intracoronary bolus injection of 1-^{11}C-palmitate can be described according to fractional distributions. Individual components of extraction and efflux are shown for each time period. Total efflux is constituted by the sum of the non-extracted (vascular) component X_1, ^{11}C-palmitate back-diffusion (X_2), and $^{11}CO_2$ efflux from oxidative metabolism (X_3). $X_1 + X_2 + X_3 + X_4 = 100\%$ of injected dose; with X_4 = residual myocardial ^{11}C-activity. For the time period 0 to 1 min total washout was in the form of ^{11}C-palmitate for all hearts, constituted by the throughput of non-extracted ^{11}C-palmitate and efflux of ^{11}C-P from the interstitial and intracellular spaces. With ischemia, cumulative washout ($X_1 + X_2 + X_3$) is diminished compared with control, accounting for the lower rate of clearance evident on the time activity curve; oxidation is diminished (X_3) and a relatively greater residue of ^{11}C activity remains in the tissue (X_4) (probably in the form of intracellular triglyceride) (reproduced with permission of the American Heart Association, Inc. [80]).

[88,89]. Clearly, repeated studies of perfusion and metabolism using PET provide a promising approach for characterization of the natural history of myocardium subjected to persistent or transitory ischemia. Furthermore, it provides a useful tool for assessing the effects on the heart of pharmacologic interventions including coronary thrombolysis, designed to protect ischemic myocardium.

Myocardial ischemia and coronary stenosis

Regional clearance of myocardial radioactivity detectable after an intravenous injection of ^{11}C-palmitate is consistent and homogenous throughout myocardium under conditions of rest [88,89,133]. When coronary stenosis of less than 70% in a cross-sectional area is induced, clearance of the tracer in the regions supplied by the partially occluded vessel is unaltered when the heart is functioning under conditions of rest [133]. However, when stenosis of greater than 70% is induced, regional clearance of radioactivity is decreased in zones supplied by the stenotic coronary artery [133]. These findings are consistent with those from isolated perfused hearts and open chest dogs in which clearance of ^{11}C-palmitate is reduced markedly under conditions of ischemia [80-86].

Clinical tomographic differentiation of ischemic from nonischemic myocardium relies on estimates of regional perfusion and on extraction and clearance of labeled fatty acid [3,16,88,89]. Completed infarction [88] and nontransmural infarction are recognizable and distinguishable by virtue of the profound regional metabolic impairment associated with each [3]. Cardiac positron emission tomography after intravenous administration of ^{11}C-palmitate permits noninvasive detection of myocardium compromised metabolically by ischemia. However, differentiation of transiently ischemic myocardium from necrotic tissue or scar may require assessments under disparate conditions including dipyridamole stress, exercise, or atrial pacing [11,13-15,133,134]. Interpretation may be facilitated by concomitant measurement of myocardial perfusion [4,6,9,12,15]. Tomography before and after selected interventions should permit delineation of the extent and distribution of myocardium at risk as a result of flow limiting stenoses and assessment of the extent of myocardium exhibiting altered metabolic activity indicative of reversible or irreversible injury.

Differentiation of concordance or discordance among zones exhibiting hypoperfusion with respect to decreased substrate extraction may help to distinguish infarction and fibrosis from jeopardized but still viable myocardium. Transient or dipyridamole stress-induced abnormalities of both perfusion and substrate extraction are compatible with the behavior of tissue supplied by vessels with critical stenosis. Zones exhibiting only transiently diminished fatty acid extraction and clearance may define the extent of myocardium potentially salvageable by revascularization. Transient hypoperfusion in zones retaining metabolic activity may have the same potential [4,13-15]. Thus, serial tomography with $H_2{}^{15}O$ for assessment of perfusion in conjunction with tracers of substrate utilization is particularly attractive.

Reperfusion

Cardiac PET is particularly useful for characterizing the efficacy of inter-

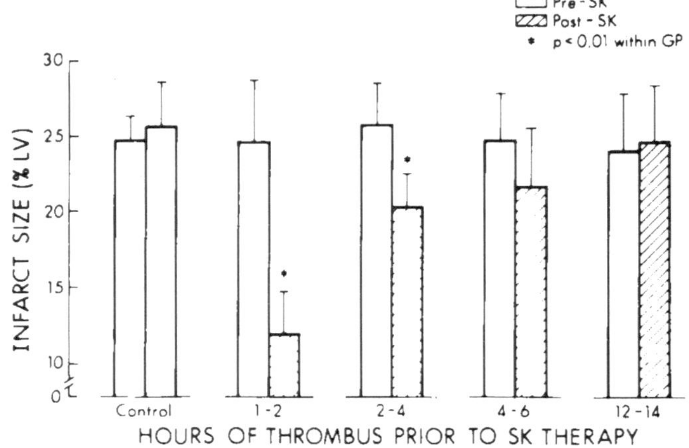

Figure 9. Histogram of tomographically estimated infarct size for control animals with sustained coronary occlusion (n=6), and animals with 1-2, (n=4), 2-4 (n=6), 4-6 (n=4) and 12-14 h of coronary occlusion prior to thrombolysis (n=3). Repeat tomography was performed 90 min after thrombolysis. Significant decreases of apparent infarct size (or increases in metabolic activity in jeopardized myocardium) occurred only in animals subjected to reperfusion within 4 h of occlusion (values indicate means ± SD) SK = steptokinase. The results illustrate the utility of PET for sequential characterization of myocardium before and after an intervention (reproduced with permission of the American Journal of Medicine [135]).

ventions designed to salvage ischemic myocardium (Figures 9, 10) [9,72,91,135,136]. In closed chest dogs with coronary thrombosis induced with a thrombogenic copper coil inserted into the LAD coronary artery, PET with ^{11}C-palmitate delineates defects of accumulation of tracer corresponding to zones of myocardium compromised by ischemia. Tomograms can be corrected for blood pool activity of tracer and spillover by employing vascular pool subtraction techniques with 0-15 labeled CO (Figure 5) [9,15,72]. When thrombolysis is induced with either intracoronary or intravenous streptokinase within the first 4 h after the onset of occlusion, the extent of the tomographically detectable defect decreases (Figure 9) [135,136]. In contrast, when thrombolysis is delayed for more than 6 h after occlusion, no significant improvement of accumulation of ^{11}C-palmitate is detectable by repeat tomography despite documented restoration of patency of epicardial vessels (Figure 9) [135]. Thus, ischemic myocardium which has not yet been irreversibly injured exhibits diminished accumulation of palmitate. This decrease is ameliorated by reperfusion initiated sufficiently early after the onset of ischemia.

In analogous clinical studies with intravenously administered human tissue type plasminogen activator (t-PA) or streptokinase administered to induce coronary thrombolysis, cardiac PET was performed before and on two occasions (early and late) after thrombolysis [137]. It demonstrated improvement of myocardial metabolism in association with successful thrombolysis [137]. Restoration of the extraction of ^{11}C-palmitate was detected noninvasively

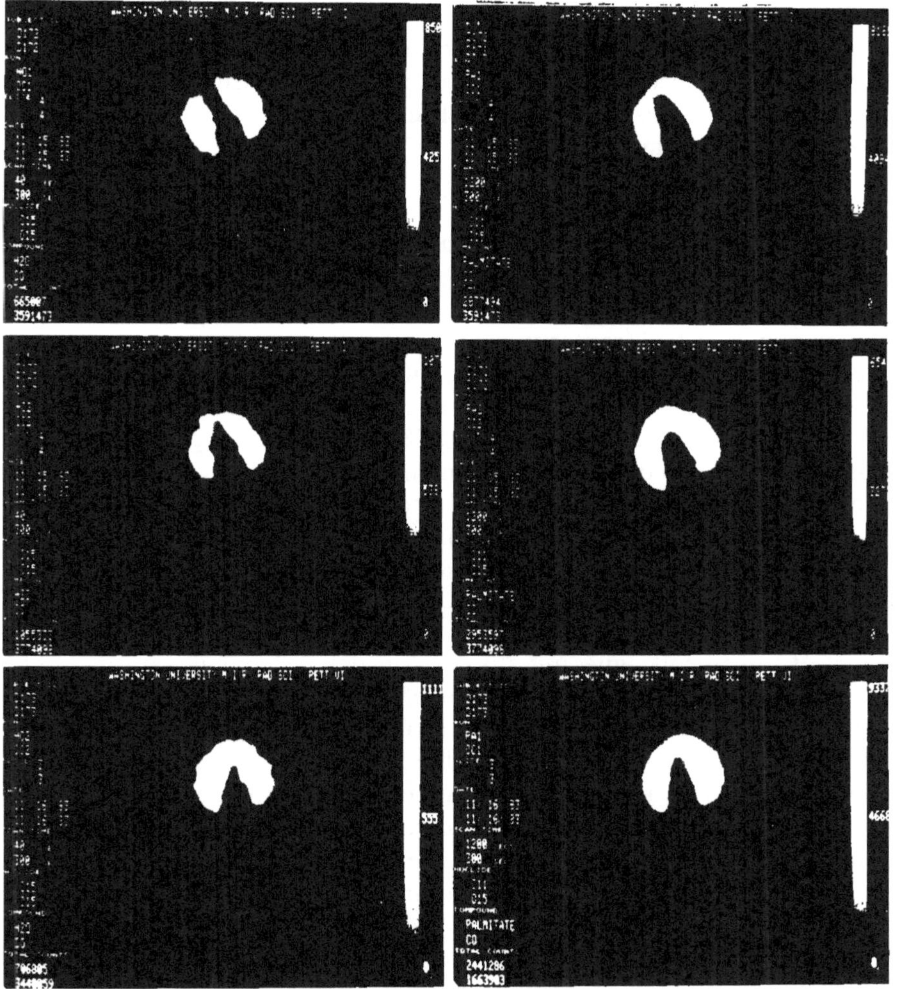

Figure 10. Tomographic reconstructions through a single midventricular plane of dog heart. All images have been corrected for activity in the vascular space with blood pool subtraction from an image obtained with $C^{15}O$. Perfusion images are on the left and were obtained with $H_2{}^{15}O$. Images on the right depict the myocardial accumulation of ^{11}C-palmitate from 4 to 10 min after intravenous administration of that tracer. A defect is seen anteriorly (arrow) in perfusion and for ^{11}C-palmitate accumulation. In the plane illustrated the transverse section passes through the mitral valve apparatus posteriorly, consistent with the lack of activity in the inferior point of the images. The uppermost images were obtained during thrombotic occlusion ofthe proximal LAD, induced with an intracoronary copper coil. Images in the center were obtained 1 h after thrombolysis induced with intracoronary streptokinase. Incomplete restoration of perfusion and restoration of palmitate extraction are demonstrated. The lower images were obtained 24 h following thrombolysis and show a further improvement in perfusion in the anterior zone but a decrease in palmitate accumulation. The example illustrates differences in the time course of recovery of extraction of fatty acid with respect to perfusion after thrombolysis. Alterations in the tissue distribution of fatty acid and the extent of oxidation may account for the differences in time course in metabolic compared with perfusion images.

providing a useful index of viable myocardium. In contrast, angiographic documentation of successful lysis of a clot does not necessarily imply salvage of myocardium [135]. Thus, when thrombolysis is late, patency is restored but the heart cannot respond favorably.

Assessment of metabolic activity with substrates other than fatty acid and with alternative tracers of metabolism

Although non-esterified free fatty acid is the primary substrate for myocardial metabolism under physiologic conditions, glucose becomes the primary source of energy in ischemic myocardium or in normoxic tissue when circulating NEFA levels are markedly depressed [75-78]. Positron tomography with ^{11}C-glucose has been limited by difficulties in differentiating the substrate from its metabolites. Incorporation of the label into metabolic intermediates or into lactate renders interpretation particularly complex. To avoid some of the difficulties encountered with C-11 glucose and its labeled metabolites, glucose analogs have been employed [4,97-101], particularly ^{18}F-2-fluoro-2-deoxy-glucose (^{18}F-2-FDG).

Sokoloff and his colleagues initially developed the "deoxy-glucose method" because of the limited temporal resolution of the available instrumentation and difficulties encountered in tracing labeled intermediates [138]. ^{18}F-2-FDG is transported across the myocardial cell, phosphorylated, protected from further metabolism via phosphofructokinase, and trapped within the cytosol because of the impermeability of sarcolemma to charged species [4,97-101,138,139]. However, some efflux can occur. Increased accumulation of ^{18}F-2-FDG in ischemic myocardium is compatible with increased anaerobic glycolytic flux and may serve as a useful predictor of myocardium potentially salvageable by revascularization. Increased accumulation has been seen in hearts of patients with Duchenne's muscular dystrophy, compatible with altered myocardial metabolism in this condition as well [17].

Although positron-emitting tracers of lactate, pyruvate, and acetate [92-94] have been employed, the rapidity with which the labeled carbon atoms in these intermediates exchange with constituents of numerous other metabolites renders interpretations complex and limits applications. Interpretation of the tomographically detectable distribution of labeled amino acids has been restricted by the relatively low extraction of these tracers. Nevertheless, studies with N-13 labeled glutamic acid, N-13 leucine, or N-13 aspartic acid may provide insight into altered metabolism handling of amino acids indicative of specific pathophysiologic conditions [95].

Interpretation of the myocardial handling of long-chain fatty acids would be facilitated by the development of suitable fatty acids analogs which undergo extraction and trapping by the myocardium. Although results of some studies of the heart with beta-methyl heptadecanoic acid are encouraging

[102,140,141], more recent results indicate that despite the reduction of beta-oxidation of the analog, efflux of the non-metabolized tracer is substantial from both ischemic and normal myocardium [103].

Recent neurological studies have employed labeled ligand agonists or antagonists for receptor binding, such as spiroperidol [142], and have raised intriguing possibilities for analogous tomographic studies of the heart. In such studies labeled agonists or antagonists can be employed to characterize specific pathways *in vivo*. Recent neurological studies of opiate receptors *in vivo* [143] and studies of dopaminergic receptors [144] raise the possibility of noninvasive assessment of transmitter substances *in vivo* [145].

Clinical implications

The potential of positron tomography for the detection of disorders of myocardial metabolism is now well appreciated. Although substantial progress has been made the full diagnostic potential of this modality has yet to be reached. Instrumentation has developed rapidly. However, delineation of specific abnormalities of intermediary metabolism presents significant problems not only because of the requirements for adequate counting statistics for tracers with kinetics requiring high temporal resolution but also because of complexities influencing extraction and clearance of tracer in multiple pools. Unambiguous interpretation may require assessment of both perfusion and metabolism. Despite these qualifications, clinical and experimental observations with positron tomography have demonstrated the utility of the approach for assessment of myocardial metabolism and perfusion. Positron tomography offers considerable advantages over imaging modalities directed exclusively toward delineating structure or physiologic function. The ability of PET to define quantitatively the extent of myocardium at risk for myocardial necrosis has been validated experimentally, histologically, and clinically[1-4]. Its utility for assessing the impact of interventions early after the onset of acute myocardial infarction such as coronary thrombolysis has been well documented [9,72,91,135-137]. Thus, among patients in whom early thrombolysis results in angiographically documented restoration of perfusion, salutary effects on regional myocardial metabolism are clearly demonstrable [137].

Accumulation of the glucose analog ^{18}F-2-FDG in zones exhibiting relatively decreased accumulation of N-13 ammonia may identify regions subject to ischemia but potentially salvageable [4]. Increased extraction of glucose and glucose analogs in myocardium subjected to ischemia followed by reperfusion may serve as a marker of compromised but still salvageable tissue. Heterogeneity of the spatial distribution of extraction of ^{11}C-palmitate may be a useful criterion of cardiomyopathy [16], perhaps indicative of admixtures of normal and fibrotic tissue. Heterogeneity of accumulation of N-13 ammonia and ^{18}F-2-FDG in hearts of patients with Duchenne's muscular dystrophy may reflect the same phenomenon [17]. Interpretation must be judicious however, because dephosphorylation of glucose-6-phosphate and 3 methyl-glucose-6-phosphate occurs in rat brain and intact perfused rat heart. Thus, uptake of glucose analogs may not parallel glycolytic flux *per se*.

The use of dipyridamole-stress for identification of myocardium supplied by vessels with critical stenoses has been demonstrated with thallium scintigraphy [146] and positron tomography with nitrogen-13 ammonia [13,14], rubidium-82 [11] and $H_2{}^{15}O$ [15]. Observations complement those obtained with angiography and the pathophysiological impact of single stenoses and of multiple lesions and modification of their impact as a result of collateral perfusion can be ascertained.

Conclusions

Important clinical questions can now be addressed with positron tomography and the impact of interventions such as thrombolysis on myocardial perfusion and metabolism can be evaluated. The temporal dependence of salvage of myocardium on the interval of ischemia prior to reperfusion [135,137] can be delineated. The combination of positron emission tomography with dipyridamole and with other inducers of physiologic testing appears promising for noninvasive determination of the functional significance of coronary stenoses with respect to myocardial tissue perfusion and metabolism [11, 13-15,133,134].

Computerized tomography and proton magnetic resonance imaging permit excellent spatial resolution of anatomic structures. Positron tomography is uniquely well suited to characterization of the metabolic derangements ultimately responsible for the functional and structural abnormalities of myocardial disease processes. In concert and with judicious selection, these three complementary modalities will markedly improve detection and characterization of cardiac disease.

Acknowledgements

Supported in part by NIH grant HL17646, SCOR in Ischemic Heart Disease.

References

1. Weiss E S, Ahmed S A, Welch M J, Williamson J R, Ter-Pogossian M M, Sobel B E (1977) Quantification of infarction in cross sections of canine myocardium in vivo with positron emission transaxial tomography and ^{11}C-palmitate. Circulation 55: 66

2. Nichols A B, Moore R H, Cochavi S, Pohost G M, Strauss W H (1980) Quantification of myocardial infarction by computer-assisted positron emission tomography. Cardiovasc Res 14: 428
3. Geltman E M, Biello D, Welch M J, Ter-Pogossian M M, Robertson R, Sobel B E (1982) Characterization of nontransmural myocardial infarction by positron-emission tomography. Circulation 65: 747
4. Marshall R C, Tillisch J H, Phelps M E, Huang S-C, Carson R, Henze E, Schelbert H R (1983) Identification and differentiation of resting myocardial ischemia and infarction in man with positron computed tomography, ^{18}F-labeled fluorodeoxyglucose and N-13 ammonia. Circulation 67: 766
5. Beller G A, Alton W J, Cochavi S, Hnatowich D, Brownell G L (1979) Assessment of regional myocardial perfusion by positron emission tomography after intracoronary administration of gallium-68 labeled albumin microspheres. J Comput Assist Tomogr 3: 447
6. Wilson R A, Shea M J, de Landsheere C M, Turton D, Brary F, Deanfield J E, Selwyn A P (1984) Validation of quantitation of regional myocardial blood flow in vivo with ^{11}C-labeled human albumin microspheres and positron emission tomography. Circulation 70: 717
7. Budinger T F, Yano Y, Hoop B (1975) A comparison of $^{82}Rb^+$ and $^{13}NH_3$ for myocardial positron scintigraphy. J Nucl Med 16: 429
8. Phelps M E, Hoffman E J, Coleman R E, Welch M J, Raichle M E, Weiss E S, Sobel B E, Ter-Pogossian M M (1976) Tomographic images of blood pool and perfusion in brain and heart. J Nucl Med 17: 603
9. Bergmann S R, Fox K A A, Rand A L, McElvany K D, Welch M J, Markham J, Sobel B E (1984) Quantification of regional myocardial blood flow in vivo with $H_2{}^{15}O$. Circulation 70: 724
10. Mullani N A, Goldstein R A, Gould K L, Marani S K, Fisher D J, O'Brien H A, Loberg M D (1983) Myocardial perfusion with rubidium-82. I. Measurement of extraction fraction and flow with external detectors. J Nucl Med 24: 898
11. Goldstein R A, Mullani N A, Marani S K, Fisher D J, Gould K L, O'Brien H A (1983) Myocardial perfusion with rubidium-82. II. Effects of metabolic and pharmacologic interventions. J Nucl Med 24: 907
12. Huang S C, Schwaiger M, Carson R E, Carson J, Hansen H, Selin C, Hoffman E J, MacDonald N, Schelbert H R, Phelps M E (1980) Quantitative measurement of myocardial blood flow with oxygen-15 water and positron computed tomography: An assessment of potential and problems. J Nucl Med 26: 616
13. Gould K L, Schelbert H R, Phelps M E, Hoffman E J (1979) Noninvasive assessment of coronary stenoses with myocardial perfusion imaging during pharmacologic coronary vasodilation. V. Detection of 47 percent diameter coronary stenosis with intravenous nitrogen-13 ammonia and emission-computed tomography in intact dogs. Am J Cardiol 43: 200
14. Schelbert H R, Wisenberg G, Phelps M E, Gould K L, Henze E, Hoffman E J, Comes A, Kuhl D E (1982) Non-invasive assessment of coronary stenoses by myocardial imaging during pharmacologic coronary vasodilation. VI. Detection of coronary artery disease in human being with intravenous N-13 ammonia and positron computed tomography. Am J Cardiol 49: 1197
15. Knabb R M, Fox K A A, Sobel B E, Bergmann S R (1985) Characterization of the functional significance of subcritical coronary stenoses with $H_2{}^{15}O$ and positron-emission tomography. Circulation 71: 1271
16. Geltman E M, Smith J L, Beecher D, Ludbrook P A, Ter-Pogossian M M, Sobel B E (1983) Altered regional myocardial metabolism in congestive cardiomyopathy detected by positron tomography. Am J Med 74: 773

17. Perloff J K, Henze E, Schelbert H R (1984) Alterations in regional myocardial metabolism, perfusion, and wall motion in Duchenne muscular dystrophy studied by radionuclide imaging. Circulation 69: 33
18. Eisenberg J D, Sobel B E, Geltman E M. Differentiation of ischemic from nonischemic cardiomyopathy with positron emission tomography. Am J Cardiol (in press)
19. Dirac P A M (1930) On the annihilation of electrons and positrons. Proc Camridge Phil Soc 26: 361
20. Brownell G L, Sweet W H (1953) Localization of brain tumors. Nucleonics 11: 40
21. Robertson J S, Marr R B, Rosenblum M, Radeka V, Yamamoto Y L (1973) 32-Crystal positron transverse section detector. In: Freedman G S (ed) Tomographic Imaging in Nuclear Medicine. New York: Society of Nuclear Medicine
22. Anger H O (1966) Survey of radioisotope cameras. ISA Trans 5: 311
23. Ter-Pogossian M M, Raiche M E, Sobel B E (1980) Positron-emission tomography. Sci Am 243: 170
24. Budinger T F (1977) Instrumentation trends in nuclear medicine. Semin Nucl Med 7: 285
25. Ter-Pogossian M M, Ficke D C, Yamamoto M, Hood Sr J T (1982) Super-PETT I: A positron emission tomography utilizing photon time-of-flight information. IEEE Trans Med Imaging MI-1: 179
26. Mullani N, Ficke D C, Ter-Pogossian M M (1980) Cesium-11 fluoride: A new detector for positron emission tomography. IEEE Trans Nucl Sci NS-27: 11
27. Snyder D L, Thomas L J, Ter-Pogossian M M (1981) A mathematical model for positron-emission tomography systems having time-of-flight measurements. IEEE Trans Nucl Sci NS-28: 3575
28. Budinger T F, Derenzo S E, Huesman R H (1984) Instrumentation for positron emission tomography. Ann Neurol 15: S35
29. Brownell G L, Budinger T F, Lauterbur P C, McGeer P L (1982) Positron tomography and nuclear magnetic resonance imaging. Science 215: 619
30. Phelps M E, Hoffman E J, Mullani N A, Ter-Pogossian M M (1975) Application of annihilation coincidence detection to transaxial reconstruction tomography. J Nucl Med 16: 210
31. Budinger T F, Rollo F D (1977) Physics and instrumentation. Prog Cardiovasc Dis 20: 19
32. Budinger T F, Derenzo S E, Greenberg W L, Gullberg G T, Huesman R H (1978) Quantitative potentials of dynamic emission computed tomography. J Nucl Med 19: 309
33. Snyder D L, Cox J R (1977) An overview of reconstructive tomography and limitations imposed by a finite number of projections. In: Ter-Pogossian M M, Cox J R Jr, Phelps M E, Davis D O, Brownell G L, Evens R G (eds) Reconstruction Tomography in Diagnostic Radiology and Nuclear Medicine. Baltimore: University Park Press
34. Snyder D L, Politte D G (1983) Image reconstruction from list-mode data in an emission tomography system having time-of-flight measurements. IEEE Trans Nucl Sci 30: 1843
35. Eichling J O, Higgins C S, Ter-Pogossian M M (1977) Determination of radionuclide concentrations with positron CT scanning (PETT): Concise communication. J Nucl Med 18: 845
36. Hoffman E J, Huang S C, Phelps M E (1979) Quantitation in positron emission computed tomography. 1. Effect of object size. J Comput Assist Tomogr 3: 299
37. Hoffman E J, Phelps M E, Wisenberg G, Schelbert H R, Kuhl D E (1979) Electrocardiographic gating in positron emission computed tomography. J Comput Assist Tomogr 3: 733
38. Mazziotta J C, Phelps M E, Plummer D, Kuhl D E (1981) Quantitation in positron emission computed tomography. 5. Physical-anatomical effects. J Comput Assist Tomogr 5: 734
39. Ter-Pogossian M M, Bergmann S R, Sobel B E (1982) Influence of cardiac and respiratory motion on tomographic reconstructions of the heart: Implications for quantitative nuclear cardiology. J Comput Assist Tomogr 6: 1148
40. Henze E, Huang S C, Ratib O, Hoffman E, Phelps M E, Schelbert H R (1983) Measurements

of regional tissue and blood-pool radiotracer concentrations from serial tomographic images of the heart. J Nucl Med 24: 987

41. Hoffman E J, van der Stee M, Ricci A R, Phelps M E (1984) Prospects for both precision and accuracy in positron emission tomography. Ann Neurol 15: S25
42. Parodi O, Schelbert H R, Schwaiger M, Hansen H, Selin C, Hoffman E J (1984) Cardiac emission computed tomography: Underestimation of regional tracer concentrations due to wall motion abnormalities. J Comput Assist Tomogr 8: 1083
43. Green M A, Welch M J, Mathias C J, Fox K A A, Knabb R M, Huffman J C (1985) Gallium-68 1,1,1-tris (5-methoxysalicylaldiminomethyl)ethane: A potential tracer for evaluation of regional myocardial blood flow. J Nucl Med 26: 170
44. Love W D, Burch G E (1959) Influence of the rate of coronary plasma flow on the extraction of RB^{86} from coronary blood. Circ Res 7: 24
45. Moir T W (1966) Measurement of coronary blood flow in dogs with normal and abnormal myocardial oxygenation and function. Circ Res 19: 695
46. Selwyn A P, Allan R G, L'Abbate A, Horlock P, Camici P, Clark J, O'Brien H A, Grant P M (1982) Relation between regional myocradial uptake of rubidium-82 and perfusion: Absolute reduction of cation uptake in ischemia. Am J Cardiol 50: 112
47. Heymann M A, Payne B D, Hoffman J I E, Rudolph A M (1977) Blood flow measurements with radionuclide-labeled particles. Prog Cardiovasc Dis 20: 55
48. Wisenberg G, Schelbert H R, Hoffman E J, Phelps M E, Robinson Jr G D, Selin C E, Child J, Skorton D, Kuhl D E (1981) In vivo quantitation of regional myocardial blood flow by positron-emission computed tomography. Circulation 63: 1248
49. Selwyn A P, Shea M J, Foale R, Deanfield J E, Wilson R, Brookes D, DeLandsheere C, Brady F, Turton D, Pike V (1984) Myocardial flow in patients with infarction. Circulation 70(Suppl II): II - 23
50. Yoshida S, Akizuki S, Gowski D, Downey J M (1985) Discrepancy between microsphere and diffusible tracer estimates of perfusion to ischemic myocardium. Am J Physiol 249: H255
51. Sapirstein L A (1958) Regional blood flow by fractional distribution of indicators. Am J Physiol 193: 161
52. Cannon P J (1975) Radioisotopic studies of the regional myocardial circulation. Circulation 51: 955
53. Bergmann S R, Hack S N, Sobel B E (1982) "Redistribution" of myocardial thallium-201 without reperfusion: Implications regarding absolute quantification of perfusion. Am J Cardiol 49: 1691 - 1698
54. Schelbert H R, Phelps M E, Hoffman E J, Huang S-C, Selin C E, Kuhl D E (1979) Regional myocardial perfusion assessed with N-13 labeled ammonia and positron emission computerized axial tomography. Am J Cardiol 43: 209
55. Bergmann S R, Hack S, Tewson T, Welch M J, Sobel B E (1980) The dependence of accumulation of quantitative assessment of perfusion. Circulation 61: 34
56. Rauch B, Helus F, Grunze M, Braunwell E, Mall G, Hasselbach W, Kubler W (1985) Kinetics of ^{13}N-ammonia uptake in myocardial single cells indicating potential limitations in its applicability as a marker of myocardial blood flow. Circulation 71: 387
57. Gould K L (1978) Noninvasive assessment of coronary stenoses by myocardial perfusion imaging during pharmacologic coronary vasodilation. I. Physiologic basis and experimental validation. Am J Cardiol 41: 276
58. Kety S S, Schmidt C F (1945) The determination of cerebral blood flow in man by the use of nitrous oxide in low concentrations. Am J Physiol 143: 53
59. Kety S S, Schmidt C F (1945) The nitrous oxide method for the quantitative determination of cerebral blood flow in man: Theory, procedures and normal values. J Clin Invest 27: 476
60. Kety S S (1951) The theory and applications of the exchange of inert gas at the lungs and tissues. Pharm Rev 3: 1
61. Landau W M, Freygang Jr W H, Roland L P, Sokoloff L, Kety S S (1955) The local

circulation of the living brain; values in the unanesthetized and anesthetized cat. Trans Am Neurol Assoc 80: 125

62. Lenzi G L, Jones T, McKenzie C G, Buckingham P D, Clark J C, Moss S (1978) Study of regional cerebral metabolism and blood flow relationship in man using the method of continuously inhaling oxygen-15 and oxygen-15 labeled carbon dioxide. J Neurol Neurosurg Psych 41: 1
63. Subramanian R, Alpert N M, Hoop Jr B, Brownell G L, Taveras J M (1978) A model for regional cerebral oxygen distribution during continuous inhalation of $^{15}O_2$, $C^{15}O$, and $C^{15}O_2$. J Nucl Med 19: 48
64. Frackowiak R S J, Lenzi G L, Jones T, Heather J D (1980) Quantitative measurement of regional cerebral blood flow and oxygen metabolism in man using ^{15}O and positron emission tomography: Theory, procedure, and normal values. J Comput Assist Tomogr 4: 727
65. Hack S N, Eichling J O, Bergmann S R, Welch M J, Sobel B E (1980) External quantification of myocardial perfusion by exponential infusion of positron-emitting radionuclides. J Clin Invest 66: 918
66. Hack S N, Bergmann S R, Eichling J O, Sobel B E (1983) Quantification of regional myocardial perfusion by exponential infusion of ^{11}C-butanol in canine hearts *in vivo*. IEEE Trans Biomed Eng 30: 716
67. Freygang Jr W H, Sokoloff L (1958) Quantitative measurement of regional circulation in the central nervous system by the use of radioactive inert gas. Adv Biol Med Phys 6: 263
68. Herscovitch P, Markham J, Raichle M E (1983) Brain blood flow measured with intravenous $H_2{}^{15}O$. I. Theory and error analysis. J Nucl Med 24: 782
69. Ypsintoi T, Bassingthwaighte J B (1970) Circulatory transport of iodoantipyrine and water in the isolated dog heart. Circ Res 27: 461
70. Roth A C, Feigle E O (1981) Diffusional shunting in the canine myocardium. Circ Res 48: 470
71. Rose C P, Goresky C A, Bach G G (1977) The capillary and sarcolemmal barriers in the heart. An exploration of labeled water permeability. Circ Res 41: 515
72. Bergmann S R, Fox K A A, Ter-Pogossian M M, Sobel B E, Collen D (1983) Clot selective coronary thrombolysis with tissue-type plasminogen activator. Science 220: 1181
73. Knabb R M, Burnes M A, Sobel B E, Fox K A A, Bergmann S R (1984) Myocardial perfusion following coronary thrombolysis assessed with positron-emission tomography (PET) with $H_2{}^{15}O$. Fed Proc (Abstr) 43: 709
74. White C W, Wright C B, Doty D B, Hiratza L F, Eastham C L, Harrison D G, Marcus M L (1984) Does visual interpretation of the coronary arteriogram predict the physiologic importance of a coronary stenosis? N Engl J Med 310: 819
75. Neely J R, Morgan H E (1974) Relationship between carbohydrate and lipid metabolism and the energy balance of heart muscle. Ann Rev Physiol 36: 413
76. Neely J R, Rovetto M J, Oram J F (1972) Myocardial utilization of carbohydrate and lipids. Prog Cardiovasc Dis 25: 289
77. Opie L H (1976) Effects of regional ischemia on metabolism of glucose and fatty acids. Relative rates of aerobic and anaerobic energy production during myocardial infarction and comparison with effects of anoxia. Circ Res 38: I - 52
78. Brachfeld N (1976) Characterization of the ischemic process by regional metabolism. Am J Cardiol 37: 467
79. van der Wall E E (1984) Myocardial imaging with radiolabeled free fatty acids. In: Nuclear Imaging in Clinical Cardiology. Simoons M L, Reiber J H C (eds) The Hague: Martinus Nijhoff Publishers: pp 83 - 102
80. Fox K A A, Abendschein D R, Ambos H D, Sobel B E, Bergmann S R (1985) Efflux of metabolized and nonmetabolized fatty acid from canine myocardium: implications for quantifying myocardial metabolism tomographically. Circ Res 57: 232
81. Weiss E S, Hoffman E J, Phelps M E, Welch M J, Henry P D, Ter-Pogossian M M, Sobel B E

(1976) External detection and visualization of myocardial ischemia with ^{11}C-substrates in vitro and in vivo. Circ Res 39: 24

82. Bergmann S R, Clark R E, Sobel B E (1979) An improved isolated heart preparation for external assessment of myocardial metabolism. Am J Physiol 236: H644
83. Lerch R A, Ambos H D, Bergmann S R, Sobel B E, Ter-Pogossian M M (1982) Kinetics of positron emitters in vivo characterized with a beta probe. Am J Physiol 242: H62
84. Lerch R A, Bergmann S R, Ambos H D, Welch M J, Ter-Pogossian M M, Sobel B E (1982) Effect of flow-independent reduction of metabolism on regional myocardial clearance of ^{11}C-palmitate. Circulation 65: 731
85. Schon H R, Schelbert H R, Robinson G, Najafi A, Huang S C, Hansen H, Barrio J, Kuhl D E, Phelps M E (1981) C-11 labeled palmitic acid for the noninvasive evaluation of regional myocardial fatty acid metabolism with positron-computed tomography. I. Kinetics of C-11 palmitic acid in normal myocardium. Am Heart J 103: 532
86. Schon H R, Schelbert H R, Najafi A, Hansen H, Huang H, Barrio J, Phelps M E (1981) C-11 labeled palmitic acid for the noninvasive evaluation of regional myocardial fatty acid metabolism with positron-computed tomography. II. Kinetics of C-11 palmitic acid in acutely ischemic myocardium. Am Heart J 103: 548
87. Fox K A A, Nomura H, Sobel B E, Bergmann S R (1983) Consistent substrate utilization despite reduced flow in hearts with maintained work. Am J Physiol 244: H799
88. Sobel B E, Weiss E S, Welch M J, Siegel B A, Ter-Pogossian M M (19777 Detection of remote myocardial infarction in patients with positron emission transaxial tomography and intravenous ^{11}C-palmitate. Circulation 55: 853
89. Ter-Pogossian M M, Klein M S, Markham J, Roberts R, Sobel B E (1980) Regional assessment of myocardial metabolic integrity in vivo by positron-emission tomography with ^{11}C-labeled palmitate. Circulation 61: 242
90. Schwaiger M, Schelbert H R, Keen R, Vinten-Johansen J, Hansen H, Selin C, Barrio J, Huang S-C, Phelps M E (1985) Retention and clearance of C-11 palmitic acid in ischemic and reperfused canine myocardium. J Am Coll Cardiol 6: 311
91. Schwaiger M, Schelbert H R, Ellison D, Hansen H, Yeatman L, Vinten-Johansen J, Selin C, Barrio J, Phelps M E (1985) Sustained regional abnormalities in cardiac metabolism after transient ischemia in the chronic dog model. J Am Coll Cardiol 6: 336
92. Goldstein R A, Klein M S, Sobel B E (1980) Detection of myocardial ischemia before infarction, based on accumulation of labeled pyruvate. J Nucl Med 21: 1101
93. Selwyn A P, MacArthur C, Allen R, Pike V, Jones T (1980) Myocardial ischemia: Metabolic studies using positron tomography. Proc 8th Eur Congr Cardiol p194
94. Pike V W, Eakins M N, Allan R M, Selwyn A P (1982) Preparation of (1-^{11}C)acetate — an agent for the study of myocardial metabolism by positron emission tomography. Int J Appl Radiat Isot 33: 505
95. Henze E, Schelbert H R, Barrio J R, Egbert J E, Hansen H W, MacDonald N S, Phelps M E (1982) Evaluation of myocardial metabolism with N-13 and C-11-labeled amino acids and positron computed tomography. J Nucl Med 23: 671
96. Knapp H W, Helus F, Ostertag H, Tillmann H, Kubler W (1982) Uptake and turnover of L-(^{13}N)-glutamate in the normal human heart and in patients with coronary artery disease. Eur J Nucl Med 7: 211
97. Gallagher B M, Ansari A, Atkins H, Casella V, Christman D R, Fowler J S, Ido T, MacGregor R R, Som P, Wan C N, Wolf A P, Kuhl D E, Reivich M (1977) Radiopharmaceuticals XXVII. ^{18}F-labeled 2-deoxy-2-fluoro-D-glucose as a radiopharmaceutical for measuring regional myocardial glucose metabolism in vivo: Tissue distribution and imaging studies in animals. J Nucl Med 18: 990
98. Phelps M E, Hoffman E J, Selin C, Huang S C, Robinson G, MacDonald N, Schelbert H, Kuhl D E (1978) Investigation of (^{18}F)2-fluoro-2-deoxyglucose for the measure of myocardial glucose metabolism. J Nucl Med 19: 1311

99. Goodman M M, Elmaleh D R, Kearfott K J, Ackerman R H, Hoop B, Brownell G L, Alpert N M, Strauss H W (1981) F-18-labeled 3-deoxy-3-fluoro-D-glucose for the study of regional metabolism in the brain and heart. J Nucl Med 22: 138
100. Ratib O, Phelps M E, Huang S C, Henze E, Selin C E, Schelbert H R (1982) Positron tomography with deoxyglucose for estimating local myocardial glucose metabolism. J Nucl med 23: 577
101. Krivokapich J, Huang S C, Phelps M E, Barrio J R, Watanabe C R, Selin C R, Shine K I (1982) Estimation of rabbit myocardial metabolic rate for glucose using fluorodeoxyglucose. Am J Physiol 243: H884
102. Livni E, Elmaleh D R, Levy S, Brownell G L, Strauss W H (1982) Beta-methyl(1-^{11}C)heptadecanoic acid: A new myocardial metabolic tracer for positron emission tomography. J Nucl Med 23: 169
103. Abendschein D R, Fox K A A, Knabb R M, Ambos H D, Elmaleh D R, Bergmann S R (1984) The metabolic fate of ^{11}C-beta-methyl heptadecanoic acid (BMHA) in myocardium subjected to ischemia. Circulation 70(Suppl II): 148
104. Fox K A A, Bergmann S R, Rand A L, Ambos H D, Sobel B E (1983) External measurement of myocardial oxygen extraction with O-15 labeled oxygen. J Nucl Med 24: P20
105. Ter-Pogossian M M, Eichling J O, Davis D O, Welch M J (1970) The measure in vivo of regional cerebral oxygen utilization by means of oxyhemoglobin labeled with radioactive oxygen-15. J Clin Invest 49: 381
106. Mintum M A, Raichle M E, Martin W R W, Herscovitch P (1984) Brain oxygen utilization measured with O-15 radiotracers and positron emission tomography. J Nucl Med 25: 177
107. Bergmann S R, Fox K A A, Geltman E M, Sobel B E. Positron emission tomography of the heart. Prog Cardiovasc Dis (in press)
108. Fikuyama T, Nakamura M, Nakagaki O, Matsuguchi H, Mitsutake A, Kikuchi Y, Kuroiwa A (1978) Reduced reflow and diminished uptake of ^{86}Rb after temporary coronary occlusion. Am J Physiol 234: H724
109. Schelbert H R, Phelps M E, Huang S C, McDonald N S, Hansen H, Selin C, Kuhl D E (1981) N-13 ammonia as an indicator of myocardial blood flow. Circulation 63: 1259
110. Rose C P, Goresky C A (1977) Constraints on the uptake of labeled palmitate by the heart. The barriers at the capillary and sarcolemmal surfaces and the control of intracellular sequestration. Circ Res 41: 534
111. Bing R J (1965) Cardiac metabolism. Physiol Rev 45: 171
112. Shrago E, Shug A L, Sul H, Bittar N, Folts J D (1976) Control of energy production in myocardial ischemia. Circ Res 38: I - 75
113. Most A S, Brachfeld N, Gorlin R, Wahren J (1969) Free fatty acid metabolism of the human heart at rest. J Clin Invest 48: 1177
114. Liedtke A J (1981) Alterations of carbohydrate and lipid metabolism in the acutely ischemic heart. Prog Cardiovasc Dis 23: 321
115. Stein O, Stein Y (1968) Lipid synthesis, intracellular transport, and storage. III. Electron microscopic radioautographic study of the rat heart perfused with tritiated oleic acid. J Cell Biol 36: 63
116. Abumrad N A, Park J H, Park C R (1984) Permeation of long-chain fatty acid into adipocytes. Kinetics, specificity, and evidence for involvement of a membrane protein. J Biol Chem 259: 8945
117. Fournier N, Geoffroy M, Deshusses J (1978) Purification and characterization of a long-chain, fatty-acid-binding protein supplying the mitochondrial β-oxidative system in the heart. Biochem Biophys Acta 533: 457
118. Fournier N C, Zuker M, Williams R E, Smith I C P (1983) Self-association of the cardiac fatty acid binding protein. Influence on membrane-bound, fatty acid dependent enzymes. Biochemistry 22: 1863

119. Ockner R K, Manning J A, Poppenhausen R B, Ho W K L (1972) A binding protein for fatty acids in cytosol of intestinal mucosa, liver, myocardium and other tissues. Science 177: 56
120. van der Vusse G J, Roemen T H M, Prinzen F W, Coumans W A, Reneman R S (1982) Uptake and tissue content of fatty acids in dog myocardium under normoxic and ischemic conditions. Circ Res 50: 538
121. Shug A L, Tomsen J H, Folths J D, Bittar N, Klein M I, Koke J R, Huth P J (1978) Changes in tissue levels of carnitine and other metabolites during myocardial ischemia and anoxia. Arch Biochem Biophys 187: 25
122. Whitmer J T, Idell-Wenger J A, Rovetto M J, Neely J R (1978) Control of fatty acid metabolism in ischemic and hypoxic hearts. J Biol Chem 253: 4305
123. Liedtke A J, Nellis S, Neely J R (1978) Effects of excess free fatty acids on mechanical and metabolic function in normal and ischemic myocardium in swine. Circ Res 43: 652
124. Corr P B, Gross R W, Sobel B E (1984) Amphipathic metabolites and membrane dysfunction in ischemic myocardium. Circ Res 55: 135
125. Hull F E, Radloff J F, Sweely C C (1976) β-Hydroxy fatty acid production during fatty acid oxidation by heart mitochondria. In: Harris P, Bing R J, Fleckenstein A (eds) Recent Advances in Studies on Cardiac Structure and Metabolism, Vol VII. Baltimore: University Park Press
126. Moore K H, Radloff J F, Hull F E, Sweeley C C (1980) Incomplete fatty acid oxidation by ischemic heart: β-hydroxy fatty acid production. Am J Physiol 239: H257
127. Moore K H, Koen A E, Hull F E (1982) β-Hydroxy fatty acid production by ischemic rabbit heart. J Clin Invest 69: 377
128. Owens K, Kennett F F, Weglicki W B. Effects of fatty acid intermediates on Na^+—K^+—ATPase activity of cardiac sarcolemma. Am J Physiol 242: H456
129. Smidt J L, Jaffe A S, Baird T, Galie E, Sobel B E, Geltman E M (1982) The interval of evolution of infarction in patients assessed by positron emission tomography. Circulation 66: II - 87
130. Sobel B E, Geltman E M, Tiefenbrunn A J, Jaffe A S, Spadaro J J, Ter-Pogossian M M, Collen D, Ludbrook P A (1984) Improvement of regional myocardial metabolism after coronary thrombolysis induced with tissue-type plasminogen activator or streptokinase. Circulation 69: 983
131. Phelps M E, Schelbert H R, Mazziotta J C (1983) Positron computed tomography for studies of myocardial and cerebral function. Ann Intern Med 98: 339
132. Schelbert H R, Henze E, Phelps M E, Kuhl D E (1982) Assessment of regional myocardial ischemia by positron-emission computed tomography. Am Heart J 103: 588
133. Lerch R A, Ambos H D, Bergmann S R, Welch M J, Ter-Pogossian M M, Sobel B E (1981) Localization of viable, ischemic myocardium by positron-emission tomography with ^{11}C-palmitate. Circulation 64: 689
134. Schelbert H R, Phelps M E, Hoffman E, Huang S-C, Kuhl D E (1980) Regional myocardial blood flow, metabolism and function assessed noninvasively with positron emission tomography. Am J Cardiol 46: 1296
135. Bergmann S R, Lerch R A, Fox K A A, Ludbrook P A, Welch M J, Ter-Pogossian M M, Sobel B E (1982) Temporal dependence of beneficial effects of coronary thrombolysis characterized by positron tomography. Am J Med 73: 573
136. van de Werf F, Bergmann S R, Fox K A A, de Geest H, Hoyng C F, Sobel B E, Collen D (1984) Coronary thrombolysis with intravenously administered human tissue-type plasminogen activator produced by recombinant DNA technology. Circulation 69: 605
137. Sobel B E, Geltman E M, Tiefenbrunn A J, Jaffe A S, Spadaro Jr J J, Ter-Pogossian M M, Collen D, Ludbrook P A (1984) Improvement of regional myocardial metabolism after coronary thrombolysis induced with tissue-type plasminogen activator or streptokinase. Circulation 69: 983

138. Sokoloff L, Reivich M, Kennedy C, Des Rosiers M H, Patlak C S, Pettigrew K D, Sakurada O, Shinohara M (1977) The (^{14}C-)deoxyglucose method for the measurement of local cerebral glucose utilization: Theory, procedure, and normal values in the conscious and anesthetized albino rat. J Neurochem 28: 897
139. Marshall R C, Huang S C, Nash W W, Phelps M E (1983) Assessment of the (^{18}F)fluorodeoxyglucose kinetic model in calculations of myocardial glucose metabolism during ischemia. J Nucl Med 24: 1060
140. Livni E, Elmaleh D R, Levy S, Brownell G L, Strauss W H (1982) Beta-methyl(1-^{11}C)heptadecanoic acid: A new myocardial metabolic tracer for positron emission tomography. J Nucl Med 23: 169
141. Elmaleh D R, Livni E, Levy D, Varnum D, Strauss H W, Brownell G L (1983) Comparison of 11C and 14C-labeled fatty acids and their beta-methyl analogs. Int J Nucl Med Biol 10: 181
142. Coma D, Maziere M, Marazano C, Raynaud C (1975) Carbon-11 labeled psychoactive drugs. J Nucl Med 16: 521
143. Frost J J, Dannals R F, Duelfer T, Burns H D, Ravert H T, Lanstrom B, Balsubramanian V, Wagner Jr H N (1984) In vivo studies of opiate receptors. Ann Neurol 15: S85
144. Wagner Jr H N, Bruns H D, Dannals F R, Wong D F, Langstrom B, Duelfer T, Frost J J, Ravert H T, Links J M, Rosenbloom S B *et al.* (1984) Assessment of dopamine receptor densities in the human brain with carbon-11-labeled N-methylspiperone. Ann Neurol 15: S79
145. Welch M J, Raichle M E, Kilbourn M R, Mintun M A (1984) (18F)spiroperidol: a radiopharmaceutical for the in vivo study of the dopamine receptor. Ann Neurol 15: S77
146. Strauss H W, Pitt B (1977) Noninvasive detection of subcritical coronary arterial narrowing with a coronary vasodilator and myocardial perfusion imaging. Am J Cardiol 39: 403

11. Assessment of glucose utilization in normal and ischemic myocardium with positron emission tomography and 18F-deoxyglucose

C.M. de LANDSHEERE[1]

Historical review

Cardiac glucose metabolism has raised much interest for many years. In 1907, Locke and Rosenheim [1] demonstrated the presence of glucose uptake in the isolated heart preparation of Langendorff. In 1914, Evans [2] suggested that carbohydrate oxidation is responsible for only one-third of the heart's energy whereas the other two third arises from fatty acids. Later on, Randle *et al.* [3] and Neely *et al.* [4] showed that during myocardial ischemia, glucose becomes the preferential substrate of the myocardium that and anaerobic metabolism is mostly maintained by glycolysis.

Carbohydrate metabolism can be divided into (1) glucose uptake (glucose transport and hexokinase reactions), (2) glycogen metabolism i.e. synthesis and degradation (reaction between glucose-6-phosphate and glycogen), (3) glycolysis (glucose-6-phosphate to pyruvate), (4) pyruvate metabolism (pyruvate to lactate, alanine or acetyl-CoA), and lastly (5) the citrate cycle [5]. In ischemia, the rate of perfusion in the coronary circulation is reduced, but in contrast to anoxia, some oxygen delivery is maintained and the products of metabolism such as lactic acid will accumulate. The effects of ischemia on myocardial glucose metabolism have initially been said to differ from the effects induced by anoxia. These differences are likely to be more relative than absolute when based on the rates of accumulation of inhibitory products which arise from oxygen deprivation [6]. In both circumstances, the main and first adaptation of myocardial metabolism is an increase in glycolytic flux that results primarily from the breakdown of glycogen [5]. Later on, inhibition of glycolysis can occur due to the accumulation of lactate [7]. Additionally, Opie [8] and Vary *et al.* [9]

1 Clinical studies presented here were performed at the Cyclotron Research Center of Liege with the cooperation of D. Raets, L. Pierard, C. Degueldre, P. Materne, V. Mahaux, V. Legrand, P. Lempereur, C. Chevolet, D. El Allaf, P. Marcelle, L. Crochelet, M. Fastrez, G. Del Fiore, C. Lemaire, L. Quaglia, J.M. Peters, M. Guillame, D. Lamotte, P. Rigo and H.E. Kulbertus, University of Liege, Belgium.

have documented an increase in the extraction of glucose by the ischemic myocardium.

In summary, during ischemia, stimulation of glycolysis and increased extraction of glucose provide glucose to cardiac cells. The magnitude of these changes depends on the duration and severity of ischemia and has major implications for the interpretation of results obtained from clinical studies with positron emission tomography (PET) and 18-fluorine-deoxyglucose (18-FDG).

Preparation of 18-FDG

Preparation of 18-FDG consists of two main steps. The first is the production of high radioactive amounts of 18-fluorine under the electrophilic form F2 and the second is to introduce 18F2 into 3,4,5,-tri-o-acetyl-D-glucose, the precursor of deoxyglucose. At the cyclotron of Liege (Belgium), 18F2 is produced with the use of the 20Neon (d,α)18F reaction with 13 MeV deuterons (other groups used 11 MeV energy) under a 10-15 μA intensity current. Bombardment of a high pressurized (13 kg/cm^2) Neon target in a Nickel or Monel cylinder yields a production rate of 12-14 mCi/μA.h of gazeous fluorine (F2) wich can easily be extracted from the cylinder when a minimum of 0.15% of molecular fluorine is present in Neon. A typical production run is characterized at end of bombardment (EOB) by a total yield of 120 mCi of 18F (F2) with a carrier average amount of 110-120 μM of F2.

The method used in Liege for the second step of preparation by Guillaume and Lemaire (unpublished data) is derived from the original work of Ido [10] and Shiue [11] with simplification and automatisation. The double bound of the ethylene group of triacetylglucal is saturated with acetylhypofluorite (CH3OOF) leading to triacetyl-fluoro-deoxyglucose. Since CH3COOF is obtained from the reaction: F2 + CH3COONa → CH3COOF + NaF, the radiochemical yield cannot exceed 50%. Triacetyl-fluoro-deoxyglucose is then separated, purified and hydrolysed with HCl 6M to form 18-FDG which is then ready to inject. If the total radioactivity (CH3COOF+NaF) is 100 mCi at EOB, the radiochemical yield leads to 25 mCi of FDG at the end of bombardment (specific activity: 1 mCi/μM) and to 17 mCi available at the time of injection.

The UCLA experience

In the isolated perfused heart, glucose labeled with 11-carbon (11-C) has a relatively rapid turnover (half-life 20 min with early production of 11-CO2) which makes its application to animal or human studies difficult [12]. The interest was therefore turned towards molecules with slower clearance. This is the case for 18-FDG which is characterized by a clearance rate of more than 2 h in rats and dogs [13]. The UCLA Group has studied the distribution of FDG both in animal experiments and in humans. Phelps *et al.*[14] studied the myocardial uptake and retenton of FDG, its blood clearance rate, the species dependence (dog, monkey, man) of myocardial uptake and the effect of diet on the uptake of FDG in the myocardium. A kinetic model was also suggested. Their data are summarized below.

The myocardial uptake of a tracer can be calculated according to the general equation (1)

$$\text{uptake} = F \times E = \frac{Q(T)e^{\lambda t}}{\int_0^T A(t)e^{\lambda t}dt} \tag{1}$$

where F is flow, E is the tissue extraction, Q(T) is the amount in the myocardium, at time T, λ is the physical decay constant, A is the arterial concentration [15].

For the calculation of the metabolic rate of FDG, the equation is:

$$MR = \frac{K[Glu]C_T}{\int_0^T Cb(t)dt} \tag{2}$$

where MR = metabolic rate for glucose K = a constant factor for all unknown parameters (rates constant for transport, enzymatic phosphorylation, glucose-6-PO4 utilization and FDG distribution volumes); (Glu) = capillary plasma glucose concentration at time T (mean time of PET measurement) expressed in units of mg/ml, Cb(t) is the FDG capillary plasma concentration at any given time between injection and time T. Cb(t) is preferentially obtained from arterial blood, but arterialized venous blood can also be used with good approximation [16]. The tissue concentration C_t is measured from tomographic image in μCi/g [14]. The integral in the denominator of the equation (1) is the area A under the blood arterial or venous curve from O to time T in units of (μCi/ml) x time. MR is expressed in glucose utilization units of mg glucose/unit time, per gram of tissue. Therefore the equation (2) can be reduced to

$$MR = \frac{k(Glu)C_T}{A}$$

Effect of diet on myocardial uptake of FDG

If MR_1 corresponds to the metabolic rate in fasting state, and MR_2 to the metabolic rate following glucose plus insulin infusion, a ratio MR_2/MR_1 can be calculated with the advantage that k cancels out. Phelps *et al.* [14] found a ratio of 2.8±0.1. By contrast, after infusion of glucose without insulin and without previous fasting, the ratio MR2/MR1 is 0.96±0.07. Therefore, the MR index appears to be sensitive to real metabolic changes and not only to variations in substrate supply.

Whole body distribution

In dogs, 3 hours after the morning meal, the whole body distribution of 18-FDG after intravenous injection shows higher uptake in the heart (3.4±1.1% of the injected dose) than in the brain (1.8±0.4%); in contrast, the monkey shows a lower uptake in the heart (3.7±0.8%) than in the brain (5.9±0.6%). In man, the normal cerebral uptake is found to be about 4 to 8% (6.3±1.8%) of the injected dose whereas the myocardial uptake varies from 1 to 4% (3.3±1.0%).

Blood clearance of FDG

Phelps *et al.* [14] demonstrated a rapid clearance of FDG from the blood and they schematically identified three components. The first and major component has a calculated half-life of about 0.2-0.3 min in both dog and man. This component probably results from dilution of the injected FDG in the total blood pool and extraction by highly perfused tissues before equilibration is achieved. The second component has a calculated half-time of 10-13 min (11.6±1.1 min) in man, whereas the third component has a half-time of 80-95 min (88±4 min). The second and third components are related to the continued metabolic extraction and also to the clearance by the kidneys. In summary, the extraction rate is initially high due to high initial 18-FDG blood content. Then, as a result of the blood clearance, 18-FDG accumulates slowly and finally reaches a plateau.

Mechanisms of 18-FDG myocardial uptake

It is likely that, in the myocardium, 18-FDG competes for transport sites and hexokinase. FDG-6-PO4 appears to be formed and trapped in the myocardium because of its low cellular membrane permeability and the low activity of glucose-6-phosphatase [4] for conversion of FDG-6-PO4 back to FDG (which can diffuse out of the tissue into the blood). FDG does not seem to be converted into glycogen (through glucose-1-phosphate) because 2-deoxyglucose inhibits the conversion of DG-6-PO4 to DG-1-PO4 for incorporation into glycogen [17].

Kinetic model of 18-FDG metabolism

The kinetic model of FDG metabolism has been summarized by Schelbert [18]. A tracer kinetic model was proposed by Sokoloff *et al.* [19] with 14-C-deoxyglucose and autoradiographic studies in rat brain. Calculations are based on the fact that deoxyglucose is involved in the initial metabolic steps similar to glucose but is then trapped in the cell. Forward and reverse processes are summarized by a three-compartment model where the exchange between compartments is described by first-order kinetic rate constants according to:

$$\text{FDG in plasma} \underset{k_2}{\overset{k_1}{\rightleftharpoons}} \text{FDG in tissue} \underset{k_4}{\overset{k_3}{\rightleftharpoons}} \text{FDG-6-P in tissue}$$

k_1 and k_2 describe the forward and reverse transport between the vascular compartment and the tissue compartment, k_3 and k_4 the exchange between the tissue and the metabolic compartment; k_3 depends on the hexokinase activity and this exchange is virtually unidirectional. The importance of k_4 is probably minimal in normoxic conditions but seems to increase markedly during ischemia [20]. Quantification of the myocardial uptake of exogeneous glucose by a tracer kinetic model requires the knowledge of the specific rate constants for the forward and reverse tracer exchange between the three compartments. In canine myocardium, Ratib *et al.* [21,22] have shown that the exchange of 18-FDG across the membranes and its initial metabolic steps are comparable to previous studies in brain tissue.

In the isolated, arterially perfused interventricular septum of the rabbit, Marshall *et al.* [23] have studied moderate or severe demand-induced and flow-reduced ischemia. They showed that the lumped constant and k_4 in each of the four experimental conditions were not significantly different from the values obtained from the nonischemic control and from values published by Krivokapich *et al.* [26] who studied the lumped constant under nonischemic conditions in the *in vitro* septal preparation. This stability of the lumped constant during altered myocardial metabolism produced by ischemia is advantageous for the calculation of the metabolic rate during ischemia.

The absolute rate constant values for bidirectional membrane transport, phosphorylation and dephosphorylation still remain to be determined. Marshall *et al.* [24] have used 2-glucose labeled with tritium to measure directly the rate constants of bidirectional membrane transport (k_1 and k_2) and phosphorylation (k_3) of glucose. The method is based on the principle that after phosphorylation, the tritium label of 2-glucose in tissue is irreversibly transferred to water in the isomerization reaction, a condition which is similar to deoxyglucose being trapped in the myocardium following phosphorylation.

In 1984, Schwaiger *et al.* [27] determined the absolute value and variability of individual k constants in nine healthy volunteers. Rate constants were determined by fitting myocardial and plasma 18-F concentration curves. The combined rate constant $k = k_1 x k_3 / k_2 + k_3$ for transmembranous exchange and phosphorylation averaged 0.039±0.021 ml/min/g and was comparable to the value previously found in canine myocardium [21,22]. Glucose utilization rates calculated with the 18-FDG model ranged from 1.8 to 13.2 mg/min/100g with a mean value of 7.2 mg/min/100g.

In patient studies, Marshall *et al.* [25] showed that a combined study of perfusion (with 13-Nitrogen-ammonia, 13-NH_3) and of glucose utilization (with 18-FDG) *at rest* allowed to differentiate myocardial ischemia from infarction. They studied 15 patients (mean age 53 years, range 41-76 years, 12 males, 3 females) and 10 normal volunteers (24-32 years old, six females, four males). Myocardial infarction (MI) was transmural in 12 cases (three inferior, seven anterior, two anterior and inferior) and nontransmural in three cases (two lateral, one anterior). The delay between the infarction and the time of PET study varied from 2 days to 13 weeks. No patient was studied during the hyperacute stage of infarction. Electrocardiographic (ECG) evidence of post-infarction ischemia was considered to be present if there was transient ST-segment depression of more than 1 mm or if T waves during chest pain were suspect for acute myocardial ischemia. No patient experienced chest pain during the PET study. Single vessel-disease was identified in two cases, two vessel-disease in three cases and three vessel-disease in seven cases. Coronary anatomy was unknown in three cases. Tomographic imaging was initiated 1-2 h after a carbohydrate-containing breakfast and additional oral glucose (40-50 g) was given 60-90 min before administration of 18-FDG. This procedure allows better evaluation of nonischemic myocardium by increasing the ratio of normal myocardial glucose to free fatty acid utilization. Infarction was identified with PET in a defined region if there was a reduction both in 18-FDG and 13-NH_3 concentrations by more than two standard deviations (SD) below the corresponding mean value obtained from normal subjects, in at least two contiguous 30° sectors. Similarly, myocardial regions were classified as ischemic on PET images if the positive difference in FDG-NH_3 concentration exceeded the corresponding value obtained in normal subjects by at least 2 SD in two or more contiguous sectors. All transmural infarctions except two (inferior MI) were identified by a parallel reduction of perfusion and 18-FDG uptake in an area corresponding to the localization on the ECG. Regarding the presence of angina, 11 patients had symptoms of ischemia either at rest (nine cases, with typical ECG changes in five) or during mild exertional angina (two cases). A disproportionately high 18-FDG uptake in a region of decreased perfusion was observed in ten cases, of whom nine suffered from angina. Therefore, only one false-positive signal of PET abnormality was noticed in this group. No tracer discordance between FDG and NH_3 could be demonstrated in five cases with two false-negative observations. The authors concluded that the presence of angina is positively correlated with a disproportionate increase of glucose utilization relative to perfusion.

More recently, Brunken *et al.* [28] have studied the distribution of 18-FDG and flow in 20 patients with chronic Q wave infarct regions. They observed a PET infarction in 32% of the Q wave regions, a disproportionately high uptake of 18-FDG relative to flow in 19% and a normal distribution of FDG in 49%. They also showed that wall motion abnormalities do not allow the differentiation of ischemic from infarcted regions.

Schwaiger *et al.* [29] have investigated the metabolic tissue characterization in patients with an acute MI. Among a total number of 29 left ventricular segments characterized by a decreased myocardial blood flow, 17 segments (59%) revealed relative or absolute increases in exogeneous glucose utilization. Regional wall motion analysis performed at the time of the PET study and 6 weeks later showed deterioration of contractility in two segments, no change in six whereas the contractility improved in nine segments. The authors concluded that persistent exogeneous glucose utilization detected by PET early after a MI can identify viable but jeopardized myocardium and may predict subsequent functional recovery.

The Hammersmith-Pisa experience

In Pisa, L'Abbate *et al.* [30] used 14-C-deoxyglucose and an autoradiographic technique in dogs and showed a higher uptake of deoxyglucose in the left than in the right ventricle. They demonstrated also a gradient across the myocardial wall with two times more deoxyglucose in the subendocardial layers than in the epicardium. If cardiac work is increased, for instance when a balloon is placed in the pulmonary artery, the uptake of deoxyglucose in the right ventricle becomes similar to the uptake in the left ventricle. The next step was accomplished by Camici *et al.* [31-36] who used 18-FDG for the study of glucose exogeneous utilization in normal subjects and in patients with severe coronary artery disease (stable or unstable angina). In 1983, Camici *et al.* [31] studied the distribution of 18-FDG (in comparison to 82-rubidium, Rb-82) which was injected during the recovery from exercise after clinical and ECG signs of ischemia had disappeared and after the distribution of Rb-82, used as a flow tracer, was back to control. Positron tomograms were recorded in seven fasting subjects (with stable angina), 45-60 min after the injection of 18-FDG. There was a high FDG:Rb uptake ratio in the ischemic region (defined by abnormal Rb distribution) in three patients and in the other four patients, an absolute increase of FDG uptake (ranging from + 30% to 70%) in the region corresponding to the Rb defect. The authors concluded that an increase in glucose uptake occurs in the myocardium as a consequence of transient ischemic episodes.

In order to investigate the significance of the increased uptake of 18-FDG relative to flow, Camici and Bailey [32] measured the myocardial glycogen content in isolated perfused working rat hearts during control, after 15 min of global ischemia and following reperfusion. At the end of the ischemic period, glycogen content was less than 20% of control whereas, during the first 20 min of reperfusion, the quantity of exogeneous glucose incorporated into glycogen was 2.5 times higher than during control. After 50 min of reperfusion, the rate of incorporation of glucose into glycogen was not any more significantly different from control (80% of glycogen being repleted). These data suggest that the increased FDG uptake in postischemic myocardium of anginal patients mainly traces repletion of glycogen.

Comparing the distribution of 18-FDG in patients with stable or unstable angina, Camici *et al.* [33] observed a different pattern of abnormal 18-FDG distribution between the two groups of patients. In stable angina, no disproportionately high 18-FDG uptake relative to flow was observed at rest whereas abnormalities appeared in the recovery period of an exercise-induced ischemic episode. In all cases, the increased uptake of 18-FDG was observed in the same myocardial region where transient Rb uptake defects developed previously. In contrast, in all cases with unstable angina, a region of high 18-FDG uptake relative to flow was already present at rest (in the absence of pain and of acute signs of ischemia in all patients but one). The effect of isosorbide dinitrate (intravenously administered at least 4 h before the PET study) was then investigated in the group of patients with unstable angina pectoris. In all patients, 18-FDG uptake was still increased in the same region as before, although the difference relative to normal areas was considerably reduced in all cases. At rest, during fast, 18-FDG uptake was negligible and not statistically different between patients, in non-affected segments and control subjects (fractional uptake respectively of 0.11±0.03 versus 0.07±0.04). In patients characterized by a regional Rb defect induced by exercise, if 18-FDG was given during exercise, glucose uptake was similar in normal and ischemic areas [34]. Relatively to the decreased flow in the area, the uptake of 18-FDG appeared to be increased in the affected segments, even if the patient was fasting. These observations were further documented by Camici *et al.* [35] who studied eight patients with severe stable angina pectoris under three conditions: injection in all patients of 18-FDG 8-19 min after the end of exercise (time needed for normalization of clinical symptoms, ECG abnormalities and Rb distribution), 2 min after the beginning of the stress test, a different day, (three patients) or at rest, another day (four patients). In all eight patients in whom 18-FDG was injected during the recovery from exercise, tracer uptake in the ischemic area (defined by the Rb abnormality) was between 1.21 and 2.00 times higher than in the nonischemic tissue. By contrast, differences between ischemic and normal myocardium were less sticking when 18-FDG was injected during the exercise (tracer uptake 0.74 to 0.98 in the ischemic region compared to normal segments). When the uptake of 18-FDG in non-ischemic myocardium was compared after injection during exercise or in recovery, Camici *et al.* [35] always observed a higher (80-170%) uptake during exercise. At rest, myocardial 18-FDG uptake ranged from 10% to 30% of the value obtained during recovery, from nonischemic tissue.

Camici *et al.* (unpublished observations) also compared the uptake of 18-FDG relative to flow in patients with severe coronary artery disease, before and after coronary artery bypass grafting. After surgery, they observed a complete normalization of regional myocardial blood flow and regional uptake of 18-FDG in most of the asymptomatic cases. In one patient restudied later with recurrence of angina, they could document a disproportionately high 18-FDG uptake relative to flow in an area supplied by an occluded graft whereas the first postoperative control had showed complete normalization in the affected territory.

Local results (Liege)

In our Hospital in Liege, streptokinase is generally administered intravenously if the patient is admitted within 3 h after the onset of symptoms suspects for an acute MI: it is suggested that this treatment mode may induce a reduction of infarct size. Studies using radioactive flow tracers like thallium-201 have been performed to assess the perfusion consequences of infarction, comparing rest and exercise thallium distribution [37]. This approach, unfortunately, has important limitations: regional blood flow can be severely depressed but focal areas of remaining viable myocardium can be preserved. As shown by the UCLA group, the combined study of regional myocardial blood flow and glucose metabolism with positron emission tomography allows to differentiate zones of infarcted myocardium without residual viability from zones with viable but compromised myocardium [25]. We have used FDG at rest as a metabolic tracer and 13-NH_3 or 38-potassium (38-K) as a flow indicator to test the hypothesis that early intervention of thrombolysis with intravenous streptokinase may improve myocardium viability in the area of the acute myocardial infarction [38, 39, 40]. Since we did not want to waste any time before the administration of thrombolytic therapy, no investigation with PET was obtained prior to the administration of streptokinase. In addition, since the recent literature strongly suggests that acute thrombolytic therapy is beneficial [41,42], we did not randomize patients and preferred to compare a group of patients submitted to fibrinolysis to another group of patients who did not receive streptokinase, because of contraindication to fibrinolysis or late admission.

In order to determine whether the presence of ischemia (demonstrated by single photon nuclear investigations with thallium-201) in a different area from the infarction could influence the relative distribution of regional myocardial blood flow and 18F-deoxyglucose utilization, we studied before and after coronary artery bypass grafting an additional subset of six patients who suffered from angina in the later course of the MI. This part of the investigation aimed at testing the hypothesis that, after successful improvement of flow by surgery, FDG distribution is no more disproportionately high in the affected area but becomes parallel to the distribution of flow. This suggests that the initial abnormality is due to ischemia and is of reversible nature.

Regional myocardial perfusion and glucose utilization were studied at rest in 30 patients and five control subjects. Patients were classified into two groups according to the delay between the MI and the positron emission studies. The larger group consisted of 24 patients studied early (10±4 days) after the acute event whereas a smaller group consisted of six patients referred later after the MI because of angina (83±44 days after the acute MI).

In the early group, patients were subdivided into two subgroups according to the treatment received in the coronary care unit, either with thrombolytic therapy (with intravenous streptokinase in 15 cases) or with conventional treatment without streptokinase (in 9 patients).

Characterization of patients is summarized in Table 1 which describes the location of MI and the extent of coronary artery disease. In the early group, there was a higher proportion of transmural anterior myocardial infarction compared to inferior, lateral and nontransmural MI and a 50% prevalence of multivessel disease (MVD). Patients of the "late" group were all characterized by a MVD. They suffered an anterior MI in three cases, an inferior MI in two and a lateral nontransmural infarction in one.

Positron emission tomograms were recorded at rest with a single-slice machine (ORTEC, ECAT-II). Three levels from the apex to the basis of the left ventricle were acquired. 18F-deoxyglucose (110 min half-life) was used for the study of regional myocardial exogeneous glucose utilization and compared with 13-NH_3 (10 min half-life) or K-38 (7 min half-life) used for perfusion analysis and injected prior to the administration of FDG. Perfusion data were normalized to the region of maximum cation uptake (defined as 100% of perfusion). The region considered as a reference for "normal" FDG uptake was the area corresponding to the region of maximum cation uptake.

Since uptake = flow × extraction, the ratio of FDG uptake to flow (F) is an expression of FDG extraction. This ratio DG:F will be close to 1 whether the distribution of FDG and 13N-ammonia or 38K are normal or abnormal in a

Table 1. Location of myocardial infarction and extent of coronary artery disease. T = treatment; SVD = single-vessel disease; MVD = multi-vessel disease.

Group I ("early")		
a) Thrombolytic T (n=15)	10 Anterior 5 Inferior	9 SVD; 6 MVD
b) Conventional T (n=9)	5 Anterior 1 Inferior 3 Nontransmural	4 SVD; 5 MVD
Group II ("late") (n=6)	3 Anterior 2 Inferior 1 Lateral Nontransmural	6 MVD

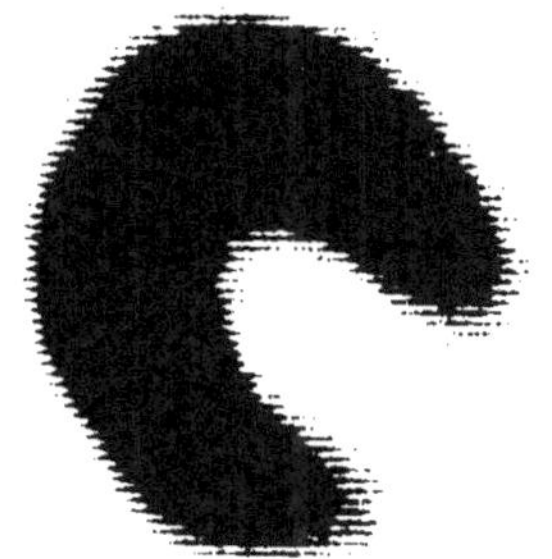
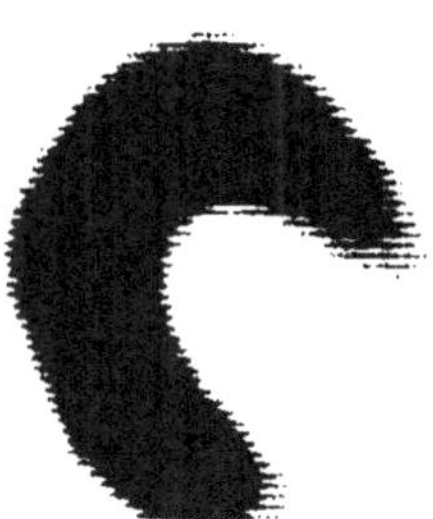

Figure 1. Regional myocardial uptake of 13N-ammonia (on the left) and 18F-deoxyglucose (on the right) are displayed in a transverse slice of the left ventricle (normal young subject). From left to right, the free wall, the anterior wall and the septum show homogeneous and similar distribution of both tracers.

similar proportion. In contrast, the ratio DG:F will increase if FDG uptake is disproportionately high in a region of decreased flow.

In normal subjects, FDG and perfusion indicators were uniformly and similarly distributed with a DG:F ratio of 1.13 +/— 0.14 (mean+/—SD). Figure 1 shows an example of tomograms recorded in a normal subject who successively received 13N-ammonia and FDG. In these transverse slices, the septum is on the right handside, the anterior wall on the top and the free wall on the left. This FDG tomogram was obtained 85 min and the 13N-ammonia scan was acquired 6 min after the injection, respectively. Distribution of both tracers is virtually identical. In this example, the DG:F ratio is 1.0 in the free wall of the left ventricle, 1.0 in the anterior wall and 0.98 in the septum.

In patients, the ratio DG:F was considered as abnormal if greater than the mean value of the ratio obtained in control subject plus two standard deviations. The threshold value of 1.50 was taken as upper limit of normal.

In the early group of patients who did not receive a thrombolytic treatment, only one out of nine — with a lateral nontransmural MI — had a high DG:F ratio (in the free wall of the left ventricle). In this untreated group, mean flow in the area of infarction was decreased to 32.5 ± 14.8% with a corresponding DG:F ratio of 1.42 ± 0.25. Figure 2 presents a mid-level left ventricular transverse slice obtained in a patient who suffered an anterior MI and did not undergo thrombolytic therapy. The 13-NH_3 tomogram is displayed on the left and 18FDG on the right. The distribution of both tracers is similar with a DG:F ratio of 0.98 in the MI region. Figure 3 illustrates corresponding profiles of

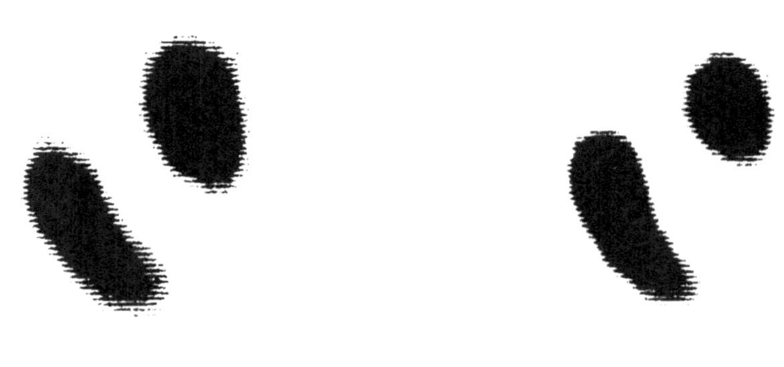

Figure 2. Regional myocardial uptake of 13N-ammonia and 18F-deoxyglucose recorded in a patient who suffered an anterior MI without thrombolytic therapy. Coronary angiography shows complete obstruction of the LAD after the first diagonal branch. The uptake of both tracers is markedly decreased, in a similar proportion, in the anterior wall of the left ventricle.

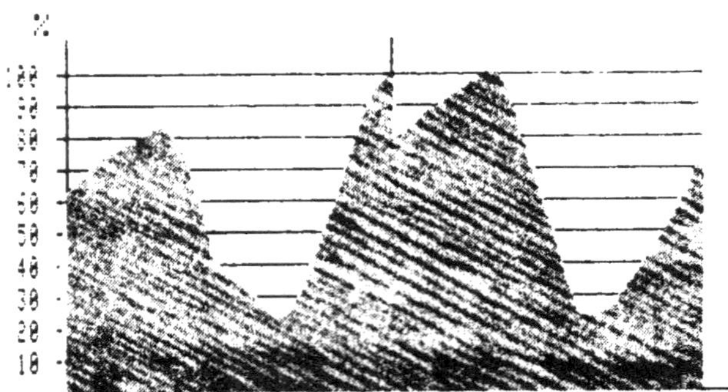

Figure 3. Profiles of activity expressed as the intrascan percentage of the maximum activity for 13-NH_3 (left) and 18-FDG (right). The uptake of both tracers is decreased to about 30% in the anterior wall.

activity from the posterior part of the free wall on the extreme left to the posterior part of the septum on the extreme right. Regional activity is expressed in percent of the maximal intrascan activity. At coronary angiography, the left anterior descending coronary artery was completely obstructed after the origin of the first diagonal branch. Ventriculography showed an anterolateral aneurysm confirmed by gated blood pool scintigraphy with a global ejection fraction of 30%. Two-dimensional (2D)-echocardiography demonstrated at mid and apical levels of anteroseptal and anterior walls a systolic wall thinning, an outward endocardial motion during systole and a diastole deformation

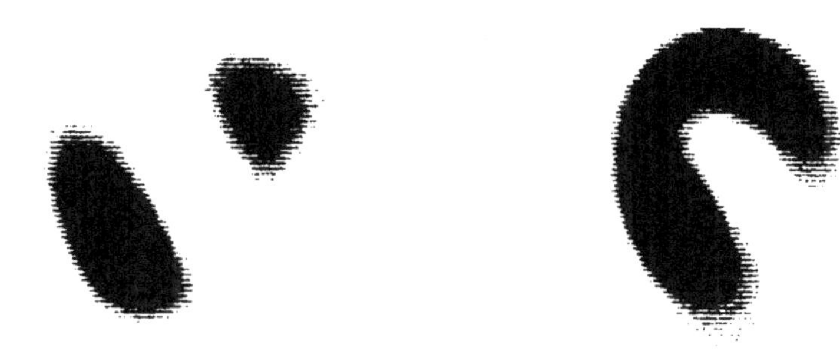

Figure 4. Discordant uptake of 13-NH_3 (left) and 18-FDG (right) in the anterior wall of a patient who suffered an anterior MI treated by 1 million units of streptokinase intravenously administered 2.5 h after the onset of pain. Coronary angiography performed after the thrombolysis reveals a 50% stenosis of the LAD after the origin of the first diagonal branch. The corresponding affected area of the myocardium is akinetic and the global ejection fraction of the left ventricle is 25%.

characteristic of aneurysmal dilatation. The conclusion of this study was anterior myocardial infarction accompanied by a left ventricular aneurysm, without demonstration of viable myocardium.

In contrast with the results of these patients untreated by thrombolysis, 13 of the 15 patients who received streptokinase had an abnormally high DG:F ratio in the area of infarction, with a mean value of 2.44 ± 0.68 related to a flow decrease of 36.7 ± 13.9%. In Figure 4, the distributions of 13-NH_3 and 18-FDG are discordant: there is a deficit of ammonia uptake in the anterior wall whereas FDG uptake demonstrates the presence of viable myocardium in this affected area. The DG:F ratio is abnormal with a ratio of 2.26 in the MI region of this patient who received one million units of streptokinase administered intravenously 2.5 h after the onset of chest pain. Figure 5 presents the NH_3 and FDG profiles of activity and illustrates the disproportionately high uptake of FDG relative to flow, in the anterior wall. Coronary angiography performed after thrombolysis revealed a 50% stenosis of the LAD after the first diagonal branch. Left ventriculography showed anterolateral and apical akinesia. Gated blood pool scintigraphy also showed akinesia in the same regions with a global ejection fraction of 25%. In 2D-echocardiography, no systolic thickening was observed in the anteroseptal segments, on the entire length of the left ventricle, in the anterior free wall (mid and apical segments) and in all apical segments.

In patients of the late group, referred for angina, the mean flow in the area of compromised myocardium localized in an area different from the site of infarction was 53.3 ± 17.7% with a corresponding abnormal DG:F ratio of 4.05 ± 0.98. All patients were operated on. In the affected area, the mean flow

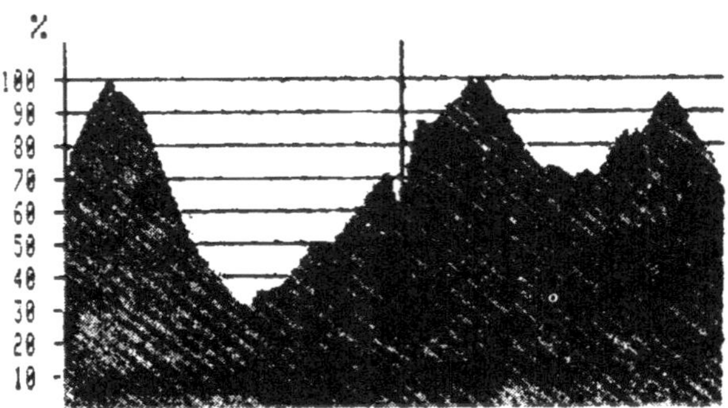

Figure 5. Profiles of activity of 13-NH_3 (left) and 18-FDG (right) demonstrate in the anterior wall (mid portion of each panel) a higher uptake of 18-FDG (in the order of 70%) than the uptake of 13-NH_3 (in the order of 30%).

increased to 79.9 ± 9.2% whereas the DG:F ratio decreased to 1.68 ± 0.22, a mean ratio which remains slightly abnormal.

In summary, in the group studied early after the onset of MI, a disproportionately high FDG uptake relative to flow was more frequently observed in patients who received streptokinase. These preliminary data therefore suggest that the thrombolytic treatment favours the salvage of jeopardized myocardium. Nevertheless, the small size sample does not allow definite conclusions. In the group that was studied later in the course of the MI because of angina, an abnormally high DG:F ratio has been demonstrated in areas different from the site of infarction. After coronary artery bypass grafting, regional myocardial blood flow was improved and the ratio DG:F was decreased. These concordant observations (six patients) seem to indicate that postoperative improvement of flow and decrease of DG:F ratio probably correspond to areas of reversible myocardial ischemia at a distance from the infarcted zone.

General discussion and future developments

Regional myocardial metabolism of fatty acid and glucose

Positron emission tomography has opened up the noninvasive access to the the study of tissue metabolism with major implications for the brain and the heart. Based on individual organ metabolism, radiotracers have been synthetized to answer specific research questions but each tracer only investigates some part of the metabolism and therefore provides limited metabolic information. In the heart, long-chain fatty acids and glucose provide the substrates for the majority of energy requirements. Long-chain fatty acids like palmitate are preferentially used under normoxic conditions and in the fasting state. Conversely, in ischemia or infarction, fatty acids are moderately or not at all extracted from blood to affected myocardium. 11C-palmitate was therefore used with positron emission tomography to quantitate the extent of infarction [43], to localize viable ischemic myocardium [44], to differentiate transmural and nontransmural infarction [45] or to assess the severity of ischemia by looking at the slowing down of palmitate clearance rate [46]. Bergmann *et al.* [47] have studied in dogs the uptake of 11C-palmitate after a thrombus induction with a copper coil and after thrombolysis induced by streptokinase injected 2.5, 4 or 7 hours after occlusion. They showed that myocardial salvage induced by thrombolysis markedly decreased (by a factor of 5) between 2.5 and 7 h after the initiation of streptokinase administration. This observation emphasizes the critical importance of the early streptokinase infusion. Beneficial effects of coronary thrombolysis were also demonstrated by Bergmann *et al.* [48] who observed in ischemic conditions either a reduction in palmitate clearance in ischemic zone ($t_{1/2}=43\pm24$ min) compared to the clearance of normal regions ($t_{1/2}=13\pm5$ min) or an accumulation of palmitate over a 20 min period. This was followed by a significant increase in the clearance of palmitate after thrombolytic treatment.

Glucose constitutes the other side of the coin: in comparison to normal areas which continue to preferentially utilize fatty acids, ischemic but still viable areas increase their extraction of glucose and are "positively" identified as a "hot" spot when a nonmetabolized glucose analogue like 18F-deoxyglucose is injected. Nevertheless, whereas the presence of ischemia is only identified by a "cold" spot after the regional distribution of palmitate, the situation is more complicated with glucose derivatives which can produce either a positive signal in moderate and mild ischemia or a negative signal in profound ischemia. At any flow rate, the regional myocardial uptake of 18-FDG depends on the product of flow X extraction. If coronary flow is reduced but still allows some delivery of the tracer, the fall in supply can be compensated by a dramatic increase of extraction responsible for a "hot" spot. If flow is further impaired, there is some evidence that the extraction also decreased, the overall result being a diminished uptake identified this time as a "cold" spot. Therefore, the proportion of FDG taken by regions of the myocardium supplied by stenotic vessels will primarily depend on the severity of reduction in regional coronary blood flow and residual potentials of glucose extraction by the affected area. This emphasizes the importance of the moment of injection in relation to the time course of ischemia: by definition, the injection of FDG will isolate a unique ischemic situation characterized by a precise flow value and a defined extraction. However, we have no idea about the exact duration of the ischemia and about the metabolic fate at the time of injection (beginning of the stimulation of the glycolytic flux? stores of glycogen completely depleted?). In other words, combined studies of flow and metabolism with positron emission tomography record a cardiac event at a definite time but do not provide any information on the temporal evolution of ischemia.

Regarding the assessment of flow changes related to the presence of ischemia, repeated studies of regional myocardial perfusion with Rb-82, at brief intervals, mainly demonstrate a prolonged recovery of flow after ischemia [49] the high frequency of changes in perfusion during spontaneous ischemia in anginal patients [50] and the importance of silent episodes of ischemia related, for instance, to mental stress [51]. The evaluation of metabolic changes over a short period of time is more difficult because, especially for glucose derivatives, for instance, the coefficient of myocardial extraction of 18-FDG is low and therefore the identification of myocardial regions is a slow process (minimal time of 45 min after the time of injection, for FDG, in fasting conditions), which excludes repeated studies at brief intervals.

The question of the time of injection

Because the combination of a flow and a metabolic signal (related to fatty acids or glucose) gives the unique opportunity to investigate the presence of regional myocardial ischemia at rest, and because the injection of FDG is more convenient and more reproducible at rest, the UCLA group and also our group have chosen this time of injection rather than the administration at peak exercise or in the early recovery. Other investigators, like the Hammersmith-Pisa group have chosen to inject FDG in the recovery time when clinical and ECG signs of ischemia have completely resolved with also normalization of regional myocardial blood flow (assessed with 82-Rubidium).

The question of the ideal time between the onset of MI and the time of the PET study

The determination of the ideal delay between the onset of infarction and the time of the PET study represents another question difficult to answer: because of the dynamic nature of infarction [52], especially during the hyperacute stage of MI, it would theoretically be more rational to investigate patients at a time when it is presumed that a stable stage is reached. It nevertheless seems more advantageous to perform a initial study with positron emission tomography as early as the hemodynamic conditions allow it: if the result demonstrates the presence of compromised but still viable myocardium, particularly in association with angina, there is no reason to waste time and the use of percutaneous transluminal coronary angioplasty or coronary artery bypass grafting can be suggested. If the result of the PET study seems to exclude the presence of viable myocardium because the flow and FDG uptake are decreased in a similar proportion, one can nevertheless argue that the myocardum is just stunned [53]. We therefore propose to repeat the study 1 or 2 weeks after the first investigation or earlier if the clinical status of the patient deteriorates, in order to determine whether the distribution of both tracers is still concordant or not. In addition, later long term follow-up PET studies are needed to compare the evolution of patients who were submitted or not to a revascularization procedure.

The question of the ideal time between CABG and the postoperative study raises an important dispute. It is likely that the slightly abnormal mean DG:F ratio (1.68), which we observed after surgery, is related to a somewhat short delay (about 6 weeks) between surgery and the PET study. Therefore, it is necessary to repeat the PET investigation at a later time, particularly in those patients with an abnormal postoperative DG:F ratio to elucidate this question.

The significance of a "hot" spot of FDG in the area of infarction

The significance of the "hot" spot identified in the area of infarction has been the subject of some controversy. In the area of an acute MI, neutrophilic leukocytes appear in large number: they may utilize glucose. This should be analyzed in relation to the timing of pathological changes: neutrophilic polymorphonuclear leukocytes have been identified at two different times: first, after 8 h, when the interstitium is oedematous with leukocytes infiltrating the muscle fibers and secondly, after 24 h, when the cytoplasm is clumping with loss of cross striations, dilatation of myocardial capillaries and accumulation of polymorphonuclear leukocytes that occurs initially at the periphery and then in the center of the infarction [54]. This progressive accumulation of leukocytes tends to last about 10 days, whereas the number of polymorphonuclear leukocytes is reduced while granulation tissue appears at the periphery. Later on, removal of necrotic muscle cells takes place, with ingrowth of blood vessels and fibroblastic activity until the fourth to sixth week following infarction [55,56]. These pathological observations have several implications: accumulation of leukocytes is a common phenomenon in the first 10 days after an MI; therefore, if this were the explanation for the disproportionate increase of FDG relative to flow in the area of infarction, all patients investigated during this period should demonstrate a "hot" spot which is, however, not the case. In addition, in the study of Marshall *et al.* [25], patients are studied later on, at a time when the accumulation of leukocytes does not exist any more and which therefore cannot explain an increase of FDG extraction. In conclusion, we believe that neutrophilic polymorphonuclear leukocytes can contribute, probably in small proportion, to the "hot" spot signal of FDG but their presence is not the primary responsible mechanism.

The compartmental model of FDG metabolism

Another source of controversy has been the validity of applying a compartmental model of quantitate glucose consumption in normal and ischemic myocardium. As pointed out earlier, it is very difficult to directly measure the k constants k_1, k_2, k_3, and k_4 involved in the rather simple metabolic fate of 18F-deoxyglucose. Discussion has been raised about the constant k_4 which can vary in relation to dephosphorylation changes. Additionally, the measurement of the total area under the blood curve can be difficult because some small components with long residency periods may be undistinguishable from background activity and still represent a significant portion of the total area. Moreover, calculations are based on the assumption that the radiolabeling of deoxyglucose with 18F gives only rise to 18F-deoxyglucose. Recent observations nevertheless suggest that the preparation is not so pure as previously considered and that 18F-mannose contaminates the final product [57,58].

Evaluation of the efficacy of thrombolysis with positron emission tomography

The evaluation of the efficacy of fibrinolytic treatment constitutes a fascinating field of research. There is evidence that this treatment completely modifies the natural course of the myocardial infarction at the level of pathological changes and hemodynamical parameters which will affect the cardiac metabolism [59]. We have to determine the proportion of salvaged myocardium related to the administration of various fibrinolytic drugs and to demonstrate which one is the most efficient without major side-effects (streptokinase, urokinase or human tissue-type plasminogen activator?). Clinicians also want to know the best procedure to apply after thrombolysis. Moreover, they like to be informed whether compromised but still viable myocardium can be demonstrated by the combined use of the flow tracer and 18F-deoxyglucose, especially in the absence of clinical signs of ischemia.

Future developments

Future developments will probably be linked to progress in physical characteristics of positron emission tomographic systems and to the preparation of new tracers. Whereas the initial machines could only acquire one slice, with an intrinsic resolution in the order of 18 mm at full width half maximum, new systems allow to record as many as 7 to 15 slices simultaneously with an intrinsic resolution in the order of 4 mm [60,61]. These advantageous physical characteristics most probably will improve the detection of smaller abnormalities in the distribution of flow and metabolic tracers. This question is important because the pattern of MI is heterogeneous. Applying the reference technique for measurement of flow i.e. 11C-microspheres (validation in dog by Wilson *et al.* [62], Selwyn *et al.* [63] demonstrated that necrosis is patchy with survival of tissue.

There is also a need to radiosynthetize new tracers of metabolism with a higher myocardial extraction and a shorter half-life than 18-FDG. In addition, receptor-binding radiotracers are being used increasingly to study the function of receptors in the brain and in the heart [64].

Among several advantages (noninvasive technique, high image resolution...), nuclear magnetic resonance can assess the amount of high energy phosphates (ATP) in the myocardial cell [65,66]. This is of major interest since the amount of ATP produced in the cells strictly reflects its metabolism [67]: in aerobic conditions, the oxidative metabolism (mitochondrial activity) provides large quantities of ATP. Once the balance between the supply and the demand of oxygen is broken, at the beginning of ischemia, glycolytic flux is enhanced and allows some ATP production. However, in comparison to oxidative phosphorylation, the rate of ATP decreases and high energy phosphate stores decline [68]. Later on, if ischemia persists, glycolysis is progressively impaired and is finally completely blocked. Therefore, with the assessment of ATP reserves [69], nuclear magnetic resonance can provide some original information about the severity and the time course of ischemia.

Without any doubt, significant progress in the noninvasive regional evaluation of ischemic heart disease can be expected from the complementary use of nuclear magnetic resonance and positron emission tomography.

Acknowledgements

We wish to express our gratitude for illustrations due to C. Degueldre and A. Marchal. We thank A.M. van Cutsem for invaluable secretarial assistance.

References

1. Locke F S, Rosenheim O (1907) Contribution to the physiology of the isolated heart. J Physiol 36: 205
2. Evans C L (1914) The effect of glucose on the gaseous metabolism of the isolated mammalian heart. J Physiol 47: 407
3. Randle P J, Garland P B, Hales C N, Newsholme E A (1963) The glucose-fatty acid cycle. Lancet i: 785 - 789
4. Neely J R, Morgan H E (1974) Relationship between carbohydrate and lipid metabolism and the energy balance of heart muscle. Annu Rev Physiol 36: 413 - 459
5. Randle P J, Tubbs P K (1979) Carbohydrate and fatty acid metabolism. In: Berner R M (ed) Handbook of Physiology, section 2: Volume 1. The heart. The cardiovascular system. Bethesda, Maryland: American Physiological Society, pp 805 - 844
6. Liedtke J A (1981) Alterations of carbohydrate and lipid metabolism in the acutely ischemic heart. Prog Cardiovasc Dis 23: 321 - 336
7. Kubler W, Spieckermann P G (1970) Regulation of glycolysis in the ischemic and the anoxic myocardium. J Mol Cell Cardiol 1: 351

8. Opie L H (1976) Effects of regional ischemia on metabolism of glucose and fatty acids. Relative rates of aerobic and anaerobic energy production during myocardial infarction and comparison with effects of anoxia. Circ Res 38(Suppl I): 52 - 58
9. Vary T C, Reibel D K, Neely J R (1981) Control of energy metabolism of heart muscle. Annu Rev Physiol 43: 419 - 439
10. Ido T, Wan C N, Fowler J S *et al.* (1977) Fluorination with F2. A convenient synthesis of 2-deoxy-fluoro-D-glucose. J Org Chem 42: 2341 - 2342
11. Shiue C Y, Salvadori P A, Wolf A P, Fowler J S, McGregor R R (1982) A new improved synthesis of 2-Deoxy-2-(18F)Fluoro-D-glucose from 18F-labeled acetyl hypofluorite. J Nucl Med 23: 899 - 903
12. Weiss E S, Hoffman E J, Phelps M E *et al.* (1976) External detection and visualization of myocardial ischemia with ^{11}C-substrates in vitro and in vivo. Circ Res 39: 24 - 32
13. Gallagher B M, Ansari A, Atkins H *et al.* (1978) Radiopharmaceuticals CCVII: 18F-labeled 2-deoxy-2-fluoro-D-glucose as a radiopharmaceutical for measuring regional myocardial glucose metabolism in vivo. Tissue distribution and imaging studies in animals. J Nucl Med 19: 635 - 647
14. Phelps M E, Hoffman E J, Selin C, Huang S C, Robinson G, MacDonald N, Schelbert H R, Kuhl D E (1978) Investigation of (^{18}F)2-fluoro-2-deoxyglucose for the measure of myocardial glucose metabolism. J Nucl Med 19: 1311 - 1319
15. Budinger T F (1979) Physiology and physics of nuclear cardiology. In: Willerson J T (ed) Nuclear Cardiology. Philadelphia: FA Davis Company, pp 9 - 78
16. Phelps M E, Huang S C, Hoffman E J, Selin C, Sokoloff L, Kuhl D E (1979) Tomographic measurement of local cerebral glucose metabolic rate in humans with (F-18)2-fluoro-2-deoxy-D-glucose: validation method. Ann Neurol 6: 371 - 388
17. Sols A, Crane R K (1954) Substrate specificity of brain hexokinase. J Biol Chem 210: 581 - 595
18. Schelbert H (1982) The heart. In: Ell P J, Holman B L (eds) Computed Emission Tomography. New York-Toronto: Oxford University Press, pp 104 - 108
19. Sokoloff L, Reivich M, Kennedy C, Des Rosiers M H, Patlak C S, Pettigrew K D, Sakurada O, Shinohara M (1977) The (14C)deoxyglucose method for the measurement of local cerebral glucose utilization. Theory, procedure, and normal values in the conscious and anesthetized albino rat. J Neurochem 28: 897
20. Hawkins R, Phelps M E, Huang S C, Kuhl D E (1981) Effect of ischemia on quantification of local cerebral metabolic rates for glucose with 2-(F-18)-fluoro-deoxyglucose studies in man. J Cereb Blood Flow Metab 1: 37 - 52
21. Ratib O, Phelps M E, Huang S C, Henze E, Selin C, Schelbert H R (1981) Determination of myocardial glucose metabolic rate (MRGlc) by positron computed tomography (PCT) and fluoro-18deoxyglucose (FDG). J Nucl Med 22: P11
22. Ratib O, Phelps M E, Huang S-C Henze E, Selin C E, Schelbert, H R (1982) Positron tomography with deoxyglucose for estimating local myocardial glucose metabolism. J Nucl Med 23: 577 - 586
23. Marshall R C, Huang S C, Nash W W, Phelps M E (1983) Assessment of the F(^{18}F)fluorodeoxyglucose kinetic model in calculations of myocardial glucose metabolism during ischemia. J Nucl Med 24: 1060 - 1064
24. Marshall R C, Huang S-C, Nash W W, Schelbert H R, Phelps M E (1983) Tracer kinetic analysis of 2-^{3}H-glucose to measure myocardial glucose transport and phosphorylation. Circulation 68: III - 67
25. Marshall R C, Tillisch J H, Phelps M E, Huang S C, Carson R, Henze E, Schelbert H R (1983) Identification and differentiation of resting myocardial ischemia and infarction in man with positron computed tomography, ^{18}F-labeled fluorodeoxyglucose and N-13 ammonia. Circulation 67: 766 - 778
26. Krivokapich J, Huang S C, Phelps M E *et al.* (1982) Determination of myocardial metabolic

rate for glucose from fluoro-18-deoxyglycose. Am J Physiol (Heart Circul Physiol) 12: H884 - H895
27. Schwaiger M, Huang S C, Phelps M E, Barrio J R, Schelbert H R (1984) Noninvasive quantitation of myocardial glucose utilization by positron-CT in man. Eur Heart J 5(Suppl I): 116
28. Brunken R, Tillisch J, Schwaiger M, Child J, Marshall R C, Phelps M, Schelbert H (1985) Identification of residual viable tissue in chronic ECG Q wave infarcts with positron emission tomography. J Nucl Med 26: p86
29. Schwaiger M, Brunken R C, Grover-McKay M, Krivokapich J, Child J S, Tillisch J H, Marshall R C, Phelps M E, Schelbert H R (1985) Metabolic tissue characterization in patients with acute myocardial infarction with positron tomography. J Nucl Med 26: p87
30. L'Abbate A, Camici P, Trivella M G, Pelosi G, Taddei L, Valli G, Placidi G (1979) Uneven myocardial glucose utilization as determined by regional 14C-deoxyglucose uptake. J Nucl Med All Sci 23: 167 - 172
31. Camici P, Kaski J C, Shea M J, Selwyn A P, Jones T, Maseri A (1983) Increased myocardial glucose utilization in exertional angina. Circulation 68(Suppl III): III - 324
32. Camici P, Bailey I (1984a) Time course of myocardial glycogen repletion following acute transient ischemia. Circulation 70: II - 85
33. Camici P, Araujo L, Spinks T, Kaski J C, Maseri A (1984b) Persistent chronic metabolic abnormalities in patients with unstable angina pectoris. Circulation 70: II - 249
34. Camici P, Kaski J C, Shea M, Lammertsma A, Selwyn A, Jones T, Maseri A (1984c) Positive identification of ischemic myocardium by F18-deoxyglucose in angina patients. Eur Heart J 5: (Suppl I): 186
35. Camici P, Kaski J C, Shea M, Lammertsma A, Araujo L, Jones T (1985a) Selective increase of glucose utilization in the postischemic myocardium of patients with stable angina. In: Maseri A (ed) Hammersmith Workshop Series. Raven Press: New-York, pp 81 - 85
36. Camici P, Spinks T, Lammertsma A A, Araujo L (1985b) Metabolic characterization of stable and unstable angina pectoris with F18-Fluorodeoxyglucose and positron emission tomography International Symposium on Preservation of Myocardial Function, Vienna, p20
37. Legrand V, De Landsheere C M, Rigo P, Pierard L, Chevigne M, Henrard L, Collignon P, Kulbertus H E (1983) Early exercise testing combined with thallium-201 scintigraphy after a first acute myocardial infarction: angiographic and prognostic implications. In: Kulbertus H E, Wellens H J J (ed) The first year after a myocardial infarction. New-York: Futura Publishing Company, pp 145 - 160
38. De Landsheere C, Raets D, Pierard L, Marcelle P, Del Fiore G, Quaglia L, Lamotte D, Kulbertus H E, Rigo P (1985) Residual metabolic abnormalities and regional viability after a myocardial infarction: a study using positron tomography, F-18 deoxyglucose and flow indicators. J Am Coll Cardiol 5: 451
39. De Landsheere C, Raets D, Pierard L, Materne P, Del Fiore G, Lemaire C, Quaglia L, Guillaume M, Peters J M, Lamotte D, Kulbertus H E, Rigo P (1986) Fibrinolysis and viable myocardium after an acute infarction: a study of regional perfusion and glucose utilization with positron emission tomography. Circulation 72: III-393
40. Rigo P, De Landsheere C, Raets D, Chevolet M, Beckers J, Lempereur P, Del Fiore G, Lemaire C, Lamotte D, Kulbertus H (1981) Demonstration by positron tomography and F-18 deoxyglucose of regional myocardial viability after myocardial infarction: influence of fibrinolysis and revascularization. J Nucl Med 26: P87
41. Relman A S (1985) Intravenous thrombolysis in acute myocardial infarction. A progress report. N Engl J Med 312: 915
42. The TIMI Study Group (1985) The thrombolysis in myocardial infarction (TIMI trial). N Engl J Med 312: 932
43. Weiss E S, Ahmed S A, Welch M J, Williamson J R, Ter-Pogossian M M, Sobel B E (1977)

Quantification of infarction in cross sections of canine myocardium in vivo with positron-emission transaxial tomography and ^{11}C-palmitate. Circulation 55: 66 - 73
44. Lerch R A, Ambos H D, Bergmann S R, Welch M J, Ter-Pogossian M M, Sobel B E (1981) Localization of viable ischemic myocardium ly positron-emission tomography with 11C-palmitate. Circulation 64: 689 - 699.
45. Geltman E M, Biello D, Welch M J, Ter-Pogossian M M, Roberts R, Sobel B E (1982) Characterization of nontransmural myocardial infarction by positron-emission tomography. Circulation 65: 747 - 755
46. Schon H R, Schelbert H R, Najafi A, Hansen H, Robinson G R, Huang S C, Barrio J, Phelps M E (1982) ^{11}C-labeled palmitic acid for the noninvasive evaluation of regional myocardial fatty acid metabolism with positron computed tomography. II. Kinetics of ^{11}C-palmitic acid in acutely ischemic myocardium. Am Heart J 103: 548
47. Bergmann S R, Lerch R A, Welch M J, Ter-Pogossian M M, Sobel B E (1981) The temporal dependence of restoration of myocardial metabolism by thrombolysis assessed with positron-emission tomography. Circulation 64: IV - 195
48. Bergmann S R, Fox K A A, Knabb R M, Burnes M A, Sobel B E (1984) Effect of coronary thrombolysis on regional myocardial perfusion and metabolism assessed with positron-emisssion tomography. Circulation 64: IV - 195
49. Selwyn A P, Allan R M, L'Abbate A, Horlock P, Camici P, Clarke J, O'Brien H, Grant P (1982) The relationship between regional myocardial uptake of Rb-82 and perfusion: absolute reduction of cation uptake in ischemia. Am J Cardiol 50: 112
50. Shea M, Deanfield J E, Wilson R, De Landsheere C M, Jonathan A, Kensett M, Maseri A, Selwyn A P (1984) Frequency of changes in perfusion during spontaneous ischemia in anginal patients. Br Heart J 51: 118
51. Deanfield J E, Shea M, Kensett M, Horlock P, Wilson R, De Landsheere C M, Selwyn A P (1984) Silent myocardial ischemia due to mental stress. Lancet ii: 1001 - 1005
52. Sobel B E, Braunwald E (1980) Limitations of infarct size in the management of acute myocardial infarction. In: Braunwald E (ed) Heart Disease, A textbook of cardiovascular medicine. Philadelphia: WB Saunders Company, p 1373
53. Braunwald E, Kloner R A (1982) The stunned myocardium: prolonged postischemic ventricular dysfunctions. Circulation 66: 1146 - 1149
54. Bouchardy B, Majno G (1974) Histopathology of early myocardial infarcts. A new approach Ann J Pathol 74: 301
55. Mallory G K, White P D, Salcedo-Salger J (1939) The speed of healing myocardial infarction: a study of the pathological anatomy in seventy-two cases. Am Heart J 18: 647
56. Fishbein M C, Maclean D, Maroko P R (1978) The histopathological evolution of myocardial infarction. Chest 73: 843
57. Bida G T, Satyamurthy N, Barrio F R (1984) The synthesis of 2-(F18)Fluoro-2-Deoxy-D-glucose using glycals. J Nucl Med 25: 1327 - 1334
58. van Rijn C J S, Herscheid J D M, Visser G W M, Hoekstra A (1985) On the stereoselectivity of the reaction of (^{18}F)acitylhypofluorite with glucals. Int J Appl Radiat Isot 36: 111 - 115
59. Ellis S G, Henschke C I, Sandor T, Wynne J, Braunwald E, Kloner R A (1983) Time course of function and biochemical recovery of myocardium salvaged by reperfusion. J Amer Coll Cardiol 1: 1047 - 1055
60. Hoffman E J, Ricci A R, van der Steel M A N, Phelps M E (1983) ECAT III — Basic design considerations. IEEE Trans Nucl Sci NS-30: 729 - 733
61. Derenzo S E, Budinger T F, Vuletich T (1983) High resolution positron emission tomography using small bismuth germanate crystals and individual photosensors. IEEE Trans Nucl Sci NS-30: 665 - 670
62. Wilson R A, Shea M J, De Landsheere C M, Turton D, Brady F, Deanfield J E, Selwyn A P

(1984) Validation of quantitation of regional myocardial blood flow in vivo with ^{11}C-labeled human albumin microspheres and positron emission tomography. Circulation 70: 717 - 723

63. Selwyn A P, Shea M, Foale R, Deanfield J E, Wilson R, De Landsheere C M, Turton D L, Brady F, Pike V W, Brookes D I. Organ blood flow in patients with myocardial infarction: necrosis is patchy with survival of tissue circulation (in press)
64. Kilbourn M R, Zalutsky M R (1985) Research and clinical potential of receptor based radiopharmaceuticals. J Mol Cell Cardiol 1: 351
65. Goldman M R, Pohost G M, Ingwall J S, Fossel E T (1980) Nuclear magnetic resonance imaging: potential cardiac applications. Am J Cardiol 46: 1278 - 1283
66. Goldman M R, Brady T J, Pykett I L, Tyler Burt C, Buonanno F S, Kistler J P, Newhouse J H, Hinshaw W S, Pohost G M (1982) Quantification of experimental myocardial infarction using nuclear magnetic resonance imaging and paramagnetic ion contrast enhancement in excised canine heart. Circulation 66: 1012 - 1016
67. Braunwald E, Sobel B E (1980) Effects of ischemia on myocardial metabolism. In: Braunwald E (ed) Heart Disease, A Text book of Cardiovascular Medicine. Philadelphia: WB Saunders Company, pp 1294 - 1297
68. Kubler W, Katz A M (1977) Mechanism of early "pump" failure of the ischemic heart: possible role of adenosine triphosphate depletion and inorganic phosphate accumulation. Am J Cardiol 40: 467 - 471
69. Flaherty J T, Weisfeldt M L, Bulkley B H, Gardner T J, Gott V L, Jacobus W E (1982) Mechanisms of ischemic myocardial cell damage assessed by Phosphorus-31 nuclear magnetic resonance. Circulation 65: 561 - 571

12. Nuclear magnetic resonance spectroscopy in experimental cardiology

C.J.A. van ECHTELD and T.J.C. RUIGROK

Nuclear magnetic resonance (NMR) spectroscopy is being used increasingly more as a tool to monitor nondestructively and, when required, noninvasively cardiac metabolism. In order to understand in what way and in what form NMR provides information on cardiac biochemistry and to be able to appreciate all the different possibilities and future applications, some basic knowledge on both the method and the instrument is required.

Every modern NMR-instrument consists of at least five important major parts:

(1) *The magnet*. The magnet has to generate a very homogeneous magnetic field. Most modern NMR magnets are liquid helium-cooled, superconducting solenoids with either a vertical or a horizontal bore of accessible diameter that may vary from 1 meter for whole human body type magnets to a few centimeters for so called high resolution type magnets. Magnetic field strengths may vary from 0.1 Tesla to 2.0 Tesla for whole body magnets and go up as high as 11.7 Tesla for high resolution magnets. (The earth's magnetic field is only 0.00005 Tesla.) When the NMR-instrument is to be used for magnetic resonance imaging too, the magnet is equipped with additional coils to generate magnetic field gradients.

(2) *The transmitter*. Once the patient, animal, tissue or sample has been placed in the centre of the magnetic field, the next step is to irradiate with short pulses of radiowaves. The frequency of this non-ionizing radiation depends both on the magnetic field strength and the atomic nucleus to be observed. Typical values range from a few megahertz (MHz) up to 500 MHz. The transmitter transmits the radiofrequency power to an antenna.

(3) *The coil*. The antenna, which transmits the radiofrequency (RF) power into the subject of investigation and subsequently detects the weak emitted RF signal is commonly referred to as the coil. It consists of a coil of wire or foil, which either surrounds the subject of investigation or is put on its surface as a flat, so called, "surface coil", depending on whether information is required from the whole subject or from a selected area.

(4) *The receiver*. The signal, which is picked up by the coil, is fed into the receiver where it gets amplified and mixed with reference signals.
(5) *The computer*. The signal finally arrives in the computer where it usually is added up to previous signals to improve the signal to noise ratio and where it is subsequently processed. Since the acquired signal normally shows a complex pattern of radiowaves with different frequencies, one of the computers main processing tasks is to unravel this complex pattern and transform it into an interpretable frequency spectrum by means of a so called "Fourier transformation". Furthermore, the computer is used to operate the entire system and is hooked up to several data output devices.

Many atomic nuclei behave, due to a property known as spin, as tiny bar magnets. When placed in a magnetic field, the tiny nuclear magnets present in the atoms that make up the many molecules of the object, will orient themselves either parallel or anti-parallel to the magnetic field. When the object is irradiated with a radiofrequency pulse, transitions between the two orientations can be induced. After the pulse the nuclei relax back to their equilibrium orientation, thereby emitting a weak radiofrequency signal. The frequency at which this so called resonance process occurs is directly proportional to the magnetic field strength and depends for a given magnetic field strength also on the type of nucleus, e.g. ^{1}H, ^{13}C, ^{31}P, etc. (see Table 1).

More precisely, the exact resonance frequency of a particular nucleus depends on the local magnetic field experienced by that nucleus. The electrons

Table 1. Resonance frequencies and NMR properties of some nuclei commonly studied in medicine and biology

Nucleus	Natural abundance (%)	Relative[a] sensitivity (%)	Resonance frequency at 1 Tesla (MHz)	
^{1}H	99.98	100.0	42.58	
^{19}F	100.0	83.0	40.05	17.237257 Pi[c]
				17.237172 CP
^{31}P	100.0	6.6	17.24	17.237131 γ-ATP
				17.237042 α-ATP
^{23}Na	100.0	9.3	11.26	17.236895 β-ATP
^{13}C[b]	1.1	1.6	10.71	

[a] Relative sensitivity is the NMR sensitivity of a number of nuclei relative to that of an equal number of protons.

[b] The most abundant isotope of carbon, ^{12}C, has zero spin and therefore produces no NMR signal, as is the case for ^{16}O.

[c] These resonance frequencies are accurate relative to one another but their absolute values depend very much on experimental conditions. They only serve the purpose of demonstrating the relative difference in resonance frequency between the different nuclei and the extent of a chemical shift range.

surrounding the nucleus shield it from the externally applied magnetic field and thereby influence the local magnetic field at the nucleus. Therefore, the resonance frequency depends on the surrounding electrons and consequently on the chemical environment of the nucleus. This property is known as "chemical shift", which reflects the separation of a resonance frequency ν_i from an arbitrarily chosen reference frequency ν_r and is defined as

$$\delta = \frac{\nu_i - \nu_r}{\nu_r} \times 10^6 \quad \text{ppm}$$

and is expressed in terms of the dimensionless unit of parts per million (ppm). It is this chemical shift that allows us to discriminate between for instance the different phosphorus nuclei, which are present in myocardial tissue, such as inorganic phosphate (P_i), phosphocreatine (PCr) and the three different phosphate groups of adenosine triphosphate (ATP), which all show up as different resonance peaks in a frequency spectrum (see also Figure 1). Since protonation of a phosphate group changes the chemical environment of the nucleus, it will also change its resonance frequency. Alternatively, determining such a resonance frequency allows us to measure intracellular pH [1-3]. Other "external" factors may also influence resonance frequencies: it could be shown from the difference in chemical shift between Mg-ATP and uncomplexed ATP that in skeletal muscle >95% of ATP is complexed to Mg^{2+}-ions [4].

Since the NMR signal is in principle proportional to the number of nuclei, that are present in the observed volume, it is evident that the NMR-technique is a powerful tool for nondestructive, quantitative determinations of myocardial metabolites and pH. Therefore it can be used to follow the metabolism of an individual heart during a series of interventions.

Unfortunately, the NMR method suffers from an inherently low sensitivity. The signal to noise ratio of a resonance peak depends on a number of factors, including:

— the type of nucleus that is observed. Table 1 gives the relative sensitivity and natural abundance of the different nuclei. Each of the mentioned nuclei has additional advantages, disadvantages and specific areas of application. The relative merits of the different nuclei for cardiac research will be discussed below;

— the strength of the magnetic field. Generally, the sensitivity increases for most nuclei when the magnetic field strength increases. ^{31}P in tissue metabolites may represent an exception, although the optimal field strength is still a matter of discussion;

— the type of molecule in which the observed nucleus is present. Narrow signals are usually only obtained from nuclei in molecules that are fairly mobile. Nuclei in large immobile molecules like ^{31}P in bone, membrane

— phospholipid or DNA give rise to very broad resonance lines underlying the narrow peaks from mobile metabolites;

measurement time. The signal to noise ratio can be improved by signal averaging. The repetition time between the individual scans is partially dictated by the time it takes for the nuclei to relax back to their equilibrium orientations, a process described by two relaxation time constants T_1 and T_2. Increasing measurement time of course decreases time resolution. However, it is possible by using NMR pulses, which are triggered by the heart beat, to obtain in a series of differently timed experiments information on tissue metabolite concentrations during several intervals of the cardiac cycle [5];

— the efficiency and type of radiofrequency coil. The, normally cylindrical, coil that completely surrounds the tissue detects signal from the enclosed cylinder. The better this cylinder is filled with the tissue of interest, the better the sensitivity. The flat, normally circular, surface coil detects as a rule signal from half a sphere subtending the coil, with the same diameter as the coil;

— the number of observed nuclei. The signal intensity is directly proportional to the number of nuclei in the sample volume. The number of nuclei can be easily increased by increasing the sample volume or amount of tissue (of course often together with an increase in coil size). However, increasing the amount of tissue will often contradict required localization.

In order to produce useful and relevant results, the NMR method has to allow for some way of localization. For the heart there are several ways to achieve this localization:

(a) Excision. The first pioneering cardiac NMR research has been done using isolated Langendorff [6] perfused rat hearts [7-9]. The perfused hearts are placed inside a cylindrical coil and are studied with a narrow bore magnet.

(b) A further refinement of this method has been achieved by using the isolated, Langendorff perfused rabbit heart with a small surface coil to detect regional ischemia [10].

(c) To study rat hearts *in situ* solenoidal coils have been surgically introduced to fit around the hearts inside the mechanically ventilated animals [11,12]. Small contributions to the signal from blood are unavoidably picked up when using this method.

(d) To allow for long-term studies and to avoid some of the adverse effects of surgery coils have also been chronically implanted around the heart. Rats were observed to tolerate the coils for up to 6 months [13].

(e) Another invasive approach has been the introduction of a small surface coil as a so called catheter coil into left and right ventricle of canine hearts. A 20 cm bore, 1.9 Tesla magnet has been used for these studies [14]. However, a surface coil used this way detects signal from both sides of the coil and localization is not easily done.

(f) Surface coils have also been straightforwardly placed on the thorax. The detected signal may contain contributions from bone, blood and skeletal muscle too, depending on the actual size and precise position of the coil. However, this approach is very easily to reconcile with clinical methods and has in fact been used as such already [15].

(g) The surface coil method has been refined by combining it with a NMR-imaging derived slice selection technique, resulting in depth resolved sur face coil spectroscopy [16]. With this method 1 cm thick slices, parallel to the coil, of dog hearts *in situ* have yielded good quality ^{31}P spectra within 20 min [17].

(h) Another NMR-imaging related method, rotating frame spectroscopic imaging, in combination with a surface coil can also give spectra from planar slices of the heart, which already has been demonstrated for the human heart [18].

(i) Narrow resonance peaks are only obtained from metabolites present in a homogeneous magnetic field. When the magnetic field is very inhomogeneous the narrow resonance peaks become very broad lines, almost indistinguishable from the baseline. In a method known as topical magnetic resonance [19] or field profiling, the magnetic field is made deliberately inhomogeneous except for a small homogeneous volume, which yields narrow resonance peaks. The method can be used with both cylindrical and surface coils. However, the sensitive volume can only be made smaller or bigger but can not be moved and it has rather poorly defined boundaries. Studies on hearts using this method have been mentioned scarcely.

(j) Final promising methods of localization are so called volume selective excitation [20] methods. These methods allow to select a volume of interest anywhere within the (cylindrical) coil boundaries, but are less sensitive than some of the previous methods and as yet no results on heart studies with this method have been published.

When comparing the different nuclei, it appears that very few NMR spectroscopic heart studies have been done with ^{19}F and ^{23}Na.

The same is true for ^{1}H, but recently substantial progress has been made in *in vivo* ^{1}H spectroscopy of other organs like brain [21,22] and skeletal muscle [23]. The major advantage of ^{1}H-NMR spectroscopy is the relatively high NMR sensitivity of the proton. Disadvantages are the relatively small chemical shift range (~ 12 ppm), which, due to the ubiquity of protons in biological molecules, sometimes results in very crowded spectra and overlapping peaks and the enormous amount of signal coming from tissue H_2O. The spectral dispersion can be increased by increasing the magnetic field strength, and overlapping peaks have been resolved by using special selective RF-pulse sequences [24]. Several powerful, sophisticated NMR-pulse methods have been applied to suppress the large water signal [21-24]. In this way it has been possible to measure in a few minutes or less, numerous metabolites like lactate, N-acetylaspartate, creatine, phosphocreatine, alanine, glutamate etc. A practical detection limit of less than 0.1 mM may well be reached. Although the motion of the heart makes it a more difficult organ to study with NMR than brain or skeletal muscle, similar results may be expected for ^{1}H-spectroscopy of myocardial tissue. When combined with some localization method, measuring tissue lactate may well become a method for determining ischemia that can also be used clinically.

Carbon-13 has a much wider chemical shift range (~ 200 ppm) and therefore gives spectra which are easier to interpret than proton spectra. Unfortunately, ^{13}C is far less sensitive than ^{1}H. In addition, the natural abundance is only 1.1% (see Table 1); the major carbon isotope ^{12}C is NMR-invisible. Therefore most of the ^{13}C *in vivo* spectroscopy is limited to those compounds that have been specifically enriched with the (nonradioactive) isotope ^{13}C. All different nuclei show, when they are close together either by chemical bond or in space, several homonuclear and heteronuclear interactions. Like the ^{1}H-^{13}C-coupling, they can show up in the NMR-spectrum as split peaks like doublets, triplets etc. By continuous irradiating with ^{1}H-frequencies this interaction can be "decoupled", thereby rendering the split peaks to single peaks, which greatly simplifies the spectra. Especially for ^{13}C this decoupling has the additional advantage of increasing the signal intensity (Nuclear Overhauser Effect). However, it introduces the necessity of a second coil for transmitting ^{1}H-frequencies next to the ^{13}C-coil making *in vivo* ^{13}C-spectroscopy more complex. Nevertheless, the method has been successfully used to study heart metabolism. Enrichment with ^{13}C has been achieved by incorporating enriched substrate in perfusate [25] or by intravenous infusion when using the open chest surface coil technique [26,27]. It has proven to be very useful method to follow many metabolic pathways including the Krebs-cycle, amino acid synthesis and particularly glycogen synthesis and glycogenolysis during anoxia [27]. Usable spectra from guinea pig hearts were obtained in 6 min.

Until now most NMR spectroscopic studies on hearts have been done using ^{31}P. The chemical shift range of biological phosphorus containing compounds (~ 30 ppm) is wider than the ^{1}H-chemical shift range and the number of phosphorus containing compounds is limited, which make the ^{31}P spectra fairly easy to interpret. Although ^{31}P has a~ 15-fold lower sensitivity than ^{1}H, ^{31}P-NMR is a very attractive method to assess tissue energetics and pH. One of the basic questions that has received some attention in experimental cardiac research is the variation of high-energy phosphate levels during the heart cycle. Using a gated NMR-method on an isolated working rat heart, a considerable variation in high-energy phosphate levels during the heart cycle has been measured [5], being maximal at minimal aortic pressure and minimal at maximal aortic pressure, whereas inorganic phosphate varied inversely with the high-energy phosphates. When a particular resonance is selectively irradiated, it may become temporaribly "saturated" and no longer produce a NMR-signal. The corresponding phosphate group thus becomes temporarily "magnetically" labeled and when this group participates in a chemical reaction

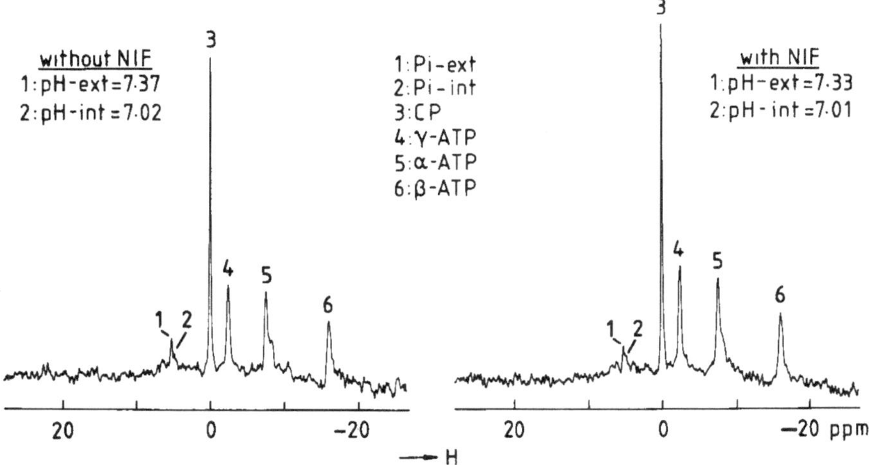

Figure 1. 81.0 MHz ^{31}P NMR spectra obtained in a 4.7 Tesla, 98 mm bore magnet between 20 and 30 min of control perfusion of an untreated heart (left) and a nifedipine-treated (NIF) (0.1 mg/l) heart (right). The spectra were obtained from 260 accumulated scans. The arrow indicates the direction of increasing field strenght or decreasing frequency. Numbered peaks include: (1) extracellular inorganic phosphate (P_i-ext), (2) intracellular inorganic phosphate (P_i-int), (3) phosphocreatine (CP), and (4), (5) and (6) the phosphate groups of adenosine triphosphate (ATP).

it can transfer its saturation. With this saturation transfer technique one can actually determine enzyme kinetics *in vivo*. Using this method it has been demonstrated in an isolated Langendorff perfused rat heart that only 2.5% of the total ATP is turned over during one heart cycle [28]. Using the implanted coil technique no difference could be detected from *in situ* rat heart spectra obtained at diastole and systole [13]. With the catheter coil approach this latter observation has been confirmed in dog hearts *in situ*, even when the rate-pressure product was increased 3-fold by right atrial pacing [29]. An explanation for the observed discrepancy may be a poor nutrient and/or oxygen supply in the isolated, working rat heart.

The calcium paradox [30], cardioplegia [31] and myocardial preservation [32] have also been studied using ^{31}P-NMR, showing the potential of this technique to evaluate different protocols.

The metabolic consequences of global or regional ischemia have been extensively investigated with ^{31}P-NMR [2,7-10,33-37]. The fast decrease of the phosphocreatine level at the onset of ischemia, followed by a slower decrease of the ATP level and a concomitant decrease of intracellular pH have been well documented. Metabolic recovery has been studied together with functional recovery, by determining left ventricular pressure, as a function of for instance the length of the ischemic period [34] or pharmacological treatment [10,37].

To illustrate this in more detail, the effects of the Calcium-antagonist drug nifedipine on intracellular pH during ischemia and reperfusion are described below.

Figure 1 shows normal ^{31}P-NMR spectra of isolated, Langendorff perfused rat hearts, obtained during control perfusion without and with nifedipine. pH values were measured from the chemical shift of the inorganic phosphate peaks. Extracellular pH (pH -ext) represents the pH of the perfusion fluid. Intracellular pH (pH-int) amounted to 7.02 in the untreated heart and to 7.01 in the nifedipine-treated heart. Table 2 shows the mean intracellular pH values of six hearts per group. Throughout the experiments the heart rate was maintained at 300 beats/min by left ventricular pacing with a KCl-wick electrode, and myocardial temperature was maintained at 37°C.

After 30 min of control perfusion, the hearts were made totally ischemic for 30 min. Severe myocardial ischemia has several important consequences, such as depletion of endogenous high-energy phosphate stores [31-38], intracellular acidosis [2,36,37,39], accumulation of calcium [40] and development of contracture [38]. Nifedipine given before or at the onset of a period of ischemia slows the rate of depletion of tissue phosphocreatine and ATP [37,41,42] and prevents calcium accumulation and contracture [40]. In addition, nifedipine prevents massive uptake of calcium during reperfusion and promotes the recovery of myocardial contractility [40]. Here we focus on the effects of nifedipine on the intracellular pH. The ^{31}P-NMR spectra in Figure 2, obtained between 20 and 30 minutes of total ischemia, show a marked increase of the intracellular inorganic phosphate peak. The corresponding intracellular pH values amounted to 6.11 in the untreated heart and 6.08 in the nifedipine-treated heart. In comparing these values with the mean intracellular pH values from six hearts (5.89 ± 0.03 and 5.92 ± 0.06, respectively) as shown in Table 2, it should be noted that the latter were derived from 130 accumulated scans,

Table 2. Intracellular pH values of untreated and nifedipine-treated hearts

	Intracellular pH (pH-int)	
	Without nifedipine	With nifedipine
Between 25 and 30 min of control perfusion	7.00 ± 0.04	7.04 ± 0.04
Between 25 and 30 min of total ischemia	5.89 ± 0.03	5.92 ± 0.06
Between 25 and 30 min of reperfusion	6.91 ± 0.04[a] 6.02 ± 0.06[a]	7.01 ± 0.12

Intracellular pH measurements were obtained from spectra made of 130 averaged scans, collected between 25 and 30 min of control perfusion, total ischemia and reperfusion, respectively. In the treated hearts, nifedipine (0.1 mg/l) was added to the perfusion fluid during the last 10 min of control perfusion.

[a] These values suggest that the untreated hearts were only partially reperfused.

Values are expressed as mean ± SD of six perfusion experiments.

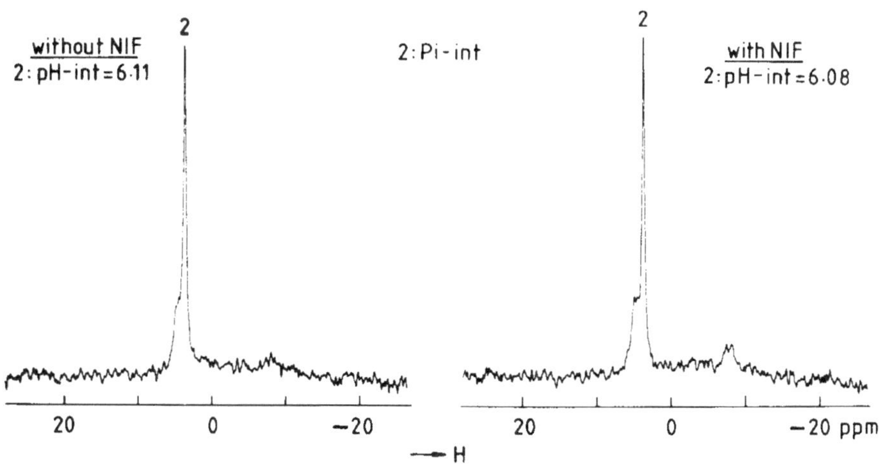

Figure 2. 81.0 MHz ^{31}P-NMR spectra obtained between 20 and 30 min of total ischemia of an untreated (left) and nifedipine-treated (NIF) (0.1 mg/l) heart (right). The spectra were obtained from 260 accumulated scans. The arrow indicates the direction of increasing field strength or decreasing frequency. Numbered peak: see legend to Figure 1.

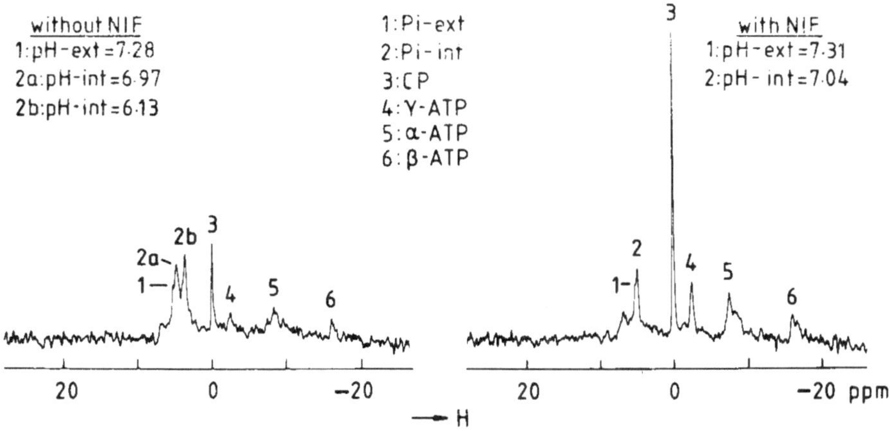

Figure 3. 81.0 MHz ^{31}P-NMR spectra obtained between 20 and 30 min of reperfusion of an untreated (left) and nifedipine-treated (NIF) (0.1 mg/l) heart (right). The spectra were obtained from 260 accumulated scans. The arrow indicates the direction of increasing field strength or decreasing frequency. Numbered peaks: see legend to Figure 1. Note the complex pattern in the inorganic phosphate region of the left spectrum.

collected later on in the ischemic period between 25 and 30 min of ischemia instead of between 20 and 30 minutes of ischemia. Although intracellular acidosis developed less rapidly in the nifedipine-treated hearts, there was no significant difference at the end of the ischemic period in intracellular pH between untreated and treated hearts.

Figure 3 shows typical ^{31}P-NMR spectra after reperfusion of untreated and nifedipine-treated hearts. During reperfusion of the nifedipine-treated heart, the intracellular pH returned to near its original value and became 7.04. There was also an almost complete return of the phosphocreatine peak. In the untreated heart, the complex pattern in the inorganic phosphate region appeared to be made up of 3 major components, corresponding to pH values of 7.28, 6.97 and 6.13. The two phosphate peaks corresponding to the lower pH values in the lefthand spectrum are attributed to two different intracellular phosphate pools. As shown in Table 2, the mean intracellular pH values of six untreated hearts after 30 min reperfusion were 6.91 ± 0.04 and 6.02 ± 0.06 and after reperfusion of six nifedipine-treated hearts pH-int was 7.01 ± 0.12.

These results show that nifedipine added to the perfusion fluid for 10 min before the onset of ischemia protects the rat heart against some of the consequences of normothermic global ischemia. Intracellular acidosis appeared to develop less rapidly and myocardial high-energy phosphate pools decreased at lower rates than in untreated hearts. More strikingly, intracellular pH returned to its original value and phosphocreatine levels increased rapidly during reperfusion of the treated hearts. In contrast, the spectra of the untreated hearts showed two phosphate peaks corresponding with intracellular pH values of 6.91 ± 0.04 and 6.02 ± 0.06. We suggest that the vasodilator effect of nifedipine facilitated reperfusion of the ischemic heart, thus improving myocardial recovery. The two phosphate peaks in the spectra of the untreated reperfused hearts, corresponding to the lower pH values suggest that these hearts were only partially reperfused. The parts that remained ischemic were responsible, in our opinion, for the lowest pH value. Similar results were reported by Bailey *et al.* [34] in a study on isolated perfused rat hearts recovering from varying periods of global ischemia.

Nunnally and Bottomley studied the effect of the calcium-antagonist verapamil on high-energy phosphate metabolism [10]. They used a small surface coil that was placed on a Langendorff perfused rabbit heart. Regional ischemia was produced by ligation of the left anterior descending coronary artery (LAD). When verapamil was added 1 h after ligation of the LAD, ^{31}P-NMR spectra indicated that the phosphocreatine level in the ischemic zone was restored. The authors suggested that the vasodilator effect of verapamil caused enhancement of collateral flow to the ischemic region.

Nayler *et al.* pretreated rabbits by subcutaneous injection of nifedipine for 4 to 5 days [41]. The rabbit hearts were then isolated and made ischemic for 90 min. The pretreatment resulted in significant preservation during normothermic ischemia of myocardial high-energy phosphate stores, as measured by the freeze clamp method. These findings are in conflict with our results which show a rapid decrease of high-energy phosphate stores and pH in both treated and untreated hearts. It is possible that nifedipine when administered for several days dissolves in the lipid phase of the sarcolemma and preserves its integrity during ischemia [43]. However the different assay techniques may also be responsible for the difference in results.

Nifedipine, like other calcium-antagonists, interferes with the excitation-induced inward displacement of calcium in smooth muscle and cardiac muscle cells. When added to a perfusate, nifedipine dilates the coronary vasculature of isolated hearts and reduces cardiac contractility. Possible mechanisms of the protective effect of nifedipine observed in our experiments, include:

(a) prevention of the no-reflow phenomenon by the vasodilator activity of the drug, which would improve myocardial recovery during reperfusion, and
(b) a slower decline in high-energy phosphate levels in consequence of the negative inotropic effect of the drug. This would leave more ATP available for maintaining intracellular calcium homeostasis during ischemia and reperfusion.

The experiments descibed above serve as an example of experimental metabolic NMR studies which have already contributed and will not cease to contribute to a better understanding of myocardial biochemistry.

In addition, as already briefly mentioned in this chapter, ^{31}P-and ^{1}H-NMR spectroscopy are on the verge of being clinically used — if they are not already — for assessing human cardiac metabolism and promise a challenging future for further diagnosis in clinical cardiology.

References

1. Moon R B, Richards J H (1973) Determination of intracellular pH by ^{31}P magnetic resonance. J Biol Chem 248: 7276 - 7278
2. Garlick P B, Radda G K, Seeley P J (1979) Studies of acidosis in the ischemic heart by phosphorus nuclear magnetic resonance. Biochem J 184: 547 - 554
3. Radda G K, Gadian D G, Ross B D (1982) Energy metabolism and cellular pH in normal and pathological conditions: A new look through ^{31}phosphorus nuclear magnetic resonance. In: Metabolic acidosis, Ciba Foundation Symposium 87, London: Pitman Books Ltd, pp 36 - 57
4. Hoult D I, Busby S J W, Gadian D G, Radda G K, Richards R E, Seeley P J (1974) Observation of tissue metabolites using ^{31}P nuclear magnetic resonance. Nature 252: 285 - 287
5. Fossel E T, Morgan H E, Ingwall J S (1980) Measurement of changes in high energy phosphates in the cardiac cycle by using gated ^{31}P nuclear magnetic resonance. Proc Natl Acad Sci USA 77: 3654 - 3658
6. Langendorff O (1895) Untersuchungen am überlebenden Saügetierherzen. Pflügers Archiv 61: 291 - 332
7. Gadian D G, Hoult D I, Radda G K, Seeley P J, Chance B, Barlow C (1976) Phosphorus nuclear magnetic resonance studies on normoxic and ischemic cardiac tissue. Proc Natl Acad Sci USA 73: 4446 - 4448
8. Jacobus W E, Taylor G J, Hollis D P, Nunnally R L (1977) Phosphorus nuclear magnetic resonance of perfused working rat hearts. Nature 265: 756 - 758
9. Garlick P B, Radda G K, Seeley P J(1977) Phosphorus NMR studies on perfused hearts. Biochem Biophys Res Commum 74: 1256 - 1262

10. Nunnally R L, Bottomley P A (1981) Assessment of pharmacological treatment of myocardial infarction by phosphorus-31 NMR with surface coils. Science 211: 177 - 180
11. Grove T H, Ackerman J J H, Radda G K, Bore P J (1980) Analysis of rat heart in vivo by phosphorus nuclear magnetic resonance. Proc Natl Acad Sci USA 77: 299 - 302
12. Neurohr K J (1984) An experimental setup for carbon-13 NMR studies of heart metabolism in live guinea pigs. J Magn Reson 59: 511 - 514
13. Koretsky A P, Wang S, Murphy-Boesch J, Klein M P, James T L, Weiner M W (1983) ^{31}P NMR spectroscopy of rat organs, in situ, using chronically implanted radiofrequency coils. Proc Natl Acad Sci USA 80: 7491 - 7495
14. Kantor H L, Briggs R W, Balaban R S (1984) In vivo ^{31}P nuclear magnetic resonance measurements in canine heart using a catheter coil. Circ Res 55: 261 - 266
15. Whitman G J R, Chance B, Bode H, Maris J, Haselgrove J, Kelley R, Clark B J, Harken A H (1985) Diagnosis and therapeutic evaluation of a pediatric case of cardiomyopathy using phosphorus-31 nuclear magnetic resonance spectroscopy. J Am Coll Cardiol 5: 745 - 749
16. Bottomley P A, Foster T B, Darrow R D (1984) Depth resolved surface-coil spectroscopy (DRESS) for in vivo ^{1}H, ^{31}P and ^{13}C NMR. J Magn Reson 59: 338 - 347
17. Bottomley P A, Herfkens R, Smith L S, Brazzamano S, Blinder R, Hedlund L, Redington R W (1985) Noninvasive detection of metabolic impairment in regionally ischemic hearts in situ using depth resolved surface coil spectroscopy (DRESS). Book of abstracts of the fourth annual meeting of the Society of Magnetic Resonance in medicine 1: 447 - 448
18. Styles P, Galloway G, Blackledge M, Radda G (1985) ^{31}P spectroscopy of human organs. Book of abstracts of the fourth annual meeting of the Society of Magnetic Resonance in medicine 1: 422 - 423
19. Gordon R E, Hanley P E, Shaw D, Gadian D G, Radda G K, Styles P, Bore P J, Chan L (1980) Localization of metabolites in animals using ^{31}P topical magnetic resonance. Nature 287: 736 -738
20. Aue W P, Müller S, Cross T A, Seelig J (1984) Volume-selective excitation. A novel approach to topical NMR. J Magn Reson 56: 350 - 354
21. Behar K L, den Hollander J A, Stromski M E, Ogino T, Shulman R G, Petroff O A, Prichard J W (1983) High resolution ^{1}H nuclear magnetic resonance study of cerebral hypoxia in vivo. Proc Natl Acad Sci USA 80: 4945 - 4948
22. Behar K L, Rothman D L, Shulman R G, Petroff O A C, Prichard J W (1984) Detection of cerebral lactate in vivo during hypoxemia by ^{1}H NMR at relatively low field strengths (1.9 T). Proc Natl Acad Sci USA 81: 2517 - 2519
23. Arús C, Bárány M, Westler W M, Markley J L (1984) ^{1}H NMR of intact muscle at 11 T. FEBS Lett 165: 231 - 237
24. Hetherington H P, Avison M J, Shulman R G (1985) ^{1}H homonuclear editing of rat brain using semiselective pulses. Proc Natl Acad Sci USA 82: 3115 - 3118
25. Bailey I A, Gadian D G, Matthews P M, Radda G K, Seeley P J (1981) Studies of metabolism in the isolated, perfused rat heart using ^{13}C NMR. FEBS Lett 123: 315 - 318
26. Neurohr K J, Barrett E J, Shulman R G (1983) In vivo carbon-13 nuclear magnetic resonance studies of heart metabolism. Proc Natl Acad Sci USA 80: 1603 - 1607
27. Neurohr K J, Gollin G, Neurohr J M, Rothman D L, Shulman R G (1984) Carbon-13 nuclear magnetic resonance studies of myocardial glycogen metabolism in live guinea pigs. Biochemistry 23: 5029 - 5035
28. Matthews P M, Bland J L, Gadian D G, Radda G K (1981) The steady state rate of ATP synthesis in the perfused rat heart measured by ^{31}P NMR saturation transfer. Biochem Biophys Res Commun 103: 1052 - 1059
29. Balaban R S, Kantor H L, Metz K R, Briggs R W (1985) Spectroscopic applications of a catheter NMR probe. Book of abstracts of the fourth annual meeting of the Society of Magnetic Resonance in Medicine 1: 417 - 418
30. Bulkley B H, Nunnally R L, Hollis D P (1978) Calcium paradox and the effect of varied

temperature on its development. Lab Invest 39: 133 - 140
31. Pernot A C, Ingwall J S, Menasche P, Grousset C, Bercot M, Mollet M, Piwnica A, Fossel E T (1981) Limitations of potassium cardioplegia during cardiac ischemic arrest, a phosporus 31 nuclear magnetic resonance study. Ann Thorac Surg 32: 536 - 545
32. Flaherty J T, Jaffin J H, Magovern G J, Kanter K R, Gardner T J, Micele M V, Jacobus W E (1984) Maintenance of aerobic metabolism during global ischemia with perfluorocarbon cardioplegia improves myocardial preservation. Circulation 69: 585 - 592
33, Hollis D P, Nunnally R L, Jacobus W E, Taylor G J (1977) Detection of regional ischaemia in perfused beating hearts by phosphorus nuclear magnetic resonance. Biochem Biophys Res Commun 75: 1086 - 1091
34. Bailey I A, Seymour A M L, Radda G K (1981) A ^{31}P NMR study of the effects of reflow on the ischemic rat heart. Biochim Biophys Acta 637: 1 - 7
35. Flaherty J T, Weisfeldt M L, Bulkley B H, Gardner T J, Gott V L, Jacobus W F (1982) Mechanisms of ischemic myocardial cell damage assessed by phosphorus-31 nuclear magnetic resonance. Circulation 65: 561 - 571
36. Bailey I A, Radda G K, Seymour A M L, Williams S R (1982) The effects of insulin on myocardial metabolism and acidosis in normoxia and ischemia. Biochem Biophys Acta 720: 17 - 27
37. Ruigrok T J C, van Echteld C J A, de Kruijff B, Borst C, Meijler F L (1983) Protective effect of nifedipine in myocardial ischemia assessed by phosphorus-31 nuclear magnetic resonance. Eur Heart J 4(Suppl C): 109 - 113
38. Hearse D J, Garlick P B, Humphrey S M (1977) Ischemic contracture of the myocardium: mechanisms and prevention. Am J Cardiol 39: 986 - 993
39. Williamson J R, Schaffer S W, Ford C, Safer B (1976) Contribution of tissue acidosis to ischemic injury in the perfused rat heart. Circulation 53: I3 - I14
40. Henry P D, Schuchleib R, Davis J, Weiss E S, Sobel B E (1977) Myocardial contracture and accumulation of mitochondrial calcium in ischemic rabbit heart. Am J Physiol 233: H677 - H684
41. Nayler W G, Ferrari R, Williams A (1980) Protective effect of pretreatment with verapamil, nifedipine and propranolol on mitochondrial function in the ischemic and reperfused myocardium. Am J Cardiol 46: 242 - 248
42. de Jong J W, Harmsen E, de Tombe P P, Keijzer E (1982) Nifedipine reduces adenine nucleotide breakdown in ischemic rat heart. Eur J Pharmacol 81: 89 - 96
43. Drake-Holland A J, Noble M I M (1983) Myocardial protection by calcium antagonist drug. Eur Heart J 4: 823 - 825

13. Nuclear magnetic resonance spectroscopy: its present and future application to studies of myocardial metabolism

E. BARRETT, R. ZAHLER and M. LAUGHLIN

Introduction

Nuclear magnetic resonance (NMR) spectroscopy is rather a latecomer among techniques for noninvasive assessment of the myocardium. Furthermore, though admittedly furnishing a method for directly examining myocardial metabolic activity, its clinical utility in providing an index of myocardial health is yet to be assessed. Despite this, the development of both hardware and experimental methods necessary to apply NMR spectroscopic analysis to myocardial tissue *in vivo* is attended by a continually increasing sense of enthusiasm. In the current chapter, we have three goals: *first*, to impart some basic sense of what biological NMR spectroscopy is about, *second*, to provide, by reviewing results of recent experimental studies, some sense of the basis for the current enthusiasm for applying NMR to biological studies, and *third*, to develop some perspective from which we might anticipate both the eventual clinical capabilities and some of the limitations of NMR spectroscopy as a clinical research and ultimately diagnostic tool. Requisite to achieving these aims is some understanding of the physical basis of NMR.

Basic physical description

We will only consider here the physical principles which underlie NMR spectroscopy at a very descriptive level. More detailed and mathematical descriptions are to be found in several texts [1,2]. The fundamental principle of NMR spectroscopy is that certain nuclei (those with an odd number of protons and/or neutrons) possess a property called "spin" which allows them to react like magnetic dipoles and orient themselves when placed in an external magnetic field. Nuclei with a spin quantum number of $\pm\frac{1}{2}$ (this includes ^{1}H-hydrogen, ^{31}P-phosphorus and ^{13}C-carbon) align either parallel or antiparallel to the applied field and precess about it. The parallel orientation has the lower energy state, and therefore a larger population of nuclear spins. This "net magnetization" that can be manipulated by pulses of very low energy radiofrequency radiation. As might be expected, the size of the energy difference and therefore the net magnetization is proportional to the strength of the applied field. During the radiofrequency pulses, the nuclei are promoted from one spin state to another. It is the absorption of energy by the small excess of nuclei in the low energy state and their subsequent relaxation back towards the preferred alignment that form the basis of signal detection in NMR spectroscopy.

Like many other forms of spectroscopy each peak of an NMR spectrum has three basic properties: height, width, and location along a frequency axis, all being a function of the position of the nucleus in the molecule of interest. In standard ultraviolet or visible light spectroscopy signals result from discrete transitions of electrons among different orbitals. NMR differs in that the transitions are among nuclear energy states created by the imposed magnetic field and these transitions require a very small amount of energy. Even in today's very strong superconducting magnets, the energy required is in the radiofrequency range, well below the ionizing electromagnetic radiation of conventional X-ray methods. The low energy non-ionizing character of the radiofrequency waves favors their use for *in vivo* biological studies.

As mentioned, increasing the strength of the imposed field results in a greater dichotomy in the population distribution of nuclear spins, which translates into an improvement in signal strength and peak height in the spectrum. Increasing field strength and homogeneity also results in significant changes in resonance frequency and peak width. To consider how this occurs, it is first necessary to consider how different signals arise within a spectrum.

The tendency for a nucleus to behave like a bar magnet when placed in an external field is expressed as its gyromagnetic ratio or γ, which is characteristic and constant for any given nucleus. Taking the simple case of the nucleus with a spin of $\pm\frac{1}{2}$, the energy difference between the orientation of the nucleus spins is given by

$$E = h\upsilon = \frac{h\gamma B}{2\pi}$$

where h is Planck's constant, B is the net magnetic field experienced at a particular nucleus, γ is the gyromagnetic ratio and υ is the resonance frequency, i.e., that frequency of electromagnetic radiation necessary to provide transition between spin states. Importantly, B differs from the applied field B_o by a very small amount due to shielding of the nucleus by the particular electronic structure around it. This can be written as $B = B_o(1\text{-}\sigma)$ where σ is referred to as the "chemical shift". It is this electronic shielding which shifts the resonance frequency from a particular nucleus slightly from that which might be attributable to the B_o field alone and determines its exact position along the frequency

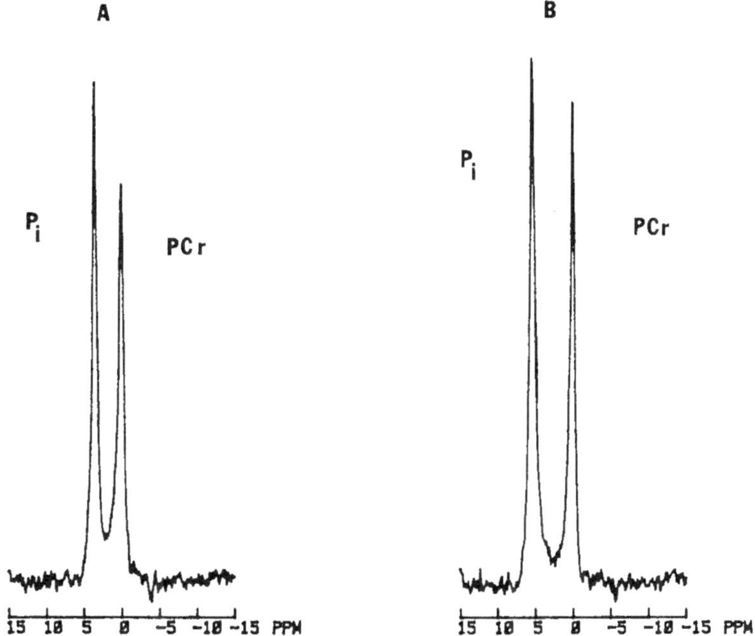

Figure 1. The ^{31}P NMR spectrum of a solution containing 100 mM inorganic phosphate and approximately 90 mM phosphocreatine. The solution was studied at pH 6 (A) and pH 8 (B). The phosphocreatine resonance is assigned a chemical shift of 0 PPM in each spectrum. Note that at pH 8 the inorganic phosphorus resonance has shifted approximately 2 PPM away from the PCr peak. This change in chemical shift can be used to measure the change in pH between the two solutions.

axis. Nuclei that are highly "shielded" by electrons will resonate at lower frequencies because the electronic currents induced in the molecules by the static magnetic field are proportional to and oppositely directed from B_o resulting in the lower local magnetic field B. As we will see, for the ^{31}P-phosphorus nucleus the resonance frequencies for each of the phosphorus atoms in ATP differ slightly from each other and from the resonance frequency of creatine phosphate and inorganic phosphate. Indeed, were it not for the effects of local electronic structure producing a chemical shift, NMR spectroscopy could provide little information since all nuclei with a particular gyromagnetic ratio would resonate at the same frequency and the spectrum would contain a single peak. The magnitude of σ will vary depending upon the chemical species in which a nucleus occurs but in all cases it is very small (10^{-5}—10^{-6}) and the chemical shift is on the order of parts per million of the imposed B_o field. The separation between peaks in a spectrum becomes greater at high magnetic fields, underlining the need for very strong magnets to improve spectral resolution.

This effect of local electronic structure can be well illustrated by changes in

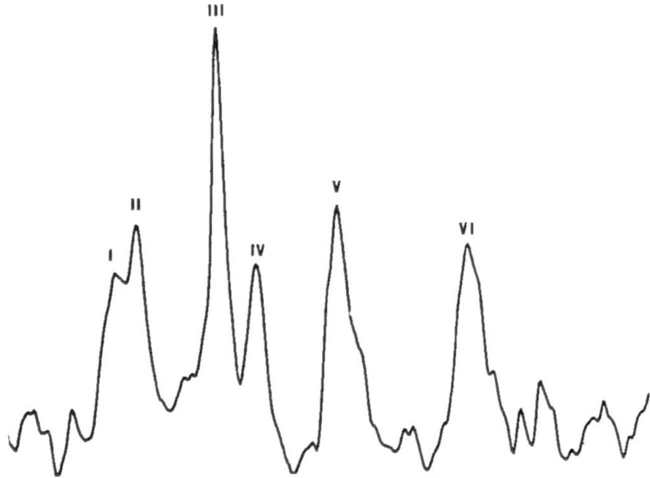

Figure 2. A typical ^{31}P NMR spectrum of the rat heart, obtained *in vivo*, by modification of the methods described in [35]. Spectra were collected in a TMR 32-200 spectrometer (Oxford Instruments) operating at 32.5 MHz, using a solenoidal receiver coil. The spectrum is the Fourier transform of 600, 10 μs pulses collected with an interpulse delay of 8 s. Peaks labeled one through six are assigned as follows: hexose monophosphate, inorganic phosphate, creatine phosphate, and the γ, α and β phosphates of ATP.

the chemical shift of inorganic phosphate as the degree of protonation increases with decreasing pH. In Figure 1, we illustrate the "chemical shift" of the inorganic phosphate resonance in a solution of K_2HPO_4 and creatine phosphate at pH 8 and pH 6. The greater protonation of phosphate at pH 6 (where $H_2PO_4^-$ is the dominant species) sufficiently alters the resultant field experienced by the ^{31}P-phosphorus nucleus that the resonance frequency is shifted by two parts per million from its position at pH 8 where $HPO_4^=$ is more abundant. The exact shift of the P_i in solution is a weighted average of the $H_2PO_4^=$ and $H_2PO_4^-$ chemical shifts due to rapid chemical exchange between the two species. This example should illustrate one of the powerful uses of NMR spectroscopy, i.e., measurement of the chemical shift of inorganic phosphate can provide a generally applicable method for measurement of pH either in free solutions, or more importantly, in intact cells, tissues or organs. A similar alteration in the chemical shift of ^{19}F within the compound (nFBAPTA) occurs when Ca^{2+} is chelated with the organic compound. Measurement of this induced change in chemical shift has been used as a method for measurement of cell Ca^{2+} concentrations [3]. With modification, this method may be applicable to studies of the intact heart.

In Figure 2, we illustrate a typical ^{31}P-phosphorus NMR spectrum of a rat heart obtained *in vivo* with the animal anesthetized and the heart exposed through a midline thoracotomy. The resonance of the nucleus in different chemical compounds or at different sites within a single compound gives rise to separate peaks. The ability to distinguish the extent of protonation of the phosphate molecule by measurement of its chemical shift, as previously illustrated, allows estimation of tissue pH. The abcissa in Figures 1 and 2 is given as parts per million (PPM) of the imposed B_0 field and emphasizes the sensitivity of the chemical shift to very small changes in field.

The chemical shift of a nucleus is also influenced by close proximity to other nuclei that possess "spin". An example is a molecule with a ^{13}C-carbon bound to a proton, ^{13}C-H. Both of these nuclei are separated into populations with different energies by the applied magnetic field (the number of populations = $\alpha|S|+1$ where S is the spin of each nucleus). The two populations of protons will create slightly different local fields at the neighboring carbon nucleus. The resonance of the carbon-13 nucleus will be "split" into 2S +1 peaks with a characteristic frequency difference (J-coupling) that depends only on the spatial relationship to the neighboring species and not on B_0. To the biochemist these "spin-spin" interactions provide a powerful tool for structural analysis, molecule identification and for tracing the movement of metabolites through metabolic pathways.

The third spectral property, peak width, is largely determined by two factors in biological systems: magnetic field homogeneity and the lifetime of the excited state. The first is most easily understood from the above discussion of chemical shift. Small variations in B_0 across a sample result in a population of resonances for a given nucleus in a single chemical species, and produces a widening or "line broadening" of the spectral peak. From this description it should be apparent that the resolution of a spectrum is critically dependent on the homogeneity and stability of the B_0 field within the region of the sample.

The relationship between the lifetime of the excited state and the width of a particular peak in a spectrum has many physical contributions. After a spin transition has occurred due to a radiofrequency pulse, the nuclei relax back to their equilibrium energy distribution due to dynamic interactions with the environment at the resonance frequency. This is termed "spin-lattice" relaxation and results in energy loss over a period characterized by a time constant T_1. The uncertainty principle dictates that the spread in E is inversely proportional to the lifetime of the E state. This leads to "lifetime broadening" of the spectral peak. A second contributing phenomenon, "spin-spin relaxation", is due to interactions between spins of like nuclei and is characterized by a time constant T_2. The effect of spin-spin relaxation on line broading can be understood by recognizing that the detection of an NMR signal is dependent on phase coherence of the precession around B_0 among the spins of the excited nuclei which resonate at a given frequency. As spin exchange takes place, no energy is lost but the relative phase of the two exchanging spins is altered and coherence is lost. This phenomenon decreases the detectable magnetization and under normal analysis conditions is the largest contribution to line width.

If a molecule has a restricted mobility in the cell, e.g., a membrane lipid, structural protein or bound enzyme substrate, the spin-spin relaxation is very efficient due to the relatively long periods of close proximity to the varying magnetic fields induced at other nuclei with similar spins. Molecules that are free in solution relax much more slowly because the time of interaction with other quickly-tumbling molecules is very short thus less spin exchange can occur. In the spectrum we see those molecules that relax very slowly have sharp lines; this serves to simplify the spectrum to include only the free metabolites and some storage molecules like fat or glycogen. Paramagnetic ions make spin-lattice relaxation much more efficient and can be used in biological studies to broaden or eliminate certain peaks.

NMR studies of heart are often hampered by a reduction in signal-to-noise due to sample and magnet inhomogeneity, and movement of perfusate or the organ itself in the magnet, and thermal noise at the elevated biological temperatures. Fourier analysis allows signal averaging over long periods of time which increases the signal to noise in spite of these limitations.

Spectral intensity and resolution is therefore ultimately dependent on the strength of the imposed magnetic field and time of accumulation; in addition the ability to detect a nucleus also depends on the natural abundance of the NMR visible isotope and on its gyromagnetic ratio, γ, which is a function of atomic weight. At the present time, the strongest wide-bore magnets can detect proton signals to $<100\,\mu M$, but compounds containing ^{31}P nuclei must be in the millimolar range. Because ^{13}C is only 1.1% of the total carbon, the metabolite pools must either be specifically enriched, or in the 100 mM range to be detected. The success of NMR spectroscopy in biological systems both in terms of sensitivity and resolution is practically limited by the state of superconducting technology which continues to give us stronger and more stable magnets.

Application of NMR spectroscopy to the heart

^{31}P-NMR – in vitro studies

The isolated perfused rat heart has been a remarkably successful *in vitro* model for study of cardiac metabolism. The importance of adenosinetriphosphate (ATP) and phosphocreatine (PCr) to the maintenance of myocardial contractile function and viability had long since been established using this model and conventional biochemical extraction techniques. The advent of wide-bore, high-field NMR spectrometers has provided a new and powerful means to study a variety of aspects of myocardial metabolism in the perfused heart. The value of the NMR method, beyond that of other biochemical analytic methods, lies in three areas: *first*, it is nondestructive, i.e., repeated measurements of ATP, PCr, inorganic phosphate or pH could be made over time in a single heart free from the destructive effects of tissue biopsy techniques. *Second*, the kinetics of certain enzyme reactions can be studied using a method called magnetization transfer. In heart, this method has been extensively applied to the study of creatine kinase which functions to catalyze the transfer of high energy phosphate between ATP and PCr. *Third*, ^{31}P-NMR has greatly facilitated the measurement of intracellular pH in the intact beating heart, a measurement which is difficult to obtain by alternate means.

The nondestructive nature of NMR analysis is not restricted to ^{31}P-NMR but, as we will see, also extends to all other NMR visible nuclei. However, the ability to make repeated measurements over time affords particular advantage in studies of the effects of oxygen deprivation, flow restriction, or workload on the myocardial content of high energy phosphate.

In the isolated perfused heart, the effects of ischemia [4-8] and anoxia [9] have been studied using ^{31}P-NMR. The results of these studies, like earlier work using conventional analytic measurements, have demonstrated a rapid decline in phosphocreatine and subsequent slower decline in cell ATP which commences with onset of ischemia or anoxia. In addition, by use of the chemical shift of inorganic phosphate both ischemia and anoxia were found to cause a rapid decline in cytosolic pH which can exceed 1 pH unit [5,6].

The ability to continuously monitor the myocardial content of high energy phosphate compounds has facilitated study of both physical and pharmacologic interventions on energy metabolism. Nearly 8 years ago, Hollis and his colleagues reported obtaining good quality ^{31}P-NMR spectra of isolated rabbit hearts which required only 30 s to accumulate [4]. These same authors followed the time course of phosphocreatine decline and progression of myocardial acidosis during global ischemia and recovery from global ischemia and correlated these changes with altered ventricular performance. In the rabbit heart, regional ischemia induced by occlusion of the left anterior descending coronary artery led to a splitting of the inorganic phosphate resonance with appearance of a second peak at a lower pH suggesting acidosis in the region of impaired perfusion [4].

Periods of ischemia lasting up to 40 min led to profound decreases in PCr and ATP accompanied by contractile dysfunction. Reperfusion leads to a prompt and complete restitution of tissue PCr. Recovery of ATP after reperfusion has been more variable in the hands of different investigators. In agreement with observations in the intact animal [10], recovery of mechanical function is impaired if the ischemic period is extended beyond 5-10 min demonstrating some discordancy between ATP availability and mechanical function.

Anoxia, like ischemia, results in a prompt marked decrease of phosphocreatine and more gradual decline in ATP. As with ischemia these changes are reversible when adequate oxygenation is resumed, provided, of course, that the anoxic period is not prolonged. Anoxia produces a lesser decline in tissue pH presumably due to "washout" of lactic acid formed during hypoxemia into the perfusion buffer [11]. Using either anoxia or ischemia as the provocative stimulus, ^{31}P-NMR has been used to follow the time course of decline of PCr,

ATP and cell pH and, in some experiments, the time course of the restitution of high energy phosphates. Using this method it has been shown that hypothermia [6], KCl arrest [4,6], and a high concentration of buffer in the perfusate slow the rate of high-energy phosphate loss while an increased work load accelerates this loss. Likewise providing substrate for purine nucleotide synthesis (ribose) speeds recovery of the ATP pool [12]. Interestingly, the decline in ATP seen in some of these studies is not accompanied by a detectable rise in adenosine-diphosphate (ADP) phosphorus resonance, suggesting that the net loss of ATP is accompanied by catabolism of nucleotide beyond ADP. Indeed, a surprising, yet consistent observation is that the free ADP concentration in a variety of tissues is below the limit of detection of the ^{31}P-NMR method. Interestingly, the content of ADP in these same tissues ranges from 0.5-1.5 mM when extracts are assayed by conventional analytic methods [13], and free ADP in solution at this concentration can be readily detected by ^{31}P-NMR. These observations support the hypothesis that a substantial fraction of ADP is not freely mobile in cell cytosol. This suggestion is consistent with the earlier conclusions of Veech *et al.* that a large fraction of cellular ADP is bound to tissue elements and does not participate freely in cytosolic reactions involving ADP [14].

Although the free ADP concentration cannot be measured directly using ^{31}P-NMR, it has been estimated indirectly from the cell concentrations of PCr, ATP, pH and creatine and the creatine kinase equilibrium constant, and is reported to be 80-100 μM in the Langendorff perfused heart [15]. It is essential for the validity of this estimate that the creatine kinase reaction be in equilibrium. As discussed below this assumption is supported by *in situ* measurement of the forward and reverse rate constants for creatine kinase using magnetization transfer NMR techniques. Thus, the cytosolic phosphate potential ([ATP]/[ADP][Pi]) is substantially higher than previously appreciated and the free energy of ATP hydrolysis is greater. In addition, in tissue like heart with an active adenylate kinase which is thought to be at equilibrium, the lower estimates of ADP concentration implies a much lower free adenosine monophosphate (AMP) than previously considered. Since ADP and AMP are each thought to be involved in the regulation of the activity through several metabolic pathways (e.g., phosphorylase, phosphofructokinase, and oxidative phosphorylation), recognition that the free concentrations of these substrates are substantially less than their total cell content has significant implications for our understanding of myocardial metabolism.

Magnetization transfer

As mentioned previously, NMR techniques have been developed which allow measurement of rate constants for certain enzyme reactions, and when coupled with measurement of the substrate concentration, the fluxes through particular reactions can be determined. In perfused heart, magnetization transfer studies have been most extensively applied to the study of the creatine kinase reaction:

$$\text{ATP} + \text{Creatine} \qquad \text{ADP} + \text{PCr} + \text{H}^+$$

Two types of magnization transfer methods have been used in these studies; saturation transfer and inversion transfer. For a detailed discussion of these methods the reader is referred to a recent review [16]. In brief, each method relies on a selective perturbation of the spin state of one nucleus in a molecule (e.g., γ-phosphorus of ATP) being retained when that nucleus is transferred to a second compound (e.g., to creatine to form phosphocreatine). Such a chemical transfer causes an attenuation in peak height of the species receiving the "spin-labeled" nucleus. Measurement of the magnitude of this effect, when the spin-labeling is introduced into either ATP or PCr, together with an estimation of the spin lattice relaxation time (T_1) of ATP and PCr, allows calculation of the forward and reverse rate constants for this reaction. From these the equilibrium constant is obtained and, if the measured substrate concentrations are available, the two unidirectional fluxes mediated by the enzyme *in situ* can be calculated.

Current results indicate that in heart the forward and reverse fluxes through creatine kinase are equal in the Langendorff perfused heart, i.e., the reaction is at equilibrium [17-19]. Of great potential interest is the observation that the flux through creatine kinase increases with increasing cardiac work [17]. Since increased work is associated with an increased ATP turnover but not an increase in ATP concentration, the rise of flux through creatine kinase is consistent with the hypothesis that phosphocreatine may participate in the "shuttling" of energy from mitochondrial sites of ATP synthesis to utilization sites on the myofilaments [20].

Magnetization transfer studies such as these offer an almost unique opportunity to probe a variety of aspects of cell energetics and may ultimately allow direct measurement of ATP synthesis rates *in vivo* in hearts under a variety of physiologic or pathologic circumstances.

^{31}P-NMR applied to measurement of heart pH

We earlier illustrated in the discussion of chemical shift how the pH of a tissue might be determined from the position of the inorganic phosphate resonance and how changes in pH might be detected by a change in chemical shift. Since a number of factors influence the chemical shift of P_i (e.g., field homogeneity, ionic strength of tissue) the absolute assignment of tissue pH in heart has an uncertainty of approximately ± 0.05 pH units. Given this, in several studies myocardial pH in a Langendorff perfused heart averages 7.1 pH units when the perfusate pH is 7.4.

As mentioned previously, ischemia, and to a lesser extent anoxia, causes a decline in tissue pH [4-6]. It is clear that in these circumstances where O_2 availability is curtailed, lactic acid generated glycolytically in the myocardium is a major contributor to acid production. Bailey *et al.* [5] have shown that pretreatment of hearts with glucose and insulin to replete heart glycogen stores results in a more marked cellular acidosis during a subsequent period of ischemia. In contrast, antecedent depletion of myocardial glycogen by perfusion with a glucose free buffer or use of acetate in place of glucose in the perfusate, blunts the cellular acidosis which accompanies ischemia or anoxia. These results support an important role for cellular glycogen as a precursor for myocardial lactic acid production. These findings are in accord with the much earlier observations of Rovetto *et al.* [11] that in perfused heart glycogenolysis is rapidly stimulated by both anoxia and ischemia and provides substrate for heart lactate production. It is of interest to consider the recent observations of Neely and Grotyohan [21] that the deterioration in myocardial function in the perfused heart was greater when glycolysis was maximally stimulated and lactate production greatest. Such observations emphasize the potentially important role of cellular pH regulation in the maintenance of contractile function. Furthermore, increasing the buffering capacity of the perfusate during anoxia blunts the decline in myocardial pH but also attenuates the fall in high energy phosphates [23].

Assessment of the precise role of myocardial pH in control of contractile function will require extensive examination of cardiac performance in a variety of circumstances where pH can be altered independently of changes in a high energy phosphate content. Experimentally this will not be a trivial matter since in the two commonly used models of myocardial acidosis, i.e., hypoxemia and ischemia, cell pH and levels of high energy phosphate change simultaneously. Application of ^{31}P-NMR to an examination of the effects of systematically altering cell pH via changes in perfusate pH and buffer composition could substantially improve our understanding of the role of cell pH in regulating myocyte function and the relationship between pH and high energy phosphate metabolism [23].

^{31}P-NMR of the heart in vivo

Since the first application of NMR to the study of cardiac high-energy phosphate metabolism in the perfused heart, it has been considered that this method might eventually offer a noninvasive technique for direct assessment of myocardial energy metabolism in man. Today this possibility appears more likely than ever, owing largely to advances in magnet design and development of methods for signal localization.

The first *in vivo* ^{31}P-NMR studies of the myocardium were those of Grove *et al.* [24]. They obtained spectra from rat heart within 8 min which had excellent signal-to-noise quality. In these studies the ratio of PCr to ATP content was approximately 5:3 (this is higher than that seen in the Langendorff perfused heart) and the PCr signal declined more rapidly than ATP when animals were made anoxic. Subsequent studies in the dog [25] and guinea pig [26] have produced similar findings. In the latter studies temporal resolution of spectra (20 s) was sufficient to examine the time course of decline of the phosphocreatine signal during a transient period of anoxia and its resynthesis following reventilation. In accord with results of studies in the perfused heart [18], the decline of heart phosphocreatine is rapid ($T_{1/2}$=54 s) and essentially complete before significant changes in ATP occur. Such observations would suggest that the resonance signal from PCr would provide a more sensitive indicator of the adequacy of myocardial oxygenation. When ischemia rather than asphyxia is examined in the heart *in vivo* the PCr signal again undergoes a more rapid and marked decline.

We emphasize that in the *in vivo* studies cited above, surgical exposure of the heart was required to obtain high quality spectra. The heart was then studied either within a solenoidal receiver coil or with a surface coil directly over the heart. In this experimental setting it can be readily demonstrated that virtually all of the PCr and most of the ATP signal arises from the myocardium. Inorganic phosphate signals (and therefore pH) and phosphomonoester and phosphodiester signals may originate either from myocardial cells, interstitial fluid or blood within the ventricular chamber.

Quite recently, Whitman *et al.* [27] have reported obtaining ^{31}P-NMR spectra from both a normal human infant and from an infant with a congenital cardiomyopathy. They observed a lower PCr/ATP ratio in both the skeletal and cardiac muscle of the child with the cardiomyopathy. The nature of the myopathic defect could not be defined in this study but perhaps the greater significance of the report lies in the demonstrated ability to obtain a spectrum from the heart of the normal child. These studies were performed using a particular variety of NMR receiver coil called a "surface coil" which is essentially a loop of copper wire with appropriate capacitance added to allow it to tune at the ^{31}P-phosphorus resonance. Similar coils have been used to study human forearm muscle [28,29].

The ability to obtain phosphorus signals originating in heart muscle was facilitated by the thin chest wall of these young children and no special techniques for signal localization were required (see below). However, as larger magnets become available and the effort to study adults and larger children progresses almost certainly some volume selection method will need to be employed to differentially stimulate nuclei within the myocardium while leaving nuclei of other tissues (e.g., lung, skeletal muscle) relatively unperturbed. Several methods of volume selection are currently available or being developed. The TMR or topical magnetic resonance method relies on use of a series of field profiling coils which serve to limit the volume of B_0 field homogeneity, and hence the volume which contributes resolvable peaks in a spectrum. When used in combination with a surface coil it has been possible to use this method to selectively monitor the ^{31}P-NMR spectrum of the liver in the intact rat [30]. Whether this technique will be suitable to study the deeper, smaller beating myocardium tissues remains speculative. A second, more recently developed technique is that of the "depth-pulse". This relies on the use of a complex series of radiofrequency pulses selected to provide a maximal shift in net magnetization of the observed nucleus at some distance from the surface coil while allowing magnetization due to the sequence of pulses at sites closer to the surface coil to cancel, resulting in no effective net magnetization [31,32]. As a result, spectra will only arise from the selected site. While this may eventually provide a broadly applicable method of volume selection, we can anticipate that extensive work will be required in phantom and experimental animal studies before application to studies in man.

Another approach to volume selection in the heart which may be applicable to eventual study of man in the "catheter-coil" device described by Kantor *et al.* [33]. With this a specially designed NMR coil is introduced into the right or left ventricular chamber via either the systemic arterial or venous tree in much the same manner that catheters are positioned during conventional left or right sided cardiac catheterization. Using such a technique ^{31}P-NMR spectra of reasonable quality could be obtained from right ventricular muscle. Greater movement artifact was encountered with the catheter in the left ventricle which degraded the quality of the spectra. However, this approach appeared encouraging and with adaptation may provide a very acceptable method for obtaining spectra selectively from the left or right ventricular muscle.

In addition to lying deep within the chest cavity it can be anticipated that intrinsic movement of the heart will complicate efforts to obtain spectra and may ultimately require that spectra accumulation be gated to the heartbeat. Such gating has proved valuable in obtaining ^{1}H-proton NMR images of the heart. It should be emphasized at this juncture that the type of localization we are discussing is, by angiographic standards, very crude indeed, i.e., we are attempting to distinguish signals from cardiac versus noncardiac tissues. It is clear that early on in the development of signal localizing methods for myocardial studies in man global myopathic disorders will be more appropriate for study than the regional or localized processes encountered in disorders like coronary atherosclerosis.

In summary, of the several nuclei which may be studied in the myocardium using NMR spectroscopic methods, phosphorus has received the greatest attention. This may be attibuted to several factors including: 1) the intrinsic interest in high energy phosphate content as a tell-tale of the health of the myocardium, 2) that the NMR sensitive isotope ^{31}P-phosphorus is the predominant natural abundant species, 3) that tissue pH can be estimated from the chemical shift of inorganic phosphate and finally 4) the tissue concentration of several phosphorus containing metabolites are sufficiently high (1-8 mM) that they can be rather readily detected by NMR spectroscopic methods.

We can anticipate that as larger bore magnets, which admit the human thorax, become available studies of human myocardial high energy phosphate metabolism will figure prominently. However, we in addition anticipate that considerable development will take place in ^{13}C-carbon and proton magnetic resonance spectroscopy and these methods will significantly contribute to the overall utility of NMR spectroscopy as a method to study heart metabolism.

^{13}C-NMR

To date there have been few studies of myocardial metabolism using the ^{13}C-nucleus either in the perfused heart [34], or *in situ* in intact animals [35]. This contrasts somewhat with the extensive investigations of intermediary metabolism in heart muscle conducted using a variety of chemical and radiochemical methods over a period of many years (see [36,37] for reviews). Indeed, the very substantial bulk of information already available on myocardial metabolism together with several spectroscopic limitations described below has served to slow the application of ^{13}C-NMR to the study of myocardial metabolism. However, as previously discussed with ^{13}P-NMR the opportunity for repetitive, nondestructive analysis of tissue metabolites makes ^{13}C-NMR an attractive experimental method to examine selected aspects of heart metabolism.

We will highlight here results of some studies which have been undertaken in the perfused heart *in vitro* and *in vivo* and briefly discuss both the limitations and potential applications of this method.

Bailey *et al.* [34] provided the initial work on ^{13}C-NMR of the perfused heart. They demonstrated that several natural abundance peaks attributable to myocardial lipids were detectable and upon addition of ^{13}C-acetate to the perfusion buffer labeling of the C-2, C-3, and C-4 carbons of glutamate, and of the C-2 and C-3 carbons of aspartate could be detected. Based upon the observed pattern of metabolite labeling they suggested that malic enzyme in perfused heart is kinetically controlled to feed carbon skeletons unidirectionally into the Krebs cycle.

Subsequently, studies have been conducted in the live guinea pig in which either ^{13}C-acetate or ^{13}C-1-glucose were infused. During acetate infusion it was possible to examine the rate of entry of labeled acetate into tricarboxylic acid cycle intermediates and to observe the migration of label in glutamate from the C-4 to the C-3 carbon. This provides a relative measure of the rate of cycling of the TCA cycle. In this same *in vivo* preparation the synthesis of glycogen by heart muscle during intravenous infusion of ^{13}C-1-glucose and insulin was serially observed, and subsequent stimulation of glycogenolysis with production of ^{13}C-3-lactate was observed [35].

^{13}C-NMR spectroscopy offers several unique features which are of particular use in studies of fuel metabolism and are well-illustrated by the previously cited studies. *First,* when a ^{13}C enriched substrate is transformed into many metabolic products (as is usually the case) the appearance of tracer in multiple products can be monitored simultaneously by measurement of absorption at their characteristic resonance frequencies. Separation and purification of each product, as is needed for conventional ^{14}C radioactive tracer techniques, is thus avoided. *Second* and even more powerfully, the NMR spectrum can assign not only which metabolic products contain ^{13}C labeled carbon, but also it can show which carbon atoms within the product are preferentially labeled. This provides a powerful tool for the analysis of specific metabolic pathways and is a capability which is not available when ^{14}C labeling techniques are used without spending enormous effort. *Third*, it has been demonstrated that by analyzing the homonuclear spin-spin coupling in ^{13}C labeled products [34], it is possible to quantitate the specific activity of the metabolite pools *in situ* in whole tissues, i.e., to measure the unlabeled and labeled fractions in a single sample. The same results can be obtained from proton NMR because ^{13}C has a coupling to the adjacent proton while ^{12}C compounds do not. An added benefit with the use of ^{13}C-NMR is that since the technique is nondestructive, it is possible to repeat measurements over time and hence follow the rate of change in levels of specific intracellular metabolites or the rate of transfer of incorporated tracer among metabolic intermediates in the same living system. This enables an animal to serve as its own control in a given experiment.

The major drawback of ^{13}C-NMR is that the ^{13}C-carbon nucleus comprises only about 1.1% of all the native carbon nuclei in a particular tissue sample. As a result it is necessary to infuse either the labeled substrate of interest, or a precursor of that substrate. These ^{13}C-enriched compounds are frequently quite expensive, a fact which is likely to limit broad application of ^{13}C-NMR metabolic studies to small laboratory animals. An additional consideration is that the sensitivity of even the ^{13}C-carbon nucleus is less than of ^{31}P-phosphorus and much less than that of the proton. As a result only compounds with a ^{13}C-carbon at a concentration of approximately 1 mM or higher are NMR visible. While this insensitivity will be a major drawback in the study of tissue metabolic intermediates (e.g., glycolytic or TCA cycle substrates) it does permit study of metabolites like glycogen, glutamate, and lactate which are present at higher concentrations. Finally this insensitivity of ^{13}C-NMR has led investigators to develop ^{1}H-NMR as a more sensitive method for *in vivo* spectroscopy.

Proton-NMR

There is a general recognition that it would be desirable to use proton NMR spectroscopy to study substrate metabolism in the heart. This is a direct consequence of the proton being the most sensitive nucleus, i.e., it produces the greatest signal relative to noise. Indeed, it is the sensitivity of the proton, coupled with its abundance in tissue water, that has led to its use in NMR imaging. However, two constraints limit immediate application of ^{1}H-NMR to spectroscopic study of the heart. These are the intense signal produced by solvent water either *in vivo* or in the isolated perfused heart and the narrow width of the proton spectrum. These factors combine to make it difficult to distinguish the resonance attributable to protons in various metabolites (e.g. lactate, glucose, glutamate, etc.) from one another and form the water protons.

Recently, several experimental approaches directed at enhancing the signals from protons in tissue metabolites relative to water have been undertaken. In the perfused heart Urgabil *et al.* [38] have reported using a Hahn spin-echo pulse sequence after presaturating the water with a Dante sequence. Signal arising from taurine, creatine, carnitine, and phosphocreatine were seen in the basal spectrum and a large lactate peak rose during ischemia. In studies of the brain tissue lactate has been observed in the ^{1}H-NMR spectrum to increase during anoxia. These studies utilized the spin-echo pulse sequence which reduced the intensity of the water resonance and diminished the contribution from resonances with a short T_2 (e.g., tissue lipids). More recently, a series of reports from Shulman's laboratory have detailed editing methods to enhance the information which can be obtained from proton spectra. In general these methods involve suppression of the water resonance either with a Hahn spin-echo pulse sequence or a semiselective Hahn spin-echo together with a decoupling pulse scheme directed at decoupling at a resonance frequency which is J-coupled to the resonance of interest. This decoupling is gated to alternate scans and hence the difference spectrum is enhanced for the resonances which are J-modulated by the decoupled resonance. Using such methods in studies of brain, high quality spectra of lactate, alanine, N-acetyl aspartate and glutamate have been obtained.

To date these editing methods have not been extended to the heart. However, we anticipate that this will be an area of active investigation within the next several years. Certainly a major impetus for this is the recognition that myocardial ischemia is accompanied by a prompt local rise in tissue lactate to concentrations up to 20-30 mmolar (this is 60-90 mM of the methyl protons of lactate). Such a high proton concentration would be expected to produce a very strong signal in comparison with the ATP or PCr signals which would be seen in the ^{31}P-NMR spectrum. As a result it is likely that proton spectroscopy may ultimately be the method of choice for noninvasive assessment of myocardial ischemia. However, as with phosphorus, considerable work remains to be done on the development of methods for signal localization in addition to further development of proton editing techniques.

Summary

We have attempted to provide some sense of the current status of NMR spectroscopy as a quantitative analytic method for studying a variety of aspects of cardiac metabolism and physiology. It should be apparent that this method has much to offer as an experimental tool. ^{31}P-NMR provides a valuable "on-line" method for continuous measurement of tissue pH and high energy phosphate content which will be invaluable in studies probing the relationship between myocardial function and tissue metabolism. ^{13}C-NMR has only begun to be applied to the study of myocardial biochemistry, but promises to provide truly unique information on the *in vivo* control of the reaction pathways involved in the synthesis and breakdown of tissue glycogen. Finally, *in vivo* proton spectroscopy of the heart, while still in the very early phases of its development, holds forth perhaps the greatest promise to serve both as a valuable analytic method to the biochemist and perhaps eventually as a diagnostic method to the clinician.

To be sure, a number of experimental obstacles remain to be overcome before NMR spectroscopy could become a useful tool to clinical cardiology. Foremost among these will be resolving issues of localization of the source of spectral information. In addition the issues of machine expense and patient safety will be continuing sources of concern and debate. However, while these questions remain, it has become increasingly clear that the interest and excitement generated by the possibility of having a noninvasive method to directly assess the biochemical behavior of the heart and other tissues has a momentum of its own. To the extent that this momentum is spent on addressing the outstanding technical and instrumental problems, it appears that the future of *in vivo* NMR spectroscopy in cardiology is bright indeed.

References

1. Gadian D G (1982) Nuclear magnetic resonance and its applications to living systems. Oxford: Oxford Univ Press
2. Gunther H (1980) NMR Spectroscopy: An Introduction. New York: Wiley
3. Smith G A, Hesketh R T, Metcalfe J C, Feeney J, Morris P G (1983) Proc Natl Acad Sci USA 80: 7178 - 7182
4. Hollis D P, Nunnally R L, Taylor G J, Weisfeldt M L, Jacobus W E (1978) J Magn Reson 29: 319 - 330
5. Bailey I A, Radda G K, Seymour A N, Williams S R (1982) Biochem Biophys Acta 720: 17 - 27
6. Flaherty J T, Weisfeldt M L, Bulkley B H, Gardner T J, Gott V L, Jacobus W E (1982) Circulation 65: 561 - 571
7. Gadian D G, Hoult D I, Radda G K, Seeley P J, Chance B, Barlow C (1976) Proc Natl Acad Sci USA 73: 4446 - 4448
8. Brooks W M, Willis R J (1983) J Mol Cell Cardiol 15: 495 - 502
9. Barbow R L, Sotak C H, Levy G C, Chan S H P (1984) Biochem 23: 6053 - 6062
10. Braunwald E, Kloner R A (1982) Circulation 66: 1146 - 1149

11. Rovetto M J, Whitmer J T, Neely J R (1973) Circ Res 32: 699 - 711
12. Ingwall J S (1982) Am J Physiol 242: H729 - H744
13. Swain J L, Sabina R L, McHale P A, Freenfield J C, Holmes E W (1982) Am J Physiol 242: H818 - H826
14. Veech R J, Lawson J W R, Cornell N W, Krebs H A (1979) J Biol Chem 254: 6538 - 6543
15. Matthews P M, Bland J L, Gadian D G, Radda G K (1983) Biochem Biophys Acta 721: 312 - 320
16. Alger J R, Shulman R G (1984) Quaterly Rev Biophys 17: 83 - 124
17. Ingwall J S, Kobuyashi K, Bittl J A (1984) Scientific Program of the Third Annual Meeting of the Society of Magnetic Resonance in Medicine, Aug 13, 1984, New York, p 369
18. Degani H, Laughlin M R, Campbell S, Ogino T, Shulman R G (1984) Scientific Program of the Third Annual Meeting of the Society of Magnetic Resonance in Medicine, Aug 13, 1984, New York, p 185
19. Ugurbil K, Petein M, Maidan R, Michurski S, Cohn J, From A (1985) Biophysical J 47: 369A
20. Saks V A, Chernousova G B, Gukovsky D E, Smirnov V N, Chazov E I (1975) Eur J Biochem 57: 273 - 290
21. Neely J R, Grotyohan L W (1984) Circ Res 55: 816 - 824
22. Garlick P B, Radda G K, Seeley P F (1979) Biochem J 184: 547 - 554
23. Steenbergen C, DeLeeuw G, Rich T, Williamson J R (1977) Circ Res 41: 849 - 858
24. Grove T H, Ackerman J J H, Radda G K, Bore P J (1980) Proc Natl Acad USA 77: 229 - 302
25. Nunnally R L (1983) Sem Nuc Med 13: 377 - 382
26. Neurohr K J, Gollin G, Barrett E, Shulman R G (1983) FEBS Lett 159: 207 - 210
27. Whitman G J R, Chance B, Bode H, Maris J, Haselgrove J, Kelley R, Clark B J, Harken A H (1985) JACC 5: 745 - 749
28. Ross B D, Radda G K, Gadian D G, Rocker G, Esiri M, Falconer-Smith J (1981) New Engl J Med 304: 1338 - 1342
29. Gadian D, Radda G, Ross B, Hockaday J, Bore P, Taylor D, Styles P (1981) Lancet 774 - 775
30. Gordon R E, Hanley P, Shaw D, Gadian D G, Radda G K, Styles P, Bore P J, Chan L (1980) Nature 287: 367 - 368
31. Bendall M R (1983) J Magn Reson 54: 149 - 152
32. Bendall M R, Gordon R E (1983) J Magn Reson 53: 365 - 385
33. Kantor H L, Briggs R W, Balaban R S (1984) Circ Res 55: 261 - 266
34. Bailey I A, Gadian D G, Matthews P M, Radda G K, Seeley P J (1981) FEBS Lett 123: 315 - 318
35. Neurohr K J, Barrett E, Shulman R (1983) Proc Natl Acad Sci USA 80: 1603 - 1607
36. Randle P J, Tubbs P K (1979) Handbook of Physiol, the Cardiovascular System I. Bethesda, MD: Am Physiol Soc, pp 805 - 844
37. Morgan H, Rannels D, McKee E (1979) Handbook of Physiol, the Cardiovascular System I. Bethesda, MD: Am Physiol Soc, pp 845 - 871
38. Ugurbil K, Petein M, Maidan R, Michurski S, Cohn J N, From A H (1984) FEBS Lett 167: 73 - 78
39. Behar K L, den Hollander J A, Stromski M E, Ogino T, Shulman R G, Petroff O H C, Prichard J W (1983) Proc Natl Acad Sci USA 80: 4945 - 4948
40. Behar K L, Rothman D L, Shulman R G, Petroff O A C, Prichard J W (1984) Proc Natl Acad Sci USA 81: 2517 - 2519
41. Rothman D L, Behar K L, Hetherington H P, Shulman R G (1984) Proc Natl Acad Sci USA 81: 6330 - 6334
42. Rothman D L, Arias Mendoza F, Shulman G I, Shulman R G. J Magn Reson (in press)
43. Hetherington H P, Avison M J, Shulman R G (1985) Proc Natl Acad Sci USA 82: 3115 - 3118

14. Metabolic imaging: PET or NMR?

A.M.J. PAANS and W. VAALBURG

Summary

With positron emission tomography (PET) in combination with compounds labeled with short-lived positron emitting radionuclides like ^{11}C, ^{13}N, ^{15}O and ^{18}F, it is possible to study regional metabolism *in vivo* quantitatively in a noninvasive way. Nuclear magnetic resonance (NMR) imaging takes advantage of the spin of protons in water molecules to measure both their number and relaxation times *in vivo*; NMR is not limited to protons but can also be used for other nuclei with a non-zero spin like ^{13}C and ^{31}P. PET can be used for metabolic imaging. The question arises if it is also possible to study metabolism by NMR in combination with ^{13}C-labeled compounds. To answer this question which method, PET or NMR, is the appropriate technique for metabolic imaging, it is important to know the sensitivity of each technique. Calculations based on the physical properties of the PET and the NMR technique show that, due to the low sensitivity of NMR, PET is the appropriate technique for metabolic imaging in most cases.

Introduction

In this chapter the sensitivity of positron emission tomography (PET) and nuclear magnetic resonance (NMR) is compared to evaluate the abilities of both techniques for the measurement of metabolic functions *in vivo* using two different carbon isotopes. These two isotopes are the radioactive carbon-11 nuclei, half-life 20.3 min, and the stable carbon-13 nuclei. Both isotopes have nuclear properties which allow the determination of their presence *in vivo* in a quantitative way by an external detection method. The importance of radionuclides like carbon-11, nitrogen-13, oxygen-15 and fluorine-18 for the measurement of metabolic parameters was already recognized at the time of their discovery in the 1930s [1]. The application of these radionuclides, however, was not possible at that time due to the lack of detection equipment and computer systems for image reconstructions. Since 1962 a number of positron imaging systems has been developed. By measuring the annihilation radiation in coincidence, the distribution of a positron emitting radiopharmaceutical can be measured regionally in a quantitative way. This means that the information is obtained in terms of amount of radioactivity per volume unit (Bq/cm^3) [2]. This regional quantitative feature in combination with the possibility of applying labeled drugs and compounds which are chemically identical to compounds normally involved in metabolism, is the strength of PET. These possibilities are even still more enforced if the carrier-free production aspect of positron emitting radionuclides is considered. The carrier-free and the non-carrier added synthesis of radiopharmaceuticals will be discussed later on.

The NMR technique exploits the fact that a large number of nuclei possesses a spin. Since the first description of NMR [3,4], this technique has been used and sophisticated to obtain structural information of molecules. The importance of NMR spectroscopy is due to the fact that the resonance frequency of a nucleus is directly proportional to the local magnetic field. This local effective field experienced by the nucleus is not the same as the applied static field, because the electrons in the molecule shield the nucleus. The result is a slight shift in the resonance frequency; the so called "chemical shift". This shift is used in chemistry to identify the structure of the molecule.

The value of NMR for diagnostic purposes was first stressed by Damadian [5], who proposed the measurement of proton resonances in small areas of the human body. Since the human body contains roughly 75% of water, the proton is the obvious nuclide to start with. Instead of a small area with a homogeneous magnetic field Lauterbur [6] suggested the use of gradient magnetic fields superposed on a extended static homogeneous magnetic field. An advantage of this approach is the much shorter imaging time required in comparison with Damadian's approach. Of course, in principle, also other nuclei like ^{13}C, ^{19}F, ^{23}Na and ^{31}P can be used for NMR imaging. If the NMR technique in combination with carbon-13 is able to provide regional quantitative information on the fate of metabolic compounds in the human body, it will be on a par with PET. To have insight in the potentials in metabolic imaging of PET and NMR it is necessary to compare the sensitivity of both techniques.

Positron emission tomography

PET uses the fact that after the decay of a radionuclide by positron emission, the positron and an electron present in its direct surrounding will annihilate after the positron has been slowed down by the surrounding material to (nearly) rest. This means that the masses of the electron-positron pair will be converted into energy according to $E=mc^2$. In virtually all cases this will be a two quanta annihilation, meaning that two gamma rays of 511 keV each will appear at a relative angle of 180°, so back-to-back or colinear. The PET technique exploits these two facts by putting a coincidence requirement on detectors which are opposing each other and by using energy discrimination on the measured gamma ray energy. A full exploit of the physical aspects of the decay by positron emission is made by those devices which not only establish a coincident event in a certain time window, but which are getting even more information by measuring the time difference between the two gamma rays within the time window. This is the so called "time of flight" (TOF) measurement [7]. From the coincidence data transverse section images are reconstructed which, after correction for the system response function, give information on the functioning of tissue and organs the human body. Which function is studied is determined by the radiopharmaceutical used. To obtain quantitative information the images have to be corrected for the attenuation of the radiation in the body. In X-ray transmission tomography (CT), the attenuation of the radiation in the object is used to extract information on the density. In single photon scintigraphy it is essentially not possible to correct the attenuation since it is never known at which depth in the body the radiation is originating from. In positron emission tomography this depth information is not important due to the use of a coincidence technique. Since both gamma rays have to be detected simultaneously to accept a disintegration for the reconstruction of a PET image, not the place (depth) of the annihilation is important but only the total size of the object between the detectors. Because of this fact the attenuation can be measured exactly by using an external positron emitting source surrounding the body. So PET is supplying regional quantitative information on the functioning of organs and tissue.

To understand the potential of PET not only the instrumental part is important, but also the way positron emitters can be produced. Radionuclides decaying by positron emission are neutron-deficient nuclides. They can be produced by removing one or more neutrons from a stable nucleus. This is in contrast to neutron-rich radionuclides which can be produced by adding one or more neutrons to a stable nucleus. This last process is normally carried out in a nuclear reactor. The most simple way to produce positron emitters is by charged particles induced reaction [8]. This involves the use of accelerators like cyclotrons, which deliver beams of energetic protons, deuterons or other charged particles. The nuclear reactions used are in most cases of the types (p,xn) or (p,α), where p means proton, n neutron and α an alpha-particle. The number of neutrons removed in the nuclear reaction is given by x and is a function of the energy of the incoming particle.

The process of the nuclear reaction can be understood in the following way. First of all: only a very few of the incoming particles on the target material will induce a nuclear reaction. To give a practical example: a proton beam is impinging on nitrogen as target material. This is commonly used system for the production of carbon-11 according to the $^{14}N(p,\alpha)^{11}C$ reaction. A nitrogen nucleus, seven protons and seven neutrons, forms together with the incoming proton a compound nucleus with now eight protons and seven neutrons. This compounds system has an energy excess and will try to get into a minimum energy configuration by emitting particles and gamma radiation. If the energy excess is high enough the first thing will be the emission of a neutron. Due to the energy balance of this particular system it is very likely that an alpha-particle will be emitted. The resulting nucleus is carbon-11 containing six protons and five neutrons. This change of element during the production is very important for the PET technique. If no carbon is present in the material to be irradiated all carbon after the irradiation will be in the form of carbon-11. This is called a carrier-free production. 1Ci of carrier-free carbon-11 nuclei has a weight of 1.2 ng. In this context the term specific activity, the amount of activity per mole, is used. The maximum theoretical specific activity for a number of important isotopes for PET is shown in Table 1. The theoretical specific activity can be calculated from the law of radioactivity:

$$N(t) = N(0)e^{-\lambda t} \tag{1}$$

with N(t) the number of radionuclides present at time t, and λ the decay constant; $\lambda = \ln 2/T_{1/2}$. In this equation is $T_{1/2}$ the half-life of the radionuclides. From eq. (1), assuming $T_{1/2} >> 1$ s, it can be shown that:

$$N(0) = A/\lambda \tag{2}$$

with A the amount of radiactive material measured in Becquerel (Bq). After production the radionuclides will be converted chemically into a radiopharmaceutical. If during the chemical processing procedure no dilution of the carbon-11 with stable carbon-12 occurs, the endproduct will never be toxic or disturb any physiological processes when administered, due to the extreme low amount, in weight, of the material.

The amount of radioactivity normally administered for a PET study is in the order of 370 MBq (10 mCi). This amount corresponds, in case of a carrier free production of the radiopharmaceuticals, with 1×10^{-12} mol of carbon-11 labeled material or 6.5×10^{11} molecules. If a uniform distribution of the radiopharmaceutical in the body is assumed, the radioactivity concentration is

Table 1. Maximum, theoretical, specific activity for some radionuclides important for PET

	Half-life	Maximum specific activity	
		(Ci/mol)	(Bq/mol)
^{11}C	20.38 min	9.2×10^{9}	3.4×10^{20}
^{13}N	9.96 min	1.9×10^{10}	7.0×10^{20}
^{15}O	2.03 min	9.2×10^{10}	3.4×10^{21}
^{18}F	109.8 min	1.7×10^{9}	6.3×10^{19}
^{75}Br	98 min	1.9×10^{9}	7.1×10^{19}

roughly 15×10^{-15} M. The carrier-free aspect of a synthesis is very important for many applications in the field of positron emission tomography. A carrier-free synthesis, however, is very hard to achieve, especially with carbon-11 where $^{11}CO_2$ is a frequently used synthetic precursor. Special precautions have to be taken to minimize the dilution with stable CO_2. Because a dilution is hard to avoid it may be better to speak of a "non-carrier-added" synthesis [9]. If the necessary precautions are taken, even with $^{11}CO_2$ as precursor, a non-carrier-added synthesis can result in radiopharmaceuticals with a very high specific activity. For rather complex syntheses specific activities in the range of 10^6-10^7 Ci/mol have been reported [10,11]. This means that the carrier dilution of the endproduct can be restricted to a factor of 10^3-10^4. This results in the administration of 10 nmol instead of 1 pmol in case of a carrier-free concentration of 1.5×10^{-10} M. It is unlikely that this amount of material will influence metabolism.

The most commonly used positron imaging devices consist of one or more detector rings. The sensitivity of these systems is 540 cps/MBq (20 cps/μCi) or more for each ring [2]. If each picture element represents a volume of $0.5 \times 0.5 \times 2.0$ cm^3 or 0.5 cm^3, there will be 4.6×10^6 carbon-11 labeled molecules present in each picture element. From a $32 \times 32 \times 2$ cm^3 volume this yields 1 million coincident events within 3 min.

NMR imaging

The NMR technique has been used extensively in chemistry as spectroscopic tool for the determination of molecular structures since 1946 [3,4]. The technique is based on the fact that many nuclei possess a spin. In absence of magnetic interactions, states of different spin orientation are degenerate. If an external magnetic field is applied to nuclei with a spin, the degeneracy in spin states is removed and 2I+1 different energy states are possible for nuclei with spin I. The value of I is dependent on the number of protons and neutrons in the nucleus and can have only integral or half-integral values. I is zero for nuclei with an even number of both protons and neutrons. So the most common carbon and oxygen isotopes, ^{12}C and ^{16}O, have a zero spin and consequently no information on these two species can be obtained by the NMR technique. I is an number for nuclei with even mass numbers and I is half-integral for nuclei with odd mass numbers. So ^1H, ^{13}C, ^{31}P have spin ½.

In a static magnetic field B_o the nucleus acquires an energy E as a result of the interaction between the field and the nuclear moment. If z, the quantitation axis, is taken to be parallel to the direction of the magnetic field, E is given by:

$$E = -\mu_z B_o = -\gamma m \hbar B_o \tag{3}$$

with γ the gyromagnetic ratio and mh the magnitude of the z-component of the nuclear angular momentum. The energy difference between the levels is given by:

$$dE = \gamma\hbar B_o \tag{4}$$

Transition between adjacent states are induced by application of a radio-frequency (rf) field, with its magnetic field vector in the x-y plane. Its frequency can be calculated from dE according to:

$$dE = \hbar v \tag{5}$$

where h is the Planck constant ($h=6.626\times10^{-34}$ Js, $h=1.055\times10^{-34}$ Js) and v is the frequency. In the following examples a magnetic field B_o with a strength of 8.46 T is assumed. For chemical spectroscopic studies this field strength is not excessive. For whole body imaging as a diagnostic medical tool a field strength of 8.46 T is excessive since up till now the field strength for this application did not exceed the 2 T limit. At a field strength of 8.46 T the frequency of the rf field is 360 MHz for protons.

The energy absorbed by the sample from the rf field depends on the population of the two possible energy states (for $I=\frac{1}{2}$). In thermal equilibrium the energy states are populated according to the Boltzmann distribution. The relative number of n^+ and n^- nuclei, spin $+\frac{1}{2}$ and $-\frac{1}{2}$ (spin up and spin down), is given by:

$$n^-/n^+ = e^{-dE/kT} \tag{6}$$

where k is the Boltzmann constant ($k=1.38\times10^{-23}$ JK^{-1}) and T is the temperature. At 8.46 T the energy difference dE amounts to 2.4×10^{-27} J or 1.5×10^{-6} eV and kT is roughly 2.5×10^{-2} eV. So the term in the exponent is very small, 5.8×10^{-5}. This means that the populations of both spin states are almost equal. At 8.46 T the ratio of the population of both states is $n^-/n^+=0.999942$. If both populations are equal, no net absorption from the rf field will occur, because there is an equal number of transition in both directions. This very small difference in the population of both states as calculated above determines the sensitivity of the NMR technique.

This calculation was based on a high magnetic field strength of 8.46 T. At this field strength no whole body NMR imaging is possible due to the skin effect. By skin effect the decreasing penetration depth of an rf pulse in the human body with increasing frequency is meant. Therefore it is not possible to increase the magnetic field, and by this the frequency ad libitum for imaging purposes [12]. The effect of a decreasing penetration depth is already obvious at a field strength of 2 T.

In the general practice of NMR spectroscopy practical rules have been developed to overcome the sensitivity problem of NMR. This has resulted in the requirement of minimal amounts of sample material. The minimum amounts to obtain a spectrum within a reasonable short time of a few minutes are 0.1 μmol for ^{1}H-NMR, 1 μmol for ^{31}P-NMR and 2 μmol for ^{13}C-NMR [13]. For ^{13}C-NMR a 2 μmol minimum amount only applies to a 100%-^{13}C-enriched compound. If isotope enrichment is not possible, 200 μmol is required. This difference between the amounts of sample material required is due to the natural abundance of the different isotopes and to the gyromagnetic ratio of the nucleus under investigation. The relative sensitivity with respect to the sensitivity for protons for a number of isotopes of interest for metabolic studies is shown in Table 2. When the rules for minimal amounts of sample material are converted to the field of NMR imaging they represent now the minimum amount of sample material which has to be present in each volume element of the object to be studied if a useful signal is to be obtained in a reasonable time. The minimum number of molecules required per volume element for whole body NMR imaging now can be calculated on basis of the following assumptions:

— the NMR imaging device is as sensitive as an NMR spectroscopy device which requires the minimum amounts of sample material as mentioned above;
— each picture element of the NMR imaging device represents a volume of $0.5 \times 0.5 \times 2.0$ cm^3, the same as used for the PET device. For NMR imaging this is a rather moderate demand on the resolution.

The minimum amount for a non-enriched-^{13}C compound of 200 μmol means that 1.2×10^{20} molecules have to be present per volume element of 0.5 cm^3. So the concentration is at least 0.4 M for a non-enriched carbon containing

Table 2. NMR properties of some nuclei of interest for metabolic imaging.

Spin	Isotope	NMR frequency (MHz)[a]	Natural abundance (%)	Relative sensitivity[b]
1/2	^{1}H	360.0	99.98	1.000
	^{13}C	90.5	1.11	1.59×10^{-2}
	^{15}N	36.5	0.365	1.04×10^{-2}
	^{19}F	338.7	100.	8.33×10^{-1}
	^{31}P	145.7	100.	6.63×10^{-2}
1	^{14}N	26.0	99.64	1.01×10^{-3}
3/2	^{23}Na	95.2	100.	9.25×10^{-2}
	^{39}K	16.8	93.26	5.08×10^{-4}
5/2	^{17}O	48.8	0.039	2.91×10^{-2}
	^{25}Mg	22.0	10.0	2.68×10^{-3}
7/2	^{43}Ca	24.2	0.135	6.40×10^{-3}

[a] At a field strength of 8.46 T.
[b] For an equal number of nuclei at a constant field.

compound. For 100%-^{13}C-enriched compounds the minimum concentration is 0.004 M.

The main parameters in the generation of contrast in NMR images are the relaxation times T_1 and T_2. If the relaxation time can be altered, the contrast can be enhanced. The use of paramagnetic ions for changing the relaxation times of the protons of water was reported already in 1946 by Bloch *et al.* [14]. The application of paramagnetic ions, mainly gadolinium compounds, is at the moment investigated for human application. The use of gadolinium-DTPA as a contrast agent has been described recently by Gadian *et al.* [15]. From these experiments it can be concluded that a minimum concentration in the range between 0.1 and 1.0 mM Gd-DTPA is required. The effect of Gd-DTPA on the relaxation time becomes prominent when the concentration reaches the level of 1 mM. The toxicity of a paramagnetic contrast agent may be decreased by using complexes of ions with chelating agents as is the case with EDTA and DTPA, but LD_{50} values between 0.6 and 10 mmol/kg for mice and rats have been reported for these chelating agents[16,17]. The use of gadolinium oxalate, an insoluble compound which passes unchanged through the gastrointestinal tract, was proposed as an oral NMR contrast agent [20]. In animal experiments a 10 mg/ml solution with a volume up to 200 cm^3 was used to image the gastrointestinal system by NMR. When these numbers are also valid for men, it means that a total of 40 g of gadolinium oxalate has to be administered to obtain the NMR images.

Comparison of PET and NMR

Brain imaging

By now we can make a comparison between PET and NMR for a few metabolic compounds. The first comparison is made for the regional tissue glucose metabolism. The normal glucose level in blood is approximately 90 mg per 100 cm^3. In brain tissue values of 50 to 80 mg per 100 cm^3 have been measured. The minimum concentration as calculated above for an NMR study of 0.4 M means that 7.2 g glucose per 100 cm^3 has to be present. So the glucose level required for an NMR study is roughly 100 times the concentration normally present in human tissue. By using 100%-^{13}C-enriched glucose, assuming it is possible to prepare this, a factor of 100 is gained. Administration of the necessary amount of this enriched glucose to the human body will result in an increase of the glucose level with a factor 2. It is questionable if this level can be reached under normal physiological and metabolic conditions since the human body will react on the extra supply of glucose. In the ideal case one should like to replace all the glucose in the body system by 100%-^{13}C-enriched glucose in order to study the glucose metabolism by an NMR imaging device as specified above. This is impossible because of the dysfunction of organs and organ systems due to kinetic isotopic effects.

Another comparison will be made for amino acids, e.g. to measure the protein synthesis rate. The free fatty acid level in plasma for most amino acids is less than 10 mg per 100 cm^3. Using 100%-^{13}C-enriched amino acids still a concentration of roughly 80 mg per 100 cm^3 is required for an NMR study according to the criteria defined before. The amino acid content in tissue may be higher than the free amino acid level in plasma, if values found in the brain of the rat [21] are also valid for the human brain, but the concentrations will be lower than those for glucose. Due to this low concentration of amino acids, the study of the amino acid metabolsim under normal physiological and metabolic conditions using an NMR imaging device is not possible.

Another field where PET and NMR have to be considered for medical application is the *in vivo* measurement of the receptor density. Again the problem of the sensitivity plays an important role since the concentration of the receptors is very low. The concentration for instance of dopamine receptors in the area of interest in the human brain is approximately 30×10^{-12} mol per gram tissue or 1.8×10^{13} receptors/cm^3. For a successful study, as previously calculated, 2.4×10^{18} molecules/cm^3 are required if a 100%-^{13}C-enriched ligand is used. The ability to study neurotransmitters and neuroreceptors as well as substrate metabolism in brain tissue is, due to the very low concentrations, only possible with PET in combination with the carrier-free, or at least non-carrier-added, prepared radiopharmaceuticals. The *in vivo* measurement of the dopamine receptor density in human brain was for the first time demonstrated in 1983 by Wagner *et al.* [22-25].

Cardiac imaging

In the field of cardiac imaging the NMR and the PET techniques are both complementary and competitive, depending on the parameters of interest. If only structures are important, as is the case with disease that produce a wall thickening or a wall thinning, the NMR technique is the technique of choice. The visualization of the wall thickness is important in the case of ischemic cardiac diseases and cardiomyopathies [26]. If the blood flow in larger vessels has to be investigated, the techniques may be competitive but not if microcirculation has to be assessed. For this application PET has to be applied to obtain regional quantitative information. The NMR signal from intravascular blood is dependent on the velocity of the flow [25]. Recently the velocity profile of blood flow in the carotid arteries has been quantitated [26]. With diffusible tracers as e.g. $^{13}NH_3$ and $^{82}RbCl$ it is possible to measure the myocardial blood flow with PET. The application of $^{13}NH_3$ as a marker for myocardial blood flow was supported by animal studies in which it was shown that myocardial flow deficits could be measured over a wide flow range [29]. To study metabolism of myocardial tissue with PET two different types of metabolic compounds are available. Since the heart can resort to different substrates to meet its energy requirements, both fluorine-18 labeled fluoro-deoxy-glucose (^{18}FDG) and carbon-11 labeled palmitic acid are used to measure metabolism *in vivo*. For the heart the fatty acid oxydation is, under aerobic conditions, the primary source of energy. When the supply of free fatty acid declines, while cardiac work and energy requirements are maintained, the heart must resort to other substrates. Although its property of using alternative substrates is preserved in normal myocardium, this ability is impaired in an ischemic area, which derives its energy primarily from glucose [31,32]. The visualization of the muscarinic receptors in the myocardium was demonstrated in baboons using carbon-11 labeled methiodide-quinuclidinyl-benzylate (^{11}C-MQNB) with a high specific activity [33].

Conclusion

NMR imaging delivers excellent images of structures by using the resonance frequency of the protons in water. In considering NMR for metabolic imaging it was shown that the number of molecules required to be present in each tissue volume element exceeds the normal concentration even if 100%-^{13}C-enriched compounds are used.

Because of the high sensitivity of PET compared to NMR, the PET technique in combination with carrier-free or very high specific active positron emitting radiopharmaceuticals is able to measure regional metabolism in quantitative terms. In conclusion: NMR is not competitive with PET for regional quantitative metabolic imaging.

References

1. Myers W G, Wagner H N Jr (1975) How it began. In: Wagner H N Jr (ed) Nuclear Medicine. New York: HP Publishing Co Inc, pp 3 - 14
2. Budinger T F, Gullberg G T, Huesman R H (1979) Emission computed tomography. In: Herman G T (ed) Image reconstructions from projections. Implementation and applications Berlin-Heidelberg-New York: Springer, pp 147 - 242
3. Bloch F, Hansen W W, Packard M (1946) Nuclear induction. Phys Rev 69: 127
4. Purcell E M, Torrey H C, Pound H V (1946) Resonance absorption by nuclear magnetic moments in a solid. Phys Rev 69: 37 - 38
5. Damadian R (1971) Tumor detection by nuclear magnetic resonance. Science 171: 1151 - 1153
6. Lauterbur P C (1973) Image formation by induced local interactions: Examples employing NMR. Nature 242: 190 - 191
7. Budinger T F (1983) Time-of-flight positron emission tomography: Status relative to conventional PET. J Nucl Med 24: 73 - 78
8. Vaalburg W, Paans A M J (1983) Short-lived positron emitting radionuclides. In: Helus F (ed) Radionuclides Production, Vol II. CRC press, Boca Raton pp 47 - 101

9. Wolf A P (1981) Synthesis of organic compounds labeled with positron emitters and the carrier problem. J Labelled Comp Radiopharm 18: 1 - 2
10. Bolster J M, Vaalburg W, van Veen W, van Dijk T, van der Molen H D, Wynberg H, Woldring M G (1983) Synthesis of no-carrier-added L- and D-(1-11C)- Dopa. Int J Appl Radiat Isot 34: 1650 - 1652
11. Berger G, Maziere M, Prenant C, Sastre J, Comar D (1984) 11C labeling of a protein: Concanavalin A. Int J Appl Radiat Isot 35: 81 - 83
12. Bottomley P A, Andrew E R (1978) RF magnetic field penetration, phase shift and power dissipation in biological tissue: Implications for NMR imaging. Phys Med Biol 23: 630 - 643
13. Gadian D G, (1982) Nuclear magnetic resonance and its application to living systems. Oxford: Clarendon Press
14. Bloch F, Hansen W W, Packard M (1946) The nuclear induction experiment. Phys Rev 70: 474 - 485
15. Gadian D G, Payne J A, Bryant D J, Young I R, Carr D H, Bydder G M (1985) Gadolinium-DTPA as a contrast agent in MR imaging — Theoretical projections and practical observations. J Comput Assist Tomogr 9: 242 - 251
16. Brown M A, Johnson G A (1984) Transition of metal chelate complexes as relaxation modifiers in nuclear magnetic resonance. Med Phys 11: 67 - 72
17. Weinmann H J, Grier H (1984) Paramagnetic contrast media in NMR tomography — basic properties and experimental studies in animals. Magn Reson Med 1: 271 - 272
18. Runge V M, Foster M A, Clanton J A, Smith F W, Lukehart C M, Hutchison J M, Mallard J R, Partain C L, James A E Jr (1985) Particulate oral NMR contrast agents. Int J Nucl Med Biol 12: 37 - 42
19. Korf J, Venema K (1983) Amino acids in substantia nigra of rats with striatal lesions produced by kainic acid. J Neurochem 40: 1171 - 1173
20. Wagner H N Jr, Burns H D, Dannals R F, Wong D F, Langstorm B, Duelfer T, Frost J J, Ravert H T, Links J M, Rosenbloom S, Lukas S E, Kramer A V, Kuhar M J (1983) Imaging dopamine receptors in the human brain by positron tomography. Science 221: 1264 - 1266
21. Wagner H N Jr, Burns H D, Dannals R F, Wond D F, Langstrom B, Duelfer T, Frost J J, Ravert H T, Links J M, Rosenbloom S, Lukas S E, Kramer A V, Kuhar M J (1984) Assessment of dopamine receptor activity in the human brain with ^{11}C-labeled N-methylspiperone. Ann Univ Turku D 17: 263 - 268
22. Wagner H N Jr (1985) Probing the chemistry of the mind. New Engl Med 312: 44 - 46
23. Kilbourn M R, Zalutsky M R (1985) Research and clinical potential of receptor based radiopharmaceuticals. J Nucl Med 26: 655 - 662
24. Higgins C B (1985) New horizons in cardiac imaging. Radiology 156: 577 - 588
25. Bradley W G Jr, Waluch V, Lai K-S, Fernandez E J, Spalter C (1984) The appearance of rapidly flowing blood on magnetic resonance images. AJR 143: 1167 - 1174
26. Feinburg D A, Crooks L, Hoenniger J, Arawaka M, Watts J (1984) Pulsatile blood velocity in human arteries displayed by magnetic resonance imaging. Radiology 153: 177 - 180
27. Gould K L, Schelbert H R, Phelps M E, Hoffman E J (1979) Noninvasive assessment of coronary stenoses with myocardial perfusion imaging during pharmacologic coronary vasodilation: V. Detection of 47 percent diameter coronary stenosis with intravenous nitrogen-13 ammonia and emission computed tomography in intact dogs. Am J Cadiol 43: 200 - 208
28. Neirinckx R D, Konauge J F, Loberg M D (1983) Evaluation of inorganic materials as adsorbents for the ^{82}Sr/^{82}Rb generator. Int J Appl Radiat Isot 34: 721 - 725
29. Schelbert H R (1983) Blood flow and substrate use in normal and diseased myocardium, 342 - 348. In: Phelps M E (moderator) Positron computed tomography for studies of myocardial and cerebral function. Ann Intern Med 98: 339 - 359
30. Schelbert H R (1984) Probing myocardial biochemistry with positron emitting tracers. Ann Univ Turku D 17: 47 - 66

31. Mazière M, Comar D, Godot J M, Collard Ph, Cepeda C, Naquet R (1981) In vivo characterization of myocardium muscarinic receptors by positron emission tomography. Life Sci 29: 2391 - 2397

Index of subjects